DEVELOPING MODERN LIVESTOCK PRODUCTION IN TROPICAL COUNTRIES

The Animal Production International Seminar (APIS) is the first international conference held by the Faculty of Animal Science, Universitas Brawijaya. APIS was held for the first time in 2010 and was repeated every three years. In 2022, the 5th APIS was organized as an online meeting. The Faculty of Animal Science, Universitas Brawijaya, is optimistic that the results of the 5th APIS will just be as successful as the 4th APIS in 2019. The theme of 5th APIS was "Developing Modern Livestock Production in Tropical Countries". The 5th APIS discussed matters related to strategies for developing modern livestock production in several tropical countries. The participants of 5th APIS, including keynote speakers and invited speakers, are from various countries (tropical and sub-tropical).

These proceedings present the selected papers from the 5th APIS conference.

PROCEEDINGS OF THE 5TH ANIMAL PRODUCTION INTERNATIONAL SEMINAR (APIS 2022), MALANG, INDONESIA, 10 NOVEMBER 2022

Developing Modern Livestock Production in Tropical Countries

Edited by

Danung Nur Adli, Muhammad Pramujo and Aulia Puspita Anugra Yekti
Faculty of Animal Science, Universitas Brawijaya, Indonesia

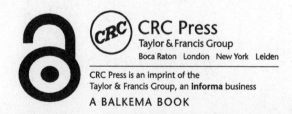

CRC Press
Taylor & Francis Group
Boca Raton   London   New York   Leiden

CRC Press is an imprint of the
Taylor & Francis Group, an **informa** business

A BALKEMA BOOK

First published 2023
by CRC Press/Balkema
4 Park Square, Milton Park, Abingdon, Oxon, OX14 4RN

and by CRC Press/Balkema
2385 NW Executive Center Drive, Suite 320, Boca Raton FL 33431

CRC Press/Balkema is an imprint of the Taylor & Francis Group, an informa business

British Library Cataloguing-in-Publication Data
A catalogue record for this book is available from the British Library

ISBN: 978-1-032-44025-5 (hbk)
ISBN: 978-1-032-44027-9 (pbk)
ISBN: 978-1-003-37004-8 (ebk)

DOI: 10.1201/9781003370048

Typeset in Times New Roman
by MPS Limited, Chennai, India

Table of contents

Preface

The authors' deep gratitude goes to the presence of God, the Great God. With his guidance, the 5th animal production international seminar (APIS) can finally get the ease and fluency in working on this book of abstracts to completion.

As a result of the 5th animal production international seminar (APIS) which was held in Malang, 10 November 2022, it was possible to present the best reviews in this book of abstracts from several topics as follows: Animal Agribusiness Related Subject, Animal Nutrition, Animal Product Technology, Animal Production, Animal Reproduction and Breeding, Animal Welfare, and Integrated Farming System.

The editors would like to thank participants who have contributed to the volume. All of the abstracts presented in this book have been passed through vigorous selection and the full paper version of the abstracts will be published separately to further disseminate into wider audiences. We would also like to express our gratitude to every staff of the Faculty of Animal Science, University of Brawijaya for the unwavering commitment as the seminar organizer and supporting organization. In the end, we are most indebted to the Fakultas Peternakan, Universitas Brawijaya press which provide the publication of this book of abstracts.

The Editors, Malang, November 2022

Committee Members

Steering Committee
Prof. Dr. Sc.Agr. Ir. Suyadi, MS., IPU., ASEAN Eng.
Prof. Dr. Muhammad Halim Natsir, S.Pt., MP., IPM., ASEAN Eng.
Prof. Dr. Ir. Budi Hartono, MS., IPU., ASEAN Eng.
Dr. Ir. Agus Susilo, S.Pt., MP., IPM., ASEAN Eng.
Prof. Dr. Ir. V. M. Ani Nurgiartiningsih, M.Sc.

Scientific Committee
Prof Erdoğan Memili, DVM, PhD. (*Prairie View, A&M University, United States*)
Prof. Martin Gierus (*Animal Nutrition, Universität für Bodenkultur Wien, Austria*)
Prof. Gatot Ciptadi (*Universitas Brawijaya, Indonesia*)
Prof. Katsuki Koh (*Shinsu University, Japan*)
Sutisa Khempaka, Ph.D. (*Suranaree University of Technology, Thailand*)
Associate Prof. Dr. Alfi Khatib (*International Islamic University Malaysia, Medical and Health Sciences*)

Organizing Committee

Chairman	Dr. Nanang Febrianto, S.Pt., MP.
Vice Chairman	Dr. Ir. Marjuki, M.Sc.
Secretary	Poespitasari Hazanah Ndaru, S.Pt. MP.
	Rahardianti Ariestya Puspita, S.Pt.
Treasurer	Aulia Puspita Anugra Yekti, S.Pt., MP., M.Sc.
	Khoiron Nisaa, S.Kom.
Secretariat	Dr. Dedes Amertaningtyas, S.Pt, MP.
	Puji Akhiroh, S.Pt., M.Sc.
	Wike Andre Septian, SPt, Msi
	Dr. Dyah Lestari Yulianti, S.Pt., MP
	Muhammad Pramujo, S.Pt., M.Si.
	Danung Nur Adli, S.Pt., M.Pt., M.Sc.
Event Division	Ria Dewi Andriani, S.Pt., M.Sc., MP.
	Rini Dwi Wahyuni, S.Pt., M.Sc.
	Yuli Frita Nuningtyas, S.Pt., M.Sc., MP.
	Dr. Herly Evanuarini, S.Pt., MP.
	Firman Jaya, S.Pt., MP.
	Zia Ul Rahman Fithron, M.B.A.
	Ahmad Khoirul Umam, S.Pt., M.Pt., M.Sc
	Ardyah Ramadhina Irsanti Putri S.Si., M.Si.
	Poppy Satya Puspita, S.Pt., M.Si.
	Mohammad Tono, A.Md.
	Muhammad Zaenal Abidin
	Arifatul Hafid Achsan
	Dita Anggraini Djumari Putri, S.Ikom.
	Kharis Izzul, S.T.P.
	Vicky Budi Hariono
	Annisa Nur C., S.Pt.
	Ahmad Eka Oktandra, S.E.
	Ari Ardiantoro, S.Si., M.Si.
	Wahdah Choe Rotunnis

Developing Modern Livestock Production in Tropical Countries – Adli et al. (eds)
© 2023 The Authors, ISBN 978-1-032-44025-5
Open Access: www.taylorfrancis.com, CC BY-NC-ND 4.0 license

Contribution of forages for the nutrient use efficiency in ruminant nutrition

M. Gierus
Institute of Animal Nutrition, Livestock Products, and Nutrition Physiology, Department for Agrobiotechnology, University of Natural Resources and Life Sciences, Vienna, Austria

ABSTRACT: High efficiency of nutrient and energy utilization is required to be in line with international commitments on greenhouse gas emissions. The focus in many regions in Europe is the N surplus, which originates from inefficient resource utilization, contributing largely to environmental pollution. In addition, large amounts protein rich concentrates are imported in EU countries, with land use changes in the producing regions worldwide like South America and South Asia. Therefore, increasing the production of home-grown proteins in Europe and quantifying their protein use efficiency is needed. In addition, alternative protein sources originating from home grown proteins in Europe should focus on factors determining the nutritive value of feedstuffs (concentrates, by-products and forages) for ruminants and its causes of variation. Focus on home grown proteins should also consider the contribution of forage production systems for the energy and protein supply of ruminants. The protein and carbohydrate fractionation is helpful for forage characterization and comparison of nutritive value.

Keywords: grass cultivar, protein fractions, CNCPS

1   INTRODUCTION

The proper feeding of ruminants is a challenging issue. Despite the nutrient and energy availability in concentrate feeds, most ruminant diets of high yielding animals are based on forages. Forages are variable in nutrient and energy content, which varies also among forage plant species, between cutting frequencies, among cutting dates (season), and forage conservation practices. Next to obtaining highest forage nutritive value and the resulting optimal animal performance, increasing issues in ruminant feeding are the efficiency of nutrient and energy utilization, the environmentally friendly production of foods of animal origin, and the expectation of consumers to obtain animal products from systems taking into consideration animal welfare issues. The main objective herein was to integrate the knowledge about evaluation of nutritive value (mainly protein) with that of grassland science to optimize the feeding of high yielding dairy cows. In this way, it should be possible to obtain a better understanding of processes influencing the variation in nutritive value of forage crops and related them to possible relevant aspects in ruminant nutrition physiology.

2   DISCUSSION

Home grown protein production – still a challenge: An increasing demand for so called "home grown proteins" is being discussed for animal feeding. Although the European Union (EU) covers its own demand for vegetable oil, the EU is protein deficient. This deficit still makes the EU the world's largest importer of soybean meal and the second-largest importer of soybeans, just behind China (Gale 2007). The import of protein sources is questioned as it is linked to additional transport and environmental costs, as well as problems with traceability and nutritive value. Farmers in Europe are facing the challenge to meet the requirements of high yielding animals, which in turn becomes difficult considering the high feed costs at the farm. The objective is to optimize the formulation of diets for high yielding dairy cows with local feed resources, for instance increasing the utilization of forage legumes or the share of high productive grasses in temporary grassland production systems (Søegaard et al. 2007). Such procedure may reduce the amount of concentrate necessary for similar milk yields, reducing the impact of nutrient losses to the environment. As the main task for most specialized dairy farms is to increase the N use efficiency, a forage production system towards cultivation of temporary grassland combines the increasing genetic potential for high yielding dairy cows with the utilization of new released cultivars of forage species or the utilization of those with high nutritive value, especially with high energy content (Gierus et al. 2005). Temporary grassland is used as alternative to optimize nutrient fluxes in the farming system, allowing the exchange between crop and livestock production to obtain higher efficiency.

Forages are important sources of proteins for high yielding dairy cows. The determination of protein quality should necessarily represent the estimation of the escape protein content of a specific feed or mixture to reduce excessive losses of intraluminal degraded protein. Different literature reports on positive influence of non-ammonia N (NAN) content in the small intestines resulting in efficient dietary N utilization when increasing amounts of escape protein available in the diet is present (Santos et al. 1998; Volden 1999). However, in the most studies concentrate with high amounts of escape protein is fed to correct for ungradable protein requirement of high yielding cows, increasing the N load in the dairy farm. Higher escape protein from forages is seldom worked out as a strategy. Due to its biological N fixation capacity, forage legumes present generally a higher protein content compared to grasses. In contrast, the available energy is lower in proportion to the protein content. Consequently, in forage legume-based production systems, the protein is poorly utilized due to energy deficiency and extensive degradation of protein in the rumen (Beever et al. 1986a; 1986b). In addition, the protein quality measured as protein fractionation varies considerably in dependence of the defoliation system in combination with the forage legume species available (Kleen et al. 2011). Furthermore, forage legume species determine the feed quality and yield of binary mixtures with perennial ryegrass (Gierus et al. 2012) in the first production year.

Protein quality of forages as breeding strategy: Plant breeding has contributed with 4–5% per decade to the increase in dry matter production, in addition to an increase of 10 g/kg DM digestibility per decade in Northwestern Europe since the 1950s (Wilkins & Humphreys 2003). However, one of the main problems in grassland-based systems is the inefficiency of ruminants to convert plant biomass into animal product, as mentioned above. Considering that only 20–30% of the ingested N can be converted to meat or milk (Dewhurst et al. 1996), ruminant feeding contributes to environmental N pollution. Considering improvement in forage quality, the high crude protein (CP) content and the fast protein degradation rate of forages in the fore stomach of the ruminant are related to inefficiency. Assuming forages as important sources of proteins for high yielding dairy cows, the determination of protein quality should necessarily represent the estimation of the escape protein content of a specific forage species or mixture to reduce excessive losses of intraluminal degraded protein and N load.

Benefits of forage legume-based systems: In forage legume-based production systems, the nutritive value of forages can be improved by increasing the amount of escape protein. In this case, forage legumes with secondary plant compound like tannins or polyphenol oxidase may be advantageous in contributing to increase the amount of escape protein of forages. Different studies demonstrated that with fast degradation rate and high losses of N in urine,

2

the absorption of amino acids in the small intestine may limit the performance of lambs, lactating ewes, and dairy cattle (Rogers *et al.* 1980; Barry 1981). In contrast, lambs grazing forage legumes with condensed tannins showed significant higher average daily gains compared to ryegrass (Speijers *et al.*, 2004). More feed protein would pass the rumen ungraded as condensed tannins are supposed to complex with proteins, protecting them from fast ruminal degradation (Kardel *et al.*, 2013).

3 CONCLUSION

Focus on home grown proteins should also consider the contribution of forage production systems for the energy and protein supply of ruminants. The protein and carbohydrate fractionation is helpful for forage characterization and comparison of nutritive value.

REFERENCES

Barry T.N. (1981). Protein Metabolism in Growing Lambs Fed on Fresh Ryegrass (Lolium Perenne)–Clover (Trifolium Repens) Pasture ad lib. 1. Protein and Energy Deposition in Response to Abomasal Infusion of Casein and Methionine. *British Journal of Nutrition*, 46(3), 521–532.

Beever D.E., Dhanoa M.S., Losada H.R., Evans R.T., Cammell S.B. and France J. (1986a). The Effect of Forage Species and Stage of Harvest on the Processes of Digestion Occurring in the Rumen of Cattle. *British Journal of Nutrition*, 56(2), 439–454.

Beever D.E., Losada H.R., Cammell S.B., Evans R.T. and Haines M.J. (1986b). Effect of Forage Species and Season on Nutrient Digestion and Supply in Grazing Cattle. *British Journal of Nutrition*, 56(1), 209–225.

Dewhurst R.J., Evans R.T., Scollan N.D., Moorby J.M., Merry R.J. and Wilkins R.J. (2003). Comparison of Grass And Legume Silages for Milk Production. 2. In Vivo and in Sacco Evaluations of Rumen Function. *Journal of Dairy Science*, 86(8), 2612–2621.

Gale F. (2007). *Economic Research Service, USDA. China's Agricultural Trade: Issues and Prospects*, 65. China.

Gierus M., Kleen J., Loges R. and Taube F. (2012). Forage Legume Species Determine the Nutritional Quality of Binary Mixtures with Perennial Ryegrass in the First Production Year. *Animal Feed Science and Technology*, 172(3–4), 150–161.

Kardel M., Taube F., Schulz H., Schütze W. and Gierus M. (2013). Different Approaches to Evaluate Tannin Content and Structure of Selected Plant Extracts-review and New Aspects. *Journal Applied Botany Food Quality*, 86(1), 154–166.

Kleen J., Taube F. and Gierus M. (2011). Agronomic Performance and Nutritive Value of Forage Legumes in Binary Mixtures with Perennial Ryegrass Under Different Defoliation Systems. *The Journal of Agricultural Science*, 149(1), 73–84.

Rogers G.L., Porter R.H.D., Clarke T. and Stewart J.A. (1980). Effect of Protected Casein Supplements on Pasture Intake, Milk Yield and Composition of Cows in Early Lactation. *Australian Journal of Agricultural Research*, 31(6), 1147–1152.

Santos F.A.P., Santos J.E.P., Theurer,C.B. and Huber J.T. (1998). Effects of Rumen-Undegradable Protein on Dairy Cow Performance: A 12-Year Literature Review. *Journal of Dairy Science*, 81(12), 3182–3213.

Søegaard K., Gierus M., Hopkins A. and Halling M. (2007). Temporary Grassland-challenges in the Future. In *Permanent and Temporary Grassland: Plant*, Environment and Economy. Proceedings of the 14th Symposium of the European Grassland Federation, Ghent, Belgium, 3–5 September 2007 (pp. 27–38). Belgian Society for Grassland and Forage Crops.

Speijers M.H., Fraser M.D., Theobald V.J. and Haresign W. (2004). The Effects of Grazing Forage Legumes on the Performance of Finishing Lambs. *The Journal of Agricultural Science*, 142(4), 483–493.

Volden H. (1999). Effects of Level of Feeding and Ruminally Undegraded Protein on Ruminal Bacterial Protein Synthesis, Escape of Dietary Protein, Intestinal Amino Acid Profile, and Performance of Dairy Cows. *Journal of Animal Science*, 77(7), 1905–1918.

Wilkins P.W. and Humphreys M.O. (2003). Progress in Breeding Perennial Forage Grasses for Temperate Agriculture. *The Journal of Agricultural Science*, 140(2), 129–150.

Developing Modern Livestock Production in Tropical Countries – Adli et al. (eds)
© 2023 The Authors, ISBN 978-1-032-44025-5
Open Access: www.taylorfrancis.com, CC BY-NC-ND 4.0 license

An approach for integrated production of mushrooms and ruminant feed

K. Koh
Shinshu University, Nagano, Japan

ABSTRACT: In the present study, we tried to produce mushrooms from agro-wastes, such as apple pomace and sweetcorn stover, and ruminant feed from the resultant spent mushroom substrate (SMS). In the first experiment, *Hypsizygus marmoreus* and *Flammulina velutipes* were cultivated on substrates containing graded levels of fermented apple pomace (FAP). The former grew successfully on the substrate containing FAP at 9%, but the latter at 15%, suggesting that the latter was more adaptable to the FAP substrate. Therefore, FAP containing SMS from *F. velutipes* was ensiled and then fed to ewes, but they consumed this silage little. In the second experiment, *F. velutipes* was cultivated on substrates containing graded levels of fermented short- and long-cut sweetcorn stover (FCS). This mushroom grew well on the substrates containing long-cut FCS at 25%. The ensiled SMS of this mushroom was consumed readily by ewes, but its function as a roughage substitute was insufficient.

Keywords: agro waste, apple pomace, ensilage, mushroom, ruminant

1 INTRODUCTION

Mushroom production is recognized to be eco-friendly agriculture because mushrooms can be produced using agro-wastes on a small land area, and the spent mushroom substrate (SMS) is returned to the soil. Japan is one of the world's leading mushroom-producing countries, but the production system there is not eco-friendly because of mass production: most substrate materials are dependent on imports, and SMS is discarded without recycling. So far, many studies have been conducted to use SMS as a ruminant feed, but such attempts have not yet been successful. The purpose of the present study was to investigate the viabilities of regional agro-wastes as materials for mushroom substrate and resultant SMS as feed for ruminants and to discuss the development of an integrated production system of mushrooms and ruminant feed. *Apple pomace:* Apple pomace was selected because this is 1) a regional agro-industrial waste in Nagano prefecture which is the second largest apple producer in Japan, 2) high in water retention which is one of the required properties of the substrate, and 3) an acceptable feedstuff (OECD 2019). When *Hypsizygus marmoreus* (Bunashimeji in Japanese) and *Flammulina velutipes* (Enokitake in Japanese) were cultivated on substrates containing graded levels of lactic fermented apple pomace (FAP), the former grew successfully on the substrate containing FAP up to 9% (DM basis) (Hiramori *et al.* 2015), but the latter 15% (DM basis), suggesting that Enokitake is more adaptable to the FAP containing substrate. This difference may be explained in part by the fact that Enokitake prefers lower substrate pH. As the next step, the adequacy of FAP-containing Enokitake SMS as a ruminant feed was evaluated. The SMS was ensiled after being heated at 90°C, because of poor fermentation when unheated. Ewes consumed this SMS silage little unless this was mixed with other feed ingredients, showing that the palatability of this SMS silage was not good.

DOI: 10.1201/9781003370048-2
This chapter has been made available under a CC BY NC ND license

2 DISCUSSION

Sweetcorn stover: As another substrate material for Enokitake, sweetcorn stover was selected because this is 1) adjustable in cutting length and 2) a regional agro-waste in Nagano which is the famous sweetcorn producer in Japan. Sweetcorn stover obtained after harvest was cut into 2 lengths (short 13mm and long 28 mm) and ensiled (FCS). Enokitake was cultivated on substrates containing graded levels of short- and long-cut FCS. Among experimental substrates, the best performance was observed in the substrate containing long-cut FCS at 25%, and hence this SMS was ensiled: the quality of this SMS silage was good. As the next step, a feeding trial using ewes was conducted to know whether this SMS silage is palatable to ewes and has physical effects such as roughage. Feed intake, eating and ruminating time, and chewing activity in ewes given this silage tended to be greater than those in ewes given conventional SMS silage. These results suggest that long-cut FCS can be used as a material for Enokitake substrate and the resultant SMS has the potential as a roughage source.

3 CONCLUSION

In conclusion, FCS is suitable for the co-production of mushrooms and ruminant feed, but the function of SMS silage containing long-cut FCS as a roughage substitute should be further improved.

REFERENCES

Hiramori C., Kurata S. and Koh K. (2021). Influence of Addition of Materials with Different Cutting Lengths to Mushroom Substrate on Productivity of Enokitake Mushroom (*Flammulina velutipes*) and the Physical Effect as Roughage of Silage Made of its Spent Substrate. *Japanese Journal of Organic Agriculture Science*, 13(2), 58–57.

Hiramori C., Uyeno Y. and Koh K. (2015). Effects of Lactic Acid Bacteria on Fermented Apple Pomace (FAP) Production and Inclusion of FAP in Medium for Bunashimeji (*Hypsizygus marmoreus*) cultivation. *Mushroom Science and Biotechnology*, 23 (3), 120–124.

OECD. (2019). *Safety assessment of foods and feeds derived from transgenic crops, Volume 3: Common bean, Rice, Cowpea and Apple Compositional Considerations, novel food and feed safety*, Paris: OECD Publishing.

Developing Modern Livestock Production in Tropical Countries – Adli et al. (eds)
© 2023 The Authors, ISBN 978-1-032-44025-5
Open Access: www.taylorfrancis.com, CC BY-NC-ND 4.0 license

The importance of conservation, commercialization, and good breeding practice of Indonesian superior ruminants for local genetics resources sustainability

G. Ciptadi
Faculty of Animal Science, Universitas Brawijaya, Malang, Indonesia

ABSTRACT: Sustainable genetic resources in a tropical country are considered very important. Various efforts have been performed to conserve and improve the productivity of ruminants by enhancing both genetics and the environment, also good breeding and artificial insemination (AI). Conservation efforts and commercialization are carried out conventionally. In Indonesia, AI is important to accelerate livestock production; this is a strategy, especially on smallholder farms. The problems of genetic resource management are as follows: How to develop and utilize research development results, the genetic impact of the implementation of AI to accelerate the improvement of genetic quality and how to manage the conservation and commercialization of local Indonesian animal genetic resources. The primary role of the AI center is to provide superior, fertile candidate males. It is time to start evaluating the genetic normality of the local breed. Molecular analysis of gen or chromosomes needs to be implemented in males for AI.

Keywords: breeding practice, ruminant, conservation, tropical, environment

1 INTRODUCTION

Indonesia has the largest germplasm wealth in the world, with hundreds or even thousands of species and local breeds that have specific advantages and characteristics in a tropical environment. Local breeds can be marginal and considered inferior with low economic value. The existence of imported superior livestock allowed by mass AI implementation should be accompanied by well-planned management of local livestock genetic resources. Good sustainable management of local genetic resources has become very strategic. The genetic resource management issues that will be discussed are the development and utilization of research or technology related to improving animal genetics and productivity, the genetic impact of biotechnology implementation to accelerate livestock genetic quality improvement, the role and importance of AI Center in conservation and semen freezing production and distribution and commercialization, and the management of conservation and commercialization of Indonesian local livestock genetic resources and its implementation in genetics and livestock breeding and reproduction.

2 DISCUSSION

Recent Development of Reproductive Biotechnology: The science of reproduction, genetics, and livestock breeding can now be understood more deeply and in detail from three levels, namely individual, cellular and molecular, for both quantitative and qualitative

DOI: 10.1201/9781003370048-3
This chapter has been made available under a CC BY NC ND license

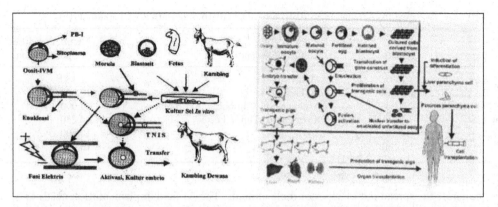

Figure 1. Implementation of cell manipulation, genetic engineering, cloning, and transgenic technology to produce non-conventional livestock products using miniature pigs and goats (Ciptadi 2019; Sato 2005).

characteristics that are hereditary and have economic value, which was then also supported by the development and innovation of Assisted Reproductive Technology, has significantly accelerated the improvement of the genetic quality of livestock. We know that the implementation of Artificial Insemination (AI) with selected males, Embryo Transfer (TE), cell nucleus transfer technology (TNS), cloning, and the birth of transgenic animals and livestock have been proven to be effective in improving genetic quality, conservation of genetic material. Each of these technologies is developing both in developed countries of the livestock industry and in developing countries (Ciptadi 2005; Sato 2003) (Figure 1).

The important history of the development of genetics, livestock breeding, biotechnology, and ART shows the very important role of science and technology in the future. The technology of freezing gametes, somatic cells, and embryos allows us not only to be used for research and development of cell conservation science (frozen) and build new theories in the cellular/molecular field but also to be used simultaneously to implement and commercialize superior genetic material or rare from livestock. The Brawijaya University research team is currently researching the actualization of cell freezing without using liquid nitrogen at a temperature of −80°C, utilizing a deep freezer (Ciptadi et al. 2017). This activity is carried out as research to develop appropriate methods (freezing) for conserving local Indonesian livestock (Ciptadi 2012). Genetic screening of livestock has been carried out in several developed countries. It is also recommended to be carried out in developing countries, including Indonesia, which is rich in specific local germplasm (Akhmad et al. 2004; Ciptadi 2018). Thus, breeder livestock is not only selected animals based on performance but should also be based on the genetic potential of superior genes and free from genetic defects. Genetic Impact of Improvement Strategies on Local Animals: The main options that can be taken related to the efforts to improve genetics are selection, purification of local animals, and cross-breeding program. Local breeder prefers to adopt AI with the semen of non-local or imported bull in some areas. Research data showed that a lower number of local breed semen used in AI was due to high-intensity semen imported breeds semen has been used.

Indonesia's major ruminant livestock population is about 47.71 million heads consisting of beef cattle, dairy cattle, buffalo, goats, and sheep (Table 1). This AI center produces as many as 20 thousand doses of cattle and goat semen per day, which is supposed to be increased continuously. Production of frozen semen, in particular of local cattle (Bali bull) from this AI center has been distributed to various regions/provinces in Indonesia, and as much as 3,000 doses of semen have been exported to three countries (Myanmar, Vietnam, and Thailand) (Ciptadi et al. 2019) as well as to Malaysia. AI center role becomes crucial to

Table 1.   Exported from semen from BBIB Singosari (BBIB Singosari 2019; Ciptadi 2019).

No.	Year	Country Destination	Number of doses of Spermatozoa
1.	2005	Malaysia	1.150
2.	2006	Malaysia	10.000
3.	2013	Afghanistan, Cambodia, Myanmar	3.000
4.	2016	Kyrgyzstan, Timor Leste	4.250
5.	2019	Kyrgyzstan	12.500
	Total		18.850

accelerate the spread out of superior male animals. The AI field implementation needs to be organized well. Typical problems in Indonesia are that AI has been performed and is too concentrated in livestock area animal production centers. In smallholder farms, there are problems of decreasing genetic quality yearly, especially because of the limited availability of superior male animals. Production of frozen semen, in particular of local cattle (Bali bull) from this AI center has been distributed to various regions/provinces in Indonesia, and as much as 3,000 doses of semen have been exported to three countries (Myanmar, Vietnam, and Thailand) (Ciptadi et al. 2019) as well as to Malaysia. Meanwhile, at the same time, the AI center of Lembang has also exported as many as 100 doses of frozen to Kinabalu, Malaysia (Table 1). The frozen semen exported abroad is beef cattle and goats for the descendants of ex-imported and local breeds. Based on the price, this export frozen cell product sells for USD 3.0 or approximately Rp. 35,000.00 per dose, while the same product is sold domestically for Rp.7,000.00 (BBIB Singosari 2019). BIB Lembang was also reported to have exported frozen cement abroad (Malaysia). The potential for frozen cement exports is very wide open. In the future, the quality of these local breeds still needs to be developed into elite male breeds whose prices can reach more than ten times (30 to 50 USD/dose). In the future, it also has the potential to be traded on a national, regional, ASEAN, and international scale. Livestock that has been conserved genetic material for the conservation and creation of new breeds (Ciptadi et al. 2019).

3 CONCLUSION

The development and innovation of new technology in animal breeding need to be continuously developed and implemented in local Indonesian livestock to accelerate productivity and genetic quality. Conservation and commercialization of genetic material of excellent Indonesian local livestock genetic resources are important and strategic things to be carried out continuously to guarantee their sustainability.

ACKNOWLEDGMENTS

Most of the data are the result of a cattle and buffalo research grant funded by the Department of Animal Husbandry Services of East Java in 2013, Hibah LPDP Rispro_kemenkeu RI, 2016–2018), and Hibah Guru Besar, 2022 no contract 827.9/UN10. F05/PN/2022, and Hibah HPU-UB, 2022 (Contract No. 975.34/UN10.C10/PN/2021).

REFERENCES

Ahmad I., Javed, K. & Sattar A. (2004). Screening of Breeding Bulls of Different Breeds through Karyotyping. *Pakistan Veterinaire Journal* 24 (4), 190–192.

BBIB Singosari. (2019). *Buku Laporan Produksi, Distribusi dan Stok Semen Beku Produksi Balai Inseminasi Buatan-Singosari Malang*, Indonesia: BBIB Singosari.

Bib Lembang. (2019). *Laporan Produksi, Distribusi dan Stok Semen Beku Minggu Ke II Bulan Juni 2019.* Indonesia: BBIB Singosari.

Ciptadi G., Putri A.R.I., Rahayu S., Wahjuningsih S., Nasich M., Rokhman F. & Budiarto A. (2018). Phenotypic and Genetic Character Variations of a New Breed of Genetic Resource of Senduro Goat, Indonesia. In *AIP Conference Proceedings, 2019*, 1

Ciptadi G., Ihsan M.N., Rahayu S., Nurgiartiningsih V.M.A., Mudawamah M. & Putri A.R.I. (2017). The Comparison of Chromosome Analysis Result by Manual and Software Cytovision Image Analysis Using Simple G-Banding. *Research Journal of Life Science*, 4(2), 106–110.

Ciptadi G. (2017). Realisasi Bank sel Gamet (Spermatozoa) Kambing dan Domba Lokal Untuk Konservasi dan Komersialisasi *Plasma Nutfah Indonesia. Laporan Penelitian. Bantuan Dana Riset Inovatif-Produktif (RISPRO) Komersial Lembaga Pengelola Dana Pendidikan (LPDP)-Kemenkeu RI*: Indonesia: LPDP.

Ciptadi G., Budiarto A. & Oktanella Y. (2019). *Genetika dan Pemuliaan: Peternakan-Veteriner.* Indonesia: Universitas Brawijaya Press.

Ciptadi G. (2012). *Bioteknologi Sel Gamet dan Kloning Hewan.* Indonesia:Universitas Brawijaya Press.

Putri A.R.I., Ciptadi G. & Warih A.P. (2018). Chromosome Characteristic of Peranakan Etawa (PE) Goat (Capra hircus Linn.) as Indonesian Local Breed. In *IOP Conference Series: Earth and Environmental Science, 119* (1), 012–032.

Sato E., Miyamoto H. and Manabe N. (2003). *Animal Frontier Sciences. Life Science Update in Animal Science.* Japan: West Wind Lab. Japan.

9

Developing Modern Livestock Production in Tropical Countries – Adli et al. (eds)
© 2023 The Authors, ISBN 978-1-032-44025-5
Open Access: www.taylorfrancis.com, CC BY-NC-ND 4.0 license

Age and individual variation affect semen quality and field fertility of Bali bulls (*Bos sondaicus*): A preliminary study

D. Heraini, D.T. Fatmila, B.P. Pardede, Y. Yudi & B. Purwantara*
School of Veterinary Medicine and Biomedical Sciences, IPB University, Bogor, West Java, Indonesia

ABSTRACT: One of the breeding strategies to increase the population of Bali cattle is through an AI program using frozen semen produced by superior Bali bulls. This research is a preliminary study examining the influence of age and individual factors on semen quality and field fertility in Bali bulls. The results of this study are expected to be the basis for further research, especially the molecular aspects that affect semen quality and fertility in Bali bulls. This study evaluated semen quality and field fertility data from eight Bali bulls. Data were analyzed based on individual factors and grouped by age (<10 years and >10 years). There were significant differences between individuals ($P<0.05$) and age ($P<0.05$) in semen quality and field fertility, except for fresh semen motility. PTM and RR were positively correlated with field fertility ($P<0.01$). Individual factors and age affect semen quality and field fertility in Bali bulls.

Keywords: age, Bali bull, individual, field fertility, semen quality

1 INTRODUCTION

Bali cattle (*Bos sondaicus*) are native Indonesian cattle with various advantages that might be an alternative to meet Indonesia's growing need for beef consumption. Bali cattle have good adaptability to different environmental conditions, poor feed, good reproductive ability, and higher carcass percentage than other local Indonesian cattle breeds (Saputra *et al.* 2017). One strategy for breeding and increasing the population of Bali cattle is through an artificial insemination (AI) program using frozen semen produced by superior Bali bulls. It must contain motile sperm to fertilize oocytes. Therefore, semen quality significantly affects bull fertility due to the critical success of AI programs (Pardede *et al.* 2020).

The failure of the AI program due to the low fertility of bulls has a significant impact on the livestock industry and economic losses, so it is necessary to predict bull fertility. Moreover, age and individual variation have been reported to affect bull fertility and semen quality (Gunes *et al.* 2016; Zhao *et al.* 2019). One of the impacts of individual variation is that bulls over ten years old are still used, provided that the semen quality and reproductive performance are still considered quite good and meet the standards. In contrast, the productive age of bulls is generally less than ten years, and there is a decline in physiological and hormonal reproductive abilities in bulls over ten years of age (Zainudin *et al.* 2014). Although semen quality still meets existing standards, it does not guarantee that fertility in the field will show optimal results (Pardede *et al.* 2022). Therefore, this study emphasizes the analysis of semen quality and field fertility, assessed from age and individual factors, to provide a new perspective on the influence of these two factors and support programs to increase the local cattle population in Indonesia.

---

*Corresponding Author: purwantara@apps.ipb.ac.id

DOI: 10.1201/9781003370048-4
This chapter has been made available under a CC BY NC ND license

2 MATERIALS AND METHODS

2.1 Data collection and animal condition

Semen quality and production data were collected from eight Bali bulls from the Regional Artificial Insemination Center, Bali Province, Indonesia, aged 6–14 years for two years. The semen quality parameters used in the study included color, consistency, pH, volume, concentration, motility of fresh and post-thawing semen (PTM), and recovery rate (RR). Field fertility is obtained through the analysis of the conception rate (CR%) collected from the data of iSIKHNAS Bali Province for two years (2020–2021) in each Bali bull.

2.2 Statistical analysis

Bali bulls were grouped into two groups based on age (<10 years and >10 years). The effect of age on semen quality and production and field fertility were analyzed using an independent t-test. In addition, an analysis of variance was conducted to examine the effect of individual variations on semen quality and production and field fertility using variance analysis (ANOVA). The data analysis was conducted by the SPSS version 25 program (IBM, Armonk, NY, USA).

3 RESULTS AND DISCUSSION

Overall, the color, consistency, and pH of the fresh semen in all bulls could be categorized as normal: milky-creamy white in color, thick consistency, and a pH of around 6.8, which has also been previously reported (Toelihere 1985).

The results showed individual variations ($P<0.05$) in semen quality, such as volume, concentration, and PTM in each bull. Meanwhile, there was no significant difference in the percentage of fresh semen motility between individuals ($P>0.05$) (Table 1). The effect of individual variations on semen quality has previously been reported in various livestock, such as bulls (Oshio et al. 2004), stallions (Loomis & Graham 2008), and rams (Ngoma et al. 2016). These differences are influenced by many factors, such as the bull's condition, the quality of the reproductive organs, secretions of the sexual glands, age, conditions of breeding management, feed, and the breed of bulls (Indriastuti et al. 2020). However, the percentage of PTM in Bali bulls used varied between bulls ($P<0.05$), and it still met the standard set in Indonesia, which was >40%. The difference in PTM values can be caused by the cryopreservation process, which can decrease semen quality and impact bull fertility (Pratalingam et al. 2006).

Table 1.   The results of the analysis of the semen quality of Bali bulls.

Bulls	Age (years)	Volume (mL)	Conc. (10^6/mL)	Motility (%)	PTM (%)
Budaparta	6	6.08 ± 0.10^b	945.89 ± 12.28^a	70.21 ± 0.19	50.81 ± 0.19^f
Badilawa	7	6.37 ± 0.16^{bc}	938.51 ± 14.73^a	70.00 ± 0.00	50.48 ± 0.16^{df}
Bangtidar	8	4.72 ± 1.03^a	1225.64 ± 21.84^b	70.24 ± 0.13	50.23 ± 0.09^{de}
Tamara	9	6.45 ± 0.28^{bcd}	982.38 ± 22.32^a	70.12 ± 0.09	49.89 ± 0.10^d
Bugamanta	12	6.53 ± 0.15^{bcd}	1000.32 ± 20.96^a	70.07 ± 0.07	45.56 ± 0.21^{bc}
Buwana Merta	12	6.88 ± 0.22^d	1390.76 ± 27.85^c	70.14 ± 0.08	45.16 ± 0.09^{ab}
Blandar	12	4.55 ± 0.10^a	985.68 ± 15.31^a	70.35 ± 0.20	45.66 ± 0.16^c
Mertasari	14	6.57 ± 0.11^{cd}	1239.07 ± 17.89^b	70.00 ± 0.00	45.04 ± 0.04^a

*PTM: post-thawing motility; [a-f] Different letters in each column are significantly different at the 0.05 level.

Significantly, the influence of individual variations (P<0.05) was also shown in the amount of frozen semen production, RR, and field fertility (Table 2). Recovery rate (RR) is the ability of sperm to recover after the cryopreservation process. It means that the sperm from each bull has different abilities in post-freezing recovery. The field fertility values of Bali bulls were classified as having good fertility, with CR reaching 65–75%. This value is supported by previous studies that states that Bali bulls have high fertility (Purwantara *et al.* 2012). The different genetic potential of each bull affects the diversity of reproductive capacity. Many factors may influence it; therefore, individual variations are not the only factor that affects the quality of semen and bull fertility. One of the factors widely studied is the effect of age because aging is an unavoidable process associated with various physiological changes, one of which is the reproductive organs (Pino *et al.* 2020). The effect of age on the decline of reproductive performance is shown in this study, where the percentage of PTM, RR, and field fertility significantly (P<0.05) decreased in the bull group >10 years (Figure 1). Physiological reproduction will reduce when aging occurs (Pardede *et al.* 2020). Li *et al.* (2011) found that although sperm concentration decreased with age, the decline was insignificant. Many factors affect the volume of semen and the concentration of spermatozoa, such as weather, storage frequency, and individual variations (Komariah *et al.* 2020). Aging results in a decrease in reproductive performance and has an impact on fertility decline (Pardede *et al.* 2020). The aging cell affects cell metabolism due to reduced cell quality and quantity. Aging will also impact histologically degenerative changes in the testis, such as morphological changes in germ cells, Sertoli, peritubular testis, and Leydig (Gunes *et al.* 2016). The concentration of reactive oxygen species (ROS) increases with age, along with a decrease in antioxidant levels (Paul & Robaire 2013). The percentage of oxidative damage in the DNA of sperm becomes higher and ultimately can cause cell death and decreased sperm fertility capacity (Pino *et al.* 2020). Based on this study, the percentage of

Table 2.   The analysis results of frozen semen production, recovery rate, and field fertility.

Bulls	Semen Production	RR (%)	Fertility (%)	Total Breeding
Budaparta	155.00 ± 3.39[b]	72.40 ± 0.29[d]	79.60[h]	10199
Badilawa	162.48 ± 5.43[bc]	72.11 ± 0.22[cd]	74.63[d]	17880
Bangtidar	153.39 ± 3.78[b]	71.54 ± 0.18[bc]	78.09[g]	11676
Tamara	167.80 ± 8.29[bc]	71.15 ± 0.17[b]	75.13[f]	3779
Bugamanta	175.38 ± 5.85[c]	65.03 ± 0.31[a]	73.43[b]	11329
Buwana Merta	265.34 ± 11.48[e]	64.40 ± 0.15[a]	74.67[e]	23296
Blandar	119.71 ± 3.57[a]	64.96 ± 0.29[a]	74.50[c]	9284
Mertasari	213.78 ± 4.57[d]	64.34 ± 0.05[a]	71.90[a]	6901

*RR: recovery rate; [a–h] Different letters in each column are significantly different at the 0.05 level.

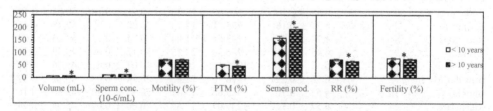

Figure 1.   The analysis results of the quality and production of semen and field fertility in Bali bulls with different age levels (<10 years and >10 years). The concentration value was converted to n 108 million/spermatozoa cell; *Significant difference compared to the <10 years group (P<0.05).

field fertility in bulls in the age group >10 years is lower. It is related to the low percentage of PTM and RR.

The results showed a positive correlation (P<0.01) of semen quality, namely PTM and RR, with the field fertility in Bali bulls (Table 3). Semen quality, including PTM, which is closely related to bull fertility, has also been previously reported (Pardede *et al.* 2022).

However, there are still many studies and relationships that have not been explained in detail. Recent gene and protein level technologies have encouraged the search for fertility biomarkers that are considered more accurate in describing the relationship between the physiological function of spermatozoa and the fertilization process. Through a more sophisticated approach, it is hoped that the mechanism of physiological decline in repro-duction at the cellular or molecular level can be explained and provide a genetic selection tool for bull fertility.

Table 3. Correlation of field fertility with semen quality parameters.

Parameters	Correlation Coefficient	P-value
%Fertility vs volume (mL)	−0.148	<0.000**
%Fertility vs sperm concentration (10^6/mL)	−0.096	<0.008**
%Fertility vs sperm motility (%)	0.049	>0.173
%Fertility vs PTM (%)	0.706	<0.000**
%Fertility vs semen production	−0.166	<0.000**
%Fertility vs RR (%)	0.678	<0.000**

*PTM: post-thawing motility; RR: recovery rate; **Means are significantly different at the P<0.01 level

4 CONCLUSION

This study found that individual and age variations affect semen quality and field fertility, except for fresh semen motility. PTM and RR are closely related to field fertility in Bali bulls.

REFERENCES

Gunes S., Hekim G.N.T., Arslan M.A. and Asci R. 2016. Effect of Aging on the Male Reproductive System. *J Assist Reprod Genet* 33(4): 441–454.

Indriastuti R., Ulum M.F., Arifiantini R.I. and Purwantara B. 2020. Individual Variation in Fresh and Frozen Semen of Bali Bulls (Bos sondaicus). *Veterinary World* 13: 840–846.

Komariah, Arifiantini R.I., Aun M. and Sukmawati E. 2020. Kualitas Semen Segar dan Produksi Semen Beku Sapi Pejantan Madura Pada Musim Yang Berbeda. *Jurnal Ilmu Produksi dan Teknologi Hasil Peternakan* 8 (1): 15–21.

Li Y., Lin H., Li Y. and Cao J. 2011. Association Between Socio-phycho-behavioral Factors and Male Semen Quality: Systematic Review and Meta-analyses. *Fertility and Sterility* 95(1): 116–123.

Loomis P.R. and Graham J.K. 2008. Commercial Semen Freezing: Individual Male Variation in Cryosurvival and the Response of Stallion Sperm to Customised Freezing Protocols. *Animal Reproduction Science* 105: 119–128.

Ngoma L., Kambulu L. and Mwanza M. 2016. Factors Influencing Goat's Semen Fertility and Storage: A Literature Review. *Journal of Human Ecology* 56(1–2): 114–125.

Oshio S., Ashizawa Y., Yotsukura M., Tohyama Y., Iwabuchi M., Adachi Y., Matsuda H., Tomomasa H., Yoshida S., Takeda K. and Umeda T. 2004. Individual Variation in Semen Parameters of Healthy Young Volunteers. *Archives of Andrology* 50: 417–425.

Pardede B.P., Agil M., Karja N.W.K., Sumantri C., Supriatna I. and Purwantara B. 2022. PRM1 Gene Expression and its Protein Abundance in Frozen-thawed Spermatozoa as Potential Fertility Markers in Breeding Bulls. *Veterinary Sciences* 9(111): 1–15.

Pardede B.P., Agil M., Yudi Y. and Supriatna I. 2020. Relationship of Frozen-thawed Semen Quality with the Fertility Rate After Being Distributed in the Brahman Cross Breeding Program. *Veterinary World* 13(12): 2649–2657.

Pardede B.P., Supriatna I., Yudi Y. and Agil M. 2020. Decreased Bull Fertility: Age-related Changes in Sperm Motility and DNA Fragmentation. *E3S Web of Conferences* 151: 1–3.

Paul C. and Robaire B. 2013. Aging of the Male Germ Line. *Nature Review Urology* 10: 227–234.

Pino V., Sanz A., Vandés N., Crosby J. and Mackenna A. 2020. The Effects of Aging on Semen Parameters and Sperm DNA Fragmentation. *JBRA Assisted Reproduction* 24(1): 82–86.

Pratalingam N.S., Holt W.V., Revell S.G., Jones S. and Watson P.F. 2006. Dilution of Spermatozoa Results in Improved Viability Following a 24h Storage Period but Decreased Acrosome Integrity Following Cryopreservation. *Animal Reproduction Science* 91(1–2): 11–22.

Purwantara B., Noor R.R., Andersson G. and Rodriguez-Martinez H. 2012. Banteng and Bali Cattle in Indonesia: Status and Forecasts. *Reprod. Domest. Anim.* 47(1): 2–6.

Saputra D.J., Ihsan M.N. and Isnaini N. 2017. Korelasi Antara Lingkar Skrotum Dengan Volume Semen, Konsentrasi Dan Motilitas Spermatozoa Pejantan Sapi Bali. *Jurnal Ternak Indonesia* 18(2): 59–68.

Toelihere M.R. 1985. *Fisiologi Reproduksi pada Ternak*. Bandung: Angkasa.

Zainudin M., Ihsan M.N. and Suyadi. 2014. Efisiensi Reproduksi Sapi Perah PFH Pada Berbagai Umur di CV. Milkindo Berka Abadi Desa Tegalsari Kecamatan Kepanjen Kabupaten Malang. *Jurnal Ilmu-Ilmu Peternakan* 24(3): 32–37.

Zhao H., Ma N., Chen Q., You X., Liu C., Wang T., Yuan D. and Zhang C. 2019. Decline in Testicular Function in Aging Rats: Changes in the Unfolded Protein Response and Mitochondrial Apoptotic Pathway. *Experimental Gerontology* 127: 1–10.

Developing Modern Livestock Production in Tropical Countries – Adli et al. (eds)
© 2023 The Authors, ISBN 978-1-032-44025-5
Open Access: www.taylorfrancis.com, CC BY-NC-ND 4.0 license

Growth performance and blood profile of IPB D1 chicken on Black Soldier Fly (BSF) larvae feed treatment

G. Ayuningtyas, P. Sembada, D. Priyambodo, F.A. Kurniawan,
S.P. Dewi & A.E.N. Syahfitri
*Livestock Management and Technology Study Program, College of Vocational Studies,
IPB University, West Java, Indonesia*

I. Kusumanti
*Technology and Management of Applied Aquaculture Hatchery Study Program, College of Vocational
Studies, IPB University, West Java, Indonesia*

A.K. Inayah
Accounting Study Program, College of Vocational Studies, IPB University, West Java, Indonesia

ABSTRACT: A study was conducted to determine the influence of feed substituted with full-fat Black Soldier Fly Larvae (BSFL) on growth performance and blood profile of IPB D1 chickens for 11 weeks. Five hundred and fifteen IPB D1 chickens were randomly divided into three treatment groups (T0, T1, and T2) comprised of one hundred and seventy-one chicks (T0), and one hundred and seventy-two chicks for each T1 and T2 treatment with three repetitions that consist of fifty-five to sixty chickens. The groups consist of control feed ration (without BSFL)/ T0), 5% BSFL (T1), and 7.5% BSFL (T2). Each treatment level was used for two kinds of diets, starter (0–7 weeks) and grower (8–11 weeks). The variable observed were feed intake, body weight, feed conversion, mortality, and blood profile (RBC, WBC, HB, leucocyte differentiation). Data collected were subjected to a One-way analysis of variance. Results show an insignificant effect ($p > 0.05$) on the growth performance parameters. Body weight at treatment T0, T1, and T2 are 609.31 ± 50.45 g/bird; 588.67 ± 8.11 g/bird; and 604.44 ± 7.70 g/bird respectively at the end of the starter period (8 weeks), and 992 ± 84.5 g/bird; 937.08 ± 15.95 g/bird; and 957.9 ± 61.49 g/bird respectively at 11 weeks. The IPB D1 Chicken fed with T2 diet (7.5% BSFL) had the best Feed Conversion Ratio (FCR) of the other treatment at the starter period and grower period. The chickens fed with T2 diet had the highest hemoglobin level than other treatments, and total RBC was at normal standard. These findings suggest that the substitution of BSFL on feed (7.5%) potential to increase feed efficiency and show a normal level of hemoglobin and RBC.

Keywords: BSF Larvae, Feed, Growth Performance, IPB-D1 Chicken

1 INTRODUCTION

Feed is an essential production input component in the poultry farming process, and at the same time, it is the dominant component of production costs, around 60–70%. On the other hand, animal feedstuff materials still depend a lot on imports such as fish meal, meat bone meal, soybean meal, and others. This condition is one of the toughest challenges related to availability, issues of domestic component level (TKDN), and also fluctuations in raw

DOI: 10.1201/9781003370048-5

material prices, affecting feed costs. The primary protein sources for animal nutrition, including soybeans, peas, and fish meal, are in increasing demand and are subsequently becoming more expensive, making their long-term use unsustainable (De Souza-Vilela et al., 2019). In connection with these challenges, it is necessary to develop locally-based alternative feed ingredients to reduce or even replace the role of these imported feed ingredients. One of the candidates is the Black Soldier Fly (BSF) larvae. The utilization of Black Soldier Fly (BSF) larvae based on research results can be processed to be used as animal feed ingredients (De Souza-Vilela et al. 2021; Harlystiarini et al. 2022) whose function is as a feed ingredient for animal protein sources. The use of non-conventional feed ingredients such as insects in animal production has the potential to increase farming efficiency and sustainability (De Souza-Vilela et al. 2021). Nowadays, the production of BSF (Hermetia illucens) larvae is getting a lot of attention and is actively being carried out because it is an approach to solving organic waste problems through the bioconversion cycle. The larvae of the BSF are rich in protein and fat and thus, are a high-value feed source. Several recent studies have shown that the use of up to 20% BSF (full fat) larvae in broiler feed still shows the best product performance and also shows better body resistance (De Souza-Vilela 2021). Feed containing BSF larvae oil has been shown to improve broiler chicken feed conversion ratio compared to corn oil and coconut oil (Kim et al. 2020). Furthermore, the substitution of soybean oil for BSF larvae fat supports performance, carcass traits, and overall meat quality (Schiavone et al. 2017). Zotte et al (2019) reported the addition of 15% defatted black soldier fly larvae meal can be an alternative to soybean meal flour in the quail production period, without a negative impact on its production performance. Research related to the use of BSF larvae in other types of poultry, for example, local chickens, still needs to be studied further and in-depth in terms of performance and also to see its effect on blood profile. The local chicken used in this study was IPB D1 chicken, which was the result of a cross between an F1 PS male (Pelung × Sentul) and an F1 female (Kampung × Cobb parent stock) (Al Habib et al. 2020). A study was conducted to determine the influence of feed substituted with full-fat Black Soldier Fly Larvae (BSFL) on the growth performance and blood profile of IPB D1 chickens for 11 weeks.

2 MATERIALS AND METHODS

2.1 Materials

Five hundred and fifteen IPB D1 chickens were obtained from a commercial hatchery. IPB D1 chickens were randomly divided into three treatment groups (T0, T1, and T2) comprised of one hundred and seventy-one chicks (T0), and one hundred and seventy-two chicks for each T1 and T2 treatment with three repetitions that consist of fifty-five to sixty chickens. The feed ingredients used in this study were maize, rice bran, crude palm oil, corn gluten meal, soybean meal, meat meal, CaCO3, sodium, DCP, L-Lysin, and premix. The BSFL meal used came from Biomagg.

2.2 Method

Feed ingredients are prepared based on SNI 7783.1.2013 regarding starter native feed requirement and SNI 7783.2:2013 regarding grower native chicken feed requirement. The process of mixing feed ingredients using an automatic feed mixer with a capacity of 100 Kg. The treatment of substitution of animal protein feed ingredients (meat bone meal) with BSF larvae meal consisted of three levels (T0, T1, T2). Five hundred and fifteen IPB D1 chickens were randomly divided into three treatment groups comprised of one hundred and seventy-one chicks (T0), and one hundred and seventy-two chicks for each T1 and T2 treatment with three repetitions. The groups consist of control feed ration (without BSFL)/ T0), 5% BSFL (T1), and 7.5% BSFL (T2). Each treatment level was used for two kinds of rations, starter (0–7 weeks) and grower (8–11 weeks). Feeding and drinking were ad libitum, and every week the growth performance will be evaluated including feed consumption, body weight, and feed conversion ratio (FCR). At the age of 10 weeks, 2 ml of blood samples were taken per bird (2 birds/block) to conduct a hematology test (blood profile). Whole blood from the brachial vein was collected and placed in 3 mL EDTA vacutainers.

2.3 *Data analysis*

The research design uses a completely randomized design. The effect of BSFL substitution in rations was analyzed using an analysis of variance with feed consumption, body weight, body weight gain, feed conversion, and also hematology as response variables. Hematology results were tested by descriptive statistics. The data analysis using Minitab 17 statistical software.

3 RESULTS AND DISCUSSION

3.1 *Growth performances*

The average IPB D1 Chicken feed consumption and body weight in fed ration with different levels of black soldier fly (BSF) larvae meal during 11 weeks of treatment can be seen in Figure 1. Table 1 presents the feed conversion ratio (FCR) of IPB D1 Chickens fed ration supplemented with different levels of BSF larvae meal. Feed consumption, body weight, and feed conversion of experimental IPB D1 chicken were similar at all feed treatments. The feed consumption and body weight increase every week, and the group T2 (7.5% BSFL meal) treatment shows the lowest cumulative feed conversion at the end of the experiment (week 11). The growth performance result indicated that the use of BSFL meal in feed has the potential to replace the role of meat bone/meat meal as a protein source feed ingredient. This is based on the similarity of growth performance between the control group and the chickens receiving 5% and 7.5% BSFL meal.

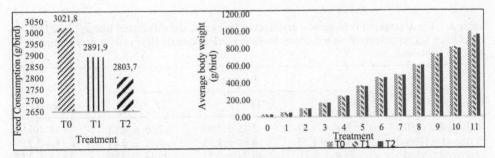

Figure 1. The average IPB D1 Chicken cumulative feed consumption and body weight in fed ration with different levels of black soldier fly (BSF) larvae meal during 11 weeks of treatment. Note: T0 = control ration/ without BSF larvae meal; T1 = ration with 5% BSF larvae meal, T2 = ration with 7.5% BSF larvae meal.

Table 1. The average IPB D1 Chicken cumulative feed conversion in fed ration with different levels of black soldier fly (BSF) larvae meal during 11 weeks of treatment.

Age (week)	Treatments		
	T0	T1	T2
1	0.97 ± 0.02	0.94 ± 0.01	1.03 ± 0.04
2	1.45 ± 0.02	1.30 ± 0.22	1.47 ± 0.04
3	1.80 ± 0.04	1.57 ± 0.30	1.79 ± 0.12
4	2.02 ± 0.08	1.81 ± 0.34	2.00 ± 0.10
5	2.06 ± 0.06	1.81 ± 0.31	2.07 ± 0.11
6	2.16 ± 0.10	2.01 ± 0.29	2.13 ± 0.07
7	2.63 ± 0.04	2.43 ± 0.36	2.58 ± 0.17
8	2.70 ± 0.24	2.56 ± 0.35	2.48 ± 0.17
9	2.86 ± 0.13	2.67 ± 0.24	2.60 ± 0.11
10	3.14 ± 0.10	2.92 ± 0.31	2.94 ± 0.10
11	3.06 ± 0.27	3.09 ± 0.30	2.93 ± 0.10

Note: T0 = control ration/ without BSF larvae meal; T1 = ration with 5% BSF larvae meal, T2 = ration with 7.5% BSF larvae meal.

3.2 Hematological parameters

Table 2 describes the hematological parameters of IPB D1 chickens. The substitution of meat meal with BSF larvae meal did not show a significant effect on the hematological profiles of IPB D1 Chickens. The chickens fed with rations supplemented with 7.5% BSFL meal showed the highest hemoglobin level compared to the other treatments. Total Erythrocytes at all treatments were in accordance with the standard (Campbell 2015), and treatment T1 has the highest level of erythrocytes. The level of leucocytes and their differentiation (lymphocyte and heterophil) were similar in all treatments. These indicate that the addition of BSFL meal in IPB-D1 chicken feed has no impact on the health and physiological conditions of IPB-D1 chickens. IPB-D's in all treatments have a higher lymphocyte percentage than their heterophile percentage. It means that the IPB-D1's has a higher ability to produce the specific immune response with forming antibody specific. The higher

Table 2. The averages of hemoglobin, erythrocyte, leucocyte, and differential leucocytes of IPB D1 chicken fed supplemented with different levels of black soldier fly (BSF) larvae meal during 10 weeks of treatment.

Variables	Treatments			Reference
	T0	T1	T2	
Hemoglobin (g/dL)	5.60 ± 1.37	5.35 ± 2.08	7,05 ± 0,83	8–101
Erythrocyte (106/μI)	3.50 ± 1.77	4.84 ± 1.35	4,62 ± 0,46	4.0–5.22
Leucocyte (103/μI)	34.4 ± 6.71	40.96 ± 2.33	35,17 ± 2,98	23.16 ± 3,103
Lymphocyte (%)	83.33 ± 6.71	81.83 ± 7.63	76,17 ± 3,44	60–731
Heterophil (%)	16.50 ± 6.80	18.17 ± 7.63	16,60 ± 3,44	9–191

Note: T0 = control ration/ without BSF larvae meal; T1 = ration with 5% BSF larvae meal, T2 = ration with 7.5% BSF larvae meal; 1 according to Simaraks (2004); 2 according to Campbell (2015); 3according to Ulupi et al. (2016).

heterophile percentage has potentially overcome the disease with a non-specific immune response through phagocytosis (Ulupi *et al.* 2016).

4 CONCLUSIONS

In this study, IPB D1 Chicken fed with T2 diet (7.5% BSFL) had the best Feed Conversion Ratio (FCR) of the other treatment at the starter period and grower period. The chickens fed with T2 diet had the highest hemoglobin level than other treatments, and total RBC (erythrocyte) was at normal standards. These findings suggest that the substitution of BSFL on feed (7.5%) potential as an alternative substitution to meat bone meal or meat meal, is based on the increased feed efficiency and hematological parameters.

REFERENCES

Al Habib M.F., Murtini S., Cyrilla L., Arief I. I., Mutia R. and Sumantri C. (2020). Performa Pertumbuhan Ayam IPB-D1 Pada Perlakuan Pakan dan Manajemen Pemeliharaan Yang Berbeda. *Jurnal Agripet*, 20(2).

Campbell T.W. and Grant K.R. (2022). *Exotic Animal Hematology and Cytology*. UK: John Wiley and Sons.

Ewald N., Vidakovic A., Langeland M., Kiessling A., Sampels S. and Lalander C. (2020). Fatty Acid Composition of Black Soldier Fly Larvae (Hermetia Illucens)–Possibilities and Limitations for Modification through Diet. *Waste Management*, 102, 40–47.

Harlystiarini H., Mutia R., Wibawan I.W.T. and Astuti D.A. (2020). Immune Responses and Egg Productions of Quails Fed Rations Supplemented with Larvae Meal of Black Soldier Fly (Hermetia Illucens). *Tropical Animal Science Journal*, 43(1), 43–49.

Mat K., Kari Z.A., Rusli N.D., Rahman M.M., Harun H.C., Al-Amsyar, S.M. and Hassan A.M. (2022). Effects of the Inclusion of Black Soldier Fly Larvae (Hermetia Illucens) Meal on Growth Performance and Blood Plasma Constituents in Broiler Chicken (Gallus Gallus Domesticus) Production. *Saudi Journal of Biological Sciences*, 29(2), 809–815.

Ulupi N., Sumantri C. and Darwati S. (2016). *Resistance Against Salmonella Pullorum in IPB-D1 Crossbreed, Kampong and Commercial Broiler Chicken*. The 1st Conference Technology on Biosciences and Social Sciences 2016.

Vilela J.D.S. Andronicos N.M. Kolakshyapati M., Hilliar M., Sibanda T.Z., Andrew N.R., and Ruhnke I. (2021). Black Soldier Fly Larvae in Broiler Diets Improve Broiler Performance and Modulate the Immune System. *Animal Nutrition*, 7(3), 695–706.

Developing Modern Livestock Production in Tropical Countries – Adli et al. (eds)

Successful pregnancy and ovarian condition in Friesian Holstein crossbred dairy cattle with reproductive disorders after single and double dosage artificial insemination

D.A. Damayanti, A.P.A. Yekti, Kuswati & T. Susilawati*
Faculty of Animal Science, Universitas Brawijaya, Malang, Indonesia

ABSTRACT: This study aimed to determine the success of pregnancy and the condition of the ovaries in Artificially Inseminated (AI) cows using single and double dosages of Friesian Holstein Crossbred cows. In this study, 100 Friesian Holstein crossbred cows were treated with single and double dosages of AI. The method was experimental, while the treatments used a single dosage at the 8th hour and double dosages at the 2nd and 8th hours after the onset of estrous. The parameters observed were non-return rate-1 (NRR1), non-return rate-2 (NRR2), conception rate, and pregnancy rate. The results showed that the values of NRR1, NRR2, CR, and PR in the single-dosage treatment were 84%, 64%, 48, and 52%, while in the double-dosage treatment, were 80%, 56%, 40, 82%, and 46.82%, respectively. In addition, the cows that experienced pregnancy failure in a single dosage treatment were normal ovaries 21 (87.5%), persistent corpus luteum 2 (8.33%), and ovarian hypofunction 1 (4.1%). While in the double dosage treatment, normal ovaries were 22 (88%), persistent corpus luteum 1 (4%), and ovarian hypofunction 2 (8%). This study concludes that pregnancy success is higher in single-dosage AI than in double-dosages. In addition, ovarian disorders do not cause pregnancy failure.

Keywords: Artificial Insemination, Friesian Holstein crossbred cow, Ovarium Condition, Reproductive Disorder

1 INTRODUCTION

Milk production in Indonesia is still insufficient to fulfill the demand for milk. Wulandari et al. (2019) mentioned that national milk production is only 20% of the total demand, and 80% is still imported to meet the deficiency. One of the causes of low milk production is the low population of Friesian Holstein dairy cows in Indonesia. Currently, the development of the dairy cattle population in Indonesia is carried out through Artificial Insemination (AI). Some factors that can influence the success of AI in cows include the female conditions, inseminator skills, detection of estrus, time of insemination, number of spermatozoa, insemination dosage, and semen composition (Hoesni 2015). Pregnancy failure in cows can be caused by poor maintenance management and the cows' hormonal conditions. Ansori et al. (2021) stated that AI using single and double dosages would give different results in pregnancy rates. The results of research conducted by Susilawati et al. (2019) using a single dosage gave a CR value of 58.10%.

Meanwhile, AI using a single dosage conducted by Wiranto et al. (2020) gave a CR value of 74.03%. Then, the research conducted by Yekti et al. (2019) using a single dosage of AI

---

*Corresponding Author: tsusilawati@ub.ac.id

DOI: 10.1201/9781003370048-6

obtained a CR value of 53.13%. The results show that many cows still fail to become pregnant. Based on the previous research, it is necessary to evaluate pregnancy failure in cows to obtain a high reproductive efficiency value.

2 MATERIALS AND METHODS

The material used in this study were 100 Friesian Holstein crossbred cows with the criteria that they had given birth at least once and had a BCS value of 2.75–4 (score 1–5). The semen was produced by the Singosari Center for Artificial Insemination (SCAI).

The research method used in this study was primary data collection using experimental methods in the field (field experiment) with AI treatment using a single dosage of frozen semen on 50 cows at the 8th hour with a total of 24 pregnancy failures. The second treatment was AI using double dosage frozen semen on 50 cows at the 2nd and 8th hours with a total failure of 25 cows. AI was carried out with double dosage at the 2nd and 8th hours after estrus (Kuswati et al. 2022). The cows were injected with 10 ml of Vitamin BIO-ATP before inseminating. The non-return rate-1 (NRR1) was observed after one cycle (days 19–20), while the non-return rate-2 (NRR2) was in the next estrus cycle (days 39–42). It was considered pregnant if the cows did not show the estrus sign. The pregnancy and ovarian condition were evaluated using ultrasound to determine the value of CR, PR, and factors of pregnancy failure experienced by the cow. The double dosage treatment gave a CR value of 44%, PR value of 64%, and NRR1 and NRR2 values of 84% and 80%, respectively (Yekti et al. 2022).

Non-return-rate (NRR) is a pregnancy detection method after artificial insemination. The NRR can be calculated using the following formula (Jainudeen & Hafez 2000):

$$NRR = \frac{\sum cows\ inseminated - \sum cows\ in\ estrus\ again}{\sum cows\ inseminated} \times 100$$

Conception rate (CR) is the number of pregnant acceptors in the 1st AI divided by the number of all acceptors multiplied by 100% (Jainudeen & Hafez 2000):

$$CR = \frac{\sum \textbf{pregnant cows in 1st AI}}{\sum \textbf{cows in AI}} \times \textbf{100\%}$$

Pregnant rate (PR) is the number of pregnant acceptors divided by acceptors multiplied by 100% (Jainudeen & Hafez 2000):

$$PR = \frac{\sum \textbf{pregnant cows}}{\sum \textbf{in AI}} \times \textbf{100\%}$$

3 RESULTS AND DISCUSSION

3.1 Non-Return Rate (NRR)

In this study, the detection of NRR was carried out twice: NRR1 within 19–22 days after AI and NRR2 within 39–42 days after AI. The NRR was evaluated based on the number of cows that did not show signs of estrus after AI, and then it was considered pregnant (Yekti et al. 2022). The results of the NRR observations are listed in Table 1.

Following the results of research that has been carried out on 100 Friesian Holstein crossbreeds, there are differences in NRR values from single-dosage and double-dosage treatments. The results of the NRR1 values with single-dosage and double-dosage treatments were 84% and 80%, respectively. At the same time, the values of NRR2 with single-dosage and double-dosage treatment were 64% and 56%, respectively. Based on Table 1, it can be seen that the NRR1 value of a single dosage is higher than that of a double dosage. This value is not better than the results of a study conducted by Yekti et al. (2019) which stated that the results showed the percentage of NRR1 and NRR2 in cows that had been inseminated using frozen semen was 90.63% and 79%.

Table 1. The value of NRR1 and NRR2 with single dosage and double dosage treatment.

	Σ Cows	NRR1(%)	NRR2 (%)
Single Dosage	50	84	64
Double Dosage	50	80	56

The absence of fertilization might cause the decrease of NRR1 to NRR2 in both treatments, no implantation after fertilization, the death of the embryo at a very young age of the embryo, silent heat, and false detection of estrus by the farmer. This follows the opinion of Wahyudi et al. (2014), where the presence of silent heat and early embryonic death causes a decrease in the value of NRR1 to NRR2. One of the factors that can be caused silent heat is stress because of hot climates (Susilawati et al. 2019).

Table 2 shows that the PR values with single and double treatment dosages were 52% and 46.82%, respectively. In contrast, the CR values with single-dosage and double-dosage treatments were 48% and 40.82%, respectively. This result is lower compared to research conducted by Efendi et al. (2015), in which the pregnancy obtained was 60% in local cattle, 83.33% in Bali cattle, and 47.37% in Ongole cattle. These results are higher than the previous result. The high PR value is influenced by several factors, including parity, age, female ovary condition, straw quality, maintenance management, inseminator skills in conducting AI, and environmental temperature (Parmar et al. 2016). A high PR value can indicate that the insemination has been successful.

Table 2. Results of changes in Conception Rate (CR) value to Pregnancy Rate (PR) with single dosage and double dosage treatment.

	Σ Cows	CR (%)	PR (%)
Single Dosage	50	48	52
Double Dosage	50	40,82	46,82

Various factors, including the cow's condition, the farmer, and the inseminator, can influence the high or low CR value. Susilawati (2011) explained that the skills of inseminators and farmers can influence the success of AI, especially in estrus detection, frozen semen handling, time of AI, semen deposition, and the quality of semen. Good-quality semen is indicated by good post-thawing motility (Kusumawati et al. 2019). The quality of estrus shown by female cows is closely related to the CR value. If the female cow does not show signs of estrus in the form of a red, swollen, warm seen on vulva, it will reduce the conception rate (Susilawati 2011).

3.2 *Causes of pregnancy failure*

Artificial insemination failure can be caused by fertilization failure, implantation failure, or early embryo death. Below is a table of causes of AI failure from 100 dairy cows in Pujon

Table 3. Factors of failure of artificial insemination in friesian holstein cows with single dosage and double dosage treatment.

Treatment	Σ Cows Failed to Get Pregnant (%)	Pregnancy Failure Factors		
		Normal Ovaries (%)	PCL (%)	Ovary Hypofunction (%)
Single Dosage	24 (48)	21 (87,5)	2 (8,33)	1 (4,1)
Double Dosage	25 (50)	22 (88)	1 (4)	2 (8)

District, Malang. These data found that the most significant cause of AI failure was in cattle with normal ovary conditions, where the single dosage was 87.5%, and the double dosage was 88%. This proves that maintenance management plays an essential role in pregnancy success. It was found that the failure of insemination in 49 out of 100 acceptor cows was mostly caused by poor rearing management. According to Putri et al. (2020), the factors that most influence the success of insemination are the cow's age, the distance from reporting to AI, and cattle feed. These three factors have a significant influence on the success of insemination.

The data show that cows failed to get pregnant 24% with single dosage treatment and 25% with the double dosage treatment. The quality of feed given to livestock has a significant effect on the nutritional adequacy of livestock. Forage is an essential source of livelihood for livestock. Table 3 lists the number and percentage of cattle that experienced AI failure due to ovarian hypofunction in Friesian Holstein crossbreds with single and double dosages of 1 and 2 dosages is 1%, and 2%, respectively. It can be seen in Table 3 that the AI failure caused by PCL was 8.33% for the single-dosage treatment and 4% for the double-dosage treatment of the total cows that experienced pregnancy failure. PCL is a condition in which the corpus luteum does not regress or lysis and remains in the ovary for a long time (Struve et al. 2013).

4 CONCLUSION

This study concludes that pregnancy success is more in single dosage AI than double dosages, namely 52%, and 46.82%, and ovarian disorders do not cause the cause of pregnancy failure but because of management in AI.

ACKNOWLEDGEMENT

The author would like to thank LPPM UB through Research Grant (HAPPU) with contract number 959.2/UN10.C10/PN/2022.

REFERENCES

Ansori A.I., Kuswati, Huda A.N., Prafitri R., Yekti A.P.A. and SusilawatI T. (2021). Tingkat Keberhasilan Inseminasi Buatan Double Dosis Pada Sapi Persilangan Ongole Dengan Kualitas Berahi Yang Berbeda. *Jurnal Ilmiah Peternakan Rekasatwa*, 3, 36–46.

Efendi M., Siregar T.N., Hamdan, Dasrul, Thasmi C.N., Razali, Sayuti A., and Panjaitan B. (2015). Angka Kebuntingan Sapi Lokal Setelah Diinduksi Dengan Protokol *Ovsynch. Jurnal Medika Veterinaria*, 9, 159–162

Hoesni F. (2015). Pengaruh Keberhasilan Inseminasi Buatan (IB) Atara Sapi Bali Dara Dengan Sapi Bali Yang Pernah Beranak di Kecamatan Pemayung Kabupaten Batanghari. *Jurnal Ilmiah Universitas Batanghari Jambi*, 15, 20–27.

Jainudeen M.R. and Hafez E.S.E. (2000). *Cattle and Buffalo in Reproduction in Farm Animals* USA, Blackwell Publishing.

Kuswati, Septian W.A., Rasyad K., Prafitri R., Huda A.N., Yekti A.P.A. and Susilawati T. (2022). The Increase of Madura Cows Reproduction Performance with Double-dosage Method of Artificial Insemination. *American Journal of Animal and Veterinary Sciences*, 17, 198–202.

Parmar S.C., Dhami A.J., Hadiya K.K. and Parmar C.P. (2016). Early Embryonic Death in Bovines: An Overview. *Raksha Technical Review*, 6, 6–12.

Putri T.D., Siregar T.N., Thasmi C.N., Melia J. and Adam M. (2020). Faktor-faktor Yang Memengaruhi Keberhasilan Inseminasi Buatan Pada Sapi di Kabupaten Asahan, Sumatera Utara. *Jurnal Ilmiah Peternakan Terpadu*, 8, 111–119.

Struve K., Herzog K., Magata F., Piechotta M., Shirasuna K., Miyamoto A. and Bollwein H. (2013). The Effect of Metritis on Luteal Function in Dairy Cows. *BMC Veterinary Research*, 9, 1–9.

Susilawati T. (2011). Tingkat Keberhasilan Inseminasi Buatan Dengan Kualitas Dan Deposisi Semen Yang Berbeda Pada Sapi Peranakan Ongole. *Jurnal Ternak Tropika*, 12, 15–24.

Susilawati T., Mahfud A., Isnaini N., Yekti A.P.A., Huda A.N., Satria A.T. and Kuswati. (2019). The Comparison of Artificial Insemination Success Between Unsexed and Sexed Sperm in Ongole Crossbred Cattle. *IOP Conf. Series: Earth and Environmental Science*, 387 (2019) 012010, 1–3.

Wahyudi L., Susilawati T. and Isnaini N. (2014). Tampilan Reproduksi Hasil Inseminasi Buatan Menggunakan Semen Beku Hasil Sexing Pada Sapi Persilangan Ongole di Peternakan Rakyat. *J. Ternak Tropika*, 15, 80–88.

Wiranto W., Kuswati K., Prafitri R., Huda A.N., Yekti A.P.A. and Susilawati T. (2020). Tingkat Keberhasilan Inseminasi Buatan Menggunakan Semen Beku Sexing Pada Bangsa Sapi Yang Berbeda. *Jurnal Agripet*, 20, 17–21.

Yekti A.P.A., Octaviani E.A., Kuswati and Susilawati T. (2019). Peningkatan Conception Rate Dengan Inseminasi Buatan Menggunakan Semen Sexing Double Dosis Pada Sapi Persilangan Ongole. *TERNAK TROPIKA Journal of Tropical Animal Production*, 20, 135–140.

Yekti A.P.A., Prafitri R., Kuswati, Huda A.N., Kusmartono and Susilawati T. (2022). The Success of Double Dosage Artificial Insemination at Different Times in Ongole Crossbred Cattle. *American Journal of Animal and Veterinary Sciences*, 17, 26–30.

Developing Modern Livestock Production in Tropical Countries – Adli et al. (eds)

The interactive influence of nano-structured encapsulation of *Moringa oleifera* leave particle size and liquid: Growth performance, and gut morphometric of Lohmann broiler

O. Sjofjan, D.N. Adli, M.H. Natsir & Y.F. Nuningtyas
Faculty of Animal Science, Universitas Brawijaya, Malang, Inonesia

ABSTRACT: The research purpose is to carry out the possible effect of *Moringa oleifera* on the growth performance, and intestinal properties of the Lohmann broiler. A total of 104 one-day-old broilers were randomly allocated to 5 dietary treatments and 4 replicates of 5 birds per cage. Four treatments used for research were dietary with control (T0), basal diet + *Moringa oleifera* 80 g (T1), drinking water + 2 mL/L *Moringa oleifera* (T2), and basal feed + *Moringa oleifera* 80 g + drinking water 2 mL/L *Moringa oleifera* (T3). The results showed that using *Moringa oleifera* presented no significant difference ($P < 0.05$) in body weight gain at 1–35 days and intestinal properties. The microstructure didn't affect its structure negatively. To sum up, the use of *Moringa oleifera* in feed gives a positive result on the broiler intestinal properties.

Keywords: crypt depth, moringa oleifera, villus height

1 INTRODUCTION

Industrial poultry faces tremendous challenges after COVID-19. The condition worsened when the inhibition and scarcity of staple feed appeared such as maize and soybean meal. This bad condition also elevated while Ukraine is facing war in 2022. Indonesia still imports the amount of wheat and staple feed for poultry feed, facing difficulty to access, challenging researchers and farmers globally to seek alternative protein sources, and increasing the quality and availability of alternative livestock feeds (Siddiqui *et al.* 2022a; Sjofjan & Adli 2020). *Moringa oleifera* is reputed for its adaptability to grow in all types of soils and to tolerate hot and dry conditions (Sugiharto *et al.* 2020). It contains negligible amounts of ant nutritional factors, has a high crude protein (CP) content, significant amounts of vitamins A, B, and C in the foliage, and contains high amounts of polyphenols, resulting in significant anti-oxidative activity (Abu *et al.* 2020). The leaves of the plant have been reported to possess many pharmacological activities which include analgesic, anti-inflammatory, antiasthmatic, antiulcer, antispasmodic, antibacterial, anti-hyperglycemic, antioxidant, anticancer, and parricidal activities (Abu *et al.* 2020). Toxicological studies on *Moringa oleifera* have shown an absence of severe hepatotoxicity and organ damage except in very high doses. After careful evaluation, the authors wish to evaluate the possible effect of the addition of *Moringa oleifera* on the growth performance and intestinal properties of the broiler.

DOI: 10.1201/9781003370048-7

2 MATERIALS AND METHODS

Experimental design. A total of 104 kg Lohmann chicken with an initial body weight (BW) of 38.13 ± 2.13 kg was used in a 5-week trial. While pens are assigned into completely randomized designs. Treatments were as follows: control (T0), basal diet + *Moringa oleifera* 80 g (T1), drinking water + 2 mL/L *Moringa oleifera* (T2), and basal feed + *Moringa oleifera* 80 g + drinking water 2 mL/L *Moringa oleifera* (T3). The facility set baby chicks and installed a semi-automated nipple drinker at the beginning periods. *Moringa oleifera* fresh leaves were sun-dried and pulverized into powder and incorporated into the basal diet. Meanwhile, the powder of *Moringa oleifera is* put down into the water to become liquid. Then, nano-structured encapsulation formulated chitosan and gum arab as much 2.542 g in acetate solution 2.0% with 250 ml and continued with trial and error comparison (w/v). The water provided was from well water, not artificial water. The water was provided in accordance to minimize the pathogenic bacteria. The data analysis was constructed using SAS online edition, using general linear models. Then, the differences among treatment means (p <0.05) were determined using Duncan's multiple-range test $Y_{ij} = B_0 + B_1 X_{ij} + e_{ij}$ (Adli *et al.* 2022; Ardiansyah *et al.* 2022).

We selected the amount of Lohmann broilers randomly for sacrifice. The body weight was weighed each week thereafter till the end of the week experiment. Feed intake was collected for the amount of feed offered and the remaining feed in the sample. The sacrificed broiler was taken as a sample at the jejunum and ileum area and immediately placed into formulated liquid following (Sjofjan & Adli 2020) formula: NA_2PO_4 2%; NA_2H_2PO4 2%, 24% Formaldehyde; and 900 ml reverse osmosis water for gut morphometric analysis. The calculated gut morphometric was accessed under a light microscope followed by a digital image software application with 200 × zooming (Sjofjan & Adli 2020).

3 RESULTS AND DISCUSSION

Data on the comparison of *Moringa oleifera* leaves and liquid in feed is shown in Table 1. Giving Red *Moringa oleifera* leaves and liquid doesn't improve ($p > 0.05$) on FI, FCR, and BWG. The increase in feed intake may be due to correlating with body weight and body weight gain, and when both of these variable growths increase, the feed intake will also increase. Mikhail *et al.* (2020) explained that the body weight of poultry would be determined by the consumption of feed with a balanced energy and protein content (Adli *et al.* 2020). In the past, the use of plants in monogastric diets was restricted because of some negative aspects of feed intake and nutrient utilization attributed to phytochemical composition that varies greatly due to variety, location, and climate (Adli 2021b). In earnest, the effect on growth performance may not be consistent, for instance, in a number of cases where plant extracts have been used, FI and FCR were not changed, although a positive effect on BW, BWG, organ weight and energy utilization was reported (Sjofjan *et al.* 2020).

Table 1. Effect of nano-structured encapsulation of *Moringa oleifera* leaves and liquid on the performance.

Item	T0	T1	T2	T3	T4	SEM
FI, g/bird	2668	2810.80	2690.80	2499	2810.80	42.10
F/G	1.48	1.54	1.58	1.49	1.45	0.37
BWG, g/bird	1411.33	1417.05	1418.86	1414.64	1416.78	21.33

FI – Feed Intake; F/G feed gain; BWG body weight gain

Table 2. Effect of nano-structured encapsulation of *Moringa oleifera* leaves and liquid in feed on the gut morphometric.

Item	T0	T1	T2	T3	T4	SEM
Villus height, μm	432.25[c]	494.25[bc]	563.50[ab]	573.25[a]	572.5[a]	5.14
Crypth depth μm	122.15[bc]	128.35[a]	128.50[ab]	133.50[ab]	127.75[a]	1.82
VH/CD ratio	5.57	7.06	6.35	6.06	5.23	0.63

VH/CD – Villus height and crypt depth ratio

Statically analysis of gut morphometrics was presented in Table 2. It is successfully impacted to increase both villus height and crypt depth. Thus, the miracle leaves pose positive results and the growth of the gut morphometric is well maintained. It means that an increase in villus may have a positive impact on the balancing of the health of broilers (Zuprizal *et al.* 2020). The quality of water was also impacted because the water consisted of antibiotics reduced the positive effect on the body of the broiler chicken (Iriyanti & Hartoyo 2019). The gut morphometric in the current study lacks linearity with the feed intake (Adli 2021a). Each treatment should be correlated in order to increase nutrient absorption (Adli *et al.* 2020). In the end, Adli *et al.* (2021b) stated that factors affecting intestinal are broiler body weight, age, broiler activity, and gender.

4 CONCLUSION

In summary, the use of *Moringa oleifera* in feed gives a positive result on the broiler intestinal properties. Furthermore, there is a need to determine correlation using polynomial contrast.

REFERENCES

Abu Hafsa S.H., Ibrahim S.A., Eid Y.Z. and Hassan A.A. (2020). Effect of Dietary *Moringa Oleifera* Leaves on the Performance, Ileal Microbiota and Antioxidative Status of Broiler Chicken *Journal of Animal Physiology and Animal Nutrition*, 104, 529–538

Adli D.N., Sjofjan O., Irawan A., Utama D.T., Sholikin M.M., Nurdianti R.R. Nurfitriani R.A., Hidayat C., Jayanegara A. and Sadarman S. (2022). Effects of Fibre-rich Ingredient Levels on Goose Growth Performance, Blood Profile, Foie Gras Quality and its Fatty Acid Profile: A Meta-analysis. *Journal of Animal and Feed Sciences*, 31(4), 301–309.

Adli D.N. (2021a). Uses Insects in Poultry Feed as Replacement Soya Bean Meal and Fish Meal in Development Countries: A Systematic Review. *Livestock Research for Rural Development*, 33(10), 1–4.

Adli D.N., Sjofjan O., Natsir M.H., Nuningtyas Y.F., Sholikah N. and Marbun A. C. (2020) The Effect of Replacing Maize with Fermented Palm Kernel Meal (FPKM) on Broiler Performance. *Livestock Research for Rural Development*, 32(7), 1–4.

Adli D.N. (2021b) The Effect of Replacing Fish Meal with Sago Larvae Meal (SLM) on Egg Production and Quality of Laying Hens. *Livestock Research for Rural Development*, 33(7), 1–8.

Ardiansyah W., Sjofjan O., Widodo E., Suyadi S. and Adli D.N. (2022). Effects of Combinations of α-Lactobacillus sp. and Curcuma Longa Flour on Production, Egg Quality, and Intestinal Profile of Mojosari Ducks. *Advance in Animal Veterinary Science*, 10(8), 1668–1677.

Iriyanti N. and Hartoyo B. (2019) Encapsulated Fermeherbafit Bioavailability and the Application to Broilers. *Journal of Agricultural Science and Technology Applied*, 9, 157–165.

Mikhail W.Z., Abd El-Samee M.O., El-Afifi T.M. and Mohammed A.R. (2020). Effect of Feeding *Moringa oleifera* Leaf Meal with or Without Enzyme on the Performance and Carcass Characteristics of Broiler Chicks. *Plant Archived*, 20, 3381–3388.

Sjofjan O. and Adli D.N. (2020) Effect of Dietary of Supplementation Mannan-Riched Fraction (MRF) and Probiotic-Enhanced Liquid Acidifier on the Growth Performance, Serum Blood Biochemistry, and Intestinal Properties of Broilers in *IOP Conference Series Earth and Envinronmental Science, 478*: 012066.

Siddiqui S.A., Asif Z., Murid M., Fernando I., Adli D.N., Blinov A.V., Golik A.B., Nugraha W.S., Ibrahim S.A. and Jafari S.M. (2022). Consumer Social and Psychological Factors Influencing the Use of Genetically Modified Foods—A Review. *Sustainability*, 14(23), 15884.

Sugiharto S., Yudiarti T., Isroli I., Widiastuti E., Wahyuni H.I. and Sartono T.A. (2020) Feeding Fermented Mixture of Cassava Pulp and *Moringa oleifera* Leaf Meal: Effect on Growth, Internal Organ and Carcass of Broiler Chickens *Agriculturae Conspectus Scientificus*, 85, 87–93.

Sjofjan O., Natsir M.H., Adli D.N., Adelina D.D. and Triana L.M. (2020) Effect of Symbiotic Flour (Lactobacillus Sp. And FOS) To the Egg Quality and Performance of Laying Hens in *OP Conference Series Earth and Envinronmental Science, 465*, 012033.

Zuprizal Z., Ningsih N. and Zulfian T.A. (2020). The Effect of Nano-Encapsulation Phaleria macrocarpa Fruits Extract in Drinking Water on the Digestive Tract and Carcass Characteristic of Broiler Chickens. *Buletin Peternakan*, 44.

Developing Modern Livestock Production in Tropical Countries – Adli et al. (eds)
© 2023 The Authors, ISBN 978-1-032-44025-5
Open Access: www.taylorfrancis.com, CC BY-NC-ND 4.0 license

Effect of chitosan as an alternative additive on preservation quality of silage: A meta-analysis

R.P. Harahap, Y. Rohayeti, D. Setiawan & D. Heraini*

Study Program of Animal Science, Faculty of Agriculture, Tanjungpura University, Pontianak, Indonesia
Animal Feed and Nutrition Modelling (AFENUE) Research Group, Faculty of Animal Science,
IPB University, Bogor, Indonesia

Sadarman

Study Program of Animal Science, Faculty of Agriculture, Tanjungpura University, Pontianak, Indonesia
Animal Feed and Nutrition Modelling (AFENUE) Research Group, Faculty of Animal Science,
IPB University, Bogor, Indonesia

Nahrowi, S. Suharti & A. Jayanegara

Department of Nutrition and Feed Technology, Faculty of Animal Science, IPB University, Bogor,
Indonesia

D.N. Adli

Faculty of Animal Science, Universitas Brawijaya, Malang, Indonesia
Animal Feed and Nutrition Modelling (AFENUE) Research Group, Faculty of Animal Science,
IPB University, Bogor, Indonesia

ABSTRACT: Chitosan is a biodegradable, antimicrobial, and antifungal polysaccharide to be used as an alternative silage additive. This study aimed to determine the effects of chitosan addition on fermentative profile, total losses, in vitro degradation of silage, and in situ digestibility. A total of eight studies of six articles that reported chitosan use as a silage feed additive were integrated into a database. Data were analysed according to a mixed model methodology in which different studies were treated as random effects and chitosan silage additive doses were treated as fixed effects. Results showed that chitosan addition was able to reduce pH, ethanol, yeast and mould of silage (P<0.05), followed by decreased effluent, gas, and total losses of silage (P<0.05). The chitosan increased lactic acid bacteria and DM recovery of silage (P<0.05). Chitosan increased concentration of lactic and acetic acid (P<0.05). Chitosan did not influence the silage's NH_3-N, propionic, and butyric (P>0.05). In contrast, adding chitosan decreased NDF in situ digestibility, besides increasing the DMD in situ digestibility of silage (P<0.05). However, chitosan addition decreased NDF and DMD in vitro degradation of silage (P<0.05). In conclusion, adding chitosan as a silage feed additive may benefit the preservation quality of silage by increasing lactic acid bacteria and DM recovery.

Keywords: additive, chitosan, digestibility, meta-analysis, silage

1 INTRODUCTION

In the tropic's country, forage deficits occur during the dry season and are expected to increase due to climate change. The high nutrient content of good quality grasses and

---

*Corresponding Author: rakhmad@faperta.untan.ac.id

DOI: 10.1201/9781003370048-8

legumes has perishable characteristics. Furthermore, the degradation of plants and the decrease in nutritional value begins with the post-harvest continuation of plant respiration leading to the hydrolysis of carbohydrates and protein proteolysis (Niderkorn & Jayanegara 2021). Therefore, forage conservation and preservation practices are urgently needed to save quantities, reduce nutrient and energy losses, and minimize spoilage. Ensilage can be used to solve the problem of wide variability in feed quality and quantity (Balehegn et al. 2022; Tufail et al. 2020). Silage is fresh forage that is preserved through anaerobic fermentation under high water content conditions, so the yield can be preserved without destroying its nutritional content. Improving the quality of silage can be done by adding silage feed additives. Silage additives generally fall into four categories based on their effect on silage preservation: fermentation stimulants, fermentation inhibitors, aerobic deterioration inhibitors, and nutrients and absorbents (Muck et al. 2018). There are alternative silage inhibitor additives derived from plant secondary metabolite compounds, namely tannins (Jayanegara et al. 2019). However, there is a potential new nomenclature for silage inhibitor additives, namely chitosan (Sirakaya & Beyzi 2022). Chitosan is a non-toxic and biodegradable biopolymer prepared by the deacetylation of chitin (Pereira et al. 2018). Chitosan is being explored for its potential as a functional feed additive agent in ruminants (Harahap et al. 2022; Jayanegara et al. 2021). Chitosan and its derivatives have been used as feed additives for their beneficial function, such as anti-bacterial, anti-fungi, and anti-inflammatory activities (Anggraeni et al. 2022). The differences among this result can be identified using study meta-analysis (Adli et al. 2022).

This study aimed to determine the effects of adding chitosan as an alternative to silage inhibitor additives on the quality of silage by using a meta-analysis.

2 MATERIALS AND METHODS

Eight studies from six papers that reported chitosan use as a feed additive in silage were integrated into a database (De Morais et al. 2021; Del Valle et al. 2018, 2020; Gandra et al. 2016, 2018; Sirakaya & Beyzi 2022). A literature search was performed on Science Direct, PubMed Central, and Google Scholar using "chitosan" and "silage" as the keywords. Treatments were categorized as control (no chitosan addition) and different doses of chitosan addition. Parameters integrated in the database were pH, NH3-N, ethanol, acetic, lactic, propionic, butyric, yeast and mould, lactic acid bacteria, effluent, gas, dry matter recovery, in situ dry matter digestibility, in situ neutral detergent fibre digestibility, in vitro dry matter degradation, in vitro neutral detergent fibre degradation. The meta-analysis was performed using mixed model analysis, considering the different chitosan doses as fixed effects and the various studies as random effects (Sauvant et al. 2008). Statistical models used for the continuous variable were p-values for intercepts and slopes; and information on root mean square error (RMSE) (Jayanegara et al. 2014). Significance was declared when p-values<0.05. The statistical analyses were performed using SAS Software version 9.1 (SAS Institute Inc., Cary, NC, USA).

3 RESULTS AND DISCUSSION

Adding chitosan additives in silage did not affect NH_3-N, propionic, and butyrate acid on fermentative profile of silage (Table 1). The results of this study showed that the addition of chitosan was able to reduce the pH, ethanol, yeast and mould silage (p <0.05), followed by increased lactic acid bacteria in silage (p <0.05). However, Table 2 showed that adding chitosan additives in silage decreased effluent, gas, and total on fermentative and effluent losses of silage (p <0.05), in contrast, increased DM recovery (p <0.05). Chitosan increased concentration of lactic and acetic acid (P <0.05). This study showed that adding chitosan

Table 1. Effects of chitosan (g/Kg DM) on fermentative profile of silage.

Parameter	Unit	n	Parameter estimates				Model statistics	
			Intercept	SE intercept	Slope	SE slope	p-Value	RMSE
pH	No unit	21	4.66	0.40	−0.009	0.024	<.0001	0.69
NH_3-N	mg/dL	11	19.51	8.72	0.607	0.383	0.111	9.05
Ethanol	g/kg DM	17	13.94	4.69	−0.588	0.631	0.025	17.63
Acetic	g/kg DM	21	13.80	3.48	0.323	0.119	0.005	3.37
Lactic	g/kg DM	21	27.40	6.81	0.298	0.805	0.005	22.96
Propionic	g/kg DM	21	1.81	1.15	0.015	0.009	0.158	0.27
Butyric	mg/kg DM	21	7.46	5.62	−0.004	0.057	0.226	1.62
Yeast and mould	log CFU/g of fresh	13	5.42	0.61	−0.152	0.124	0.001	2.56
Lactic bacteria	log CFU/g of fresh	8	6.45	0.50	0.1626	0.1687	0.000	2.87

Note: DM: dry matter, CFU: colony forming unit, SE: standard error, RMSE: root mean square error.
≤ 0.001: Significantly, $p \leq 0.05$: significant, $0.05 \leq P \leq 0.10$: tends to be significant, $p > 0.10$: insignificant

Table 2. Effects of chitosan (g/Kg DM) on fermentative and effluent losses of silage.

Parameter	Unit	n	Parameter estimates				Model statistics	
			Intercept	SE intercept	Slope	SE slope	p-Value	RMSE
Effluent	g/kg DM	17	61.01	17.70	−2.731	1.032	0.014	28.62
Gas	g/kg DM	17	104.61	24.70	−5.273	3.757	0.006	105.14
Total	g/kg DM	17	163.67	33.64	−7.302	3.649	0.003	101.68
DM recovery	g/kg DM	17	795.08	15.99	6.242	3.574	<.0001	102.29

Note: DM: dry matter, SE: standard error, RMSE: root mean square error.
$P \leq 0.001$: very significant, $P \leq 0.05$: significant, $0.05 \leq P \leq 0.10$: tends to be significant, $P > 0.10$: insignificant

decreased NDF in situ digestibility, besides increasing DMD in situ digestibility of silage (p <0.05). However, chitosan addition decreased NDF and DMD in vitro degradation of silage (p <0.05).

Chitosan act as an inhibitor during silage processed. The potential for the presence of spoilage bacteria and fungi is in the early phase of ensilage, namely the aerobic phase. This inhibition plays a role in encouraging the growth of lactic acid bacteria. The increase in lactic acid bacteria was followed by an increase in the concentration of lactic acid, resulting in a decrease in the pH value of the silage. Previous studies reported that chitosan was positively affected by chitosan on pH silage and attributed this effect to a decrease in fermentation extension (Del Valle et al. 2018; 2020). There was no butyric acid concentration effect on the silage inhibitor additive's addition, indicating that clostridia fermentation did not occur. A decrease in butyrate concentration on adding chitosan additives to alfalfa has also been reported (Sirakaya & Beyzi 2022). The addition of chitosan additives did not affect the NH_3-N concentration indicating inhibition of proteolysis in the ensilage. High silage pH, butyric acid, and NH_3-N concentration indicated poor silage preservation conditions (de Morais et al. 2021; Kung Jr et al. 2018). Adding chitosan additives can increase DM recovery, followed by a decrease in the effluent, gas, and total losses. Chitosan has reduced gas and effluent losses and increased DM recovery in sugarcane silage (Del Valle *et al.* 2018; Gandra *et al.* 2016). Several factors can affect the aerobic damage to silage after opening the silo, such as the concentration of DM, acetic acid, butyric acid, and the amount of yeast and mold (Gandra *et al.* 2018). The more extensive gas loss (g/kg natural material) in the silo treated with chitosan may be related to the results of the bacterial count (Gandra *et al.* 2018). The decreased decrease observed with intermediate levels of CHI also increased the reduced ethanol production (Del Valle *et al.* 2018).

4 CONCLUSION

Chitosan can be used as a new nomenclature for inhibitor additives in silage. It provided a beneficial effect on silage quality. Chitosan reduces fermentative losses so that it becomes positive silage preservation. In addition, chitosan increased the of DMDi in situ.

REFERENCES

Adli D.N., Sjofjan O., Irawan A., Utama D.T., Sholikin M.M., Nurdianti R.R. Nurfitriani R.A., Hidayat C., Jayanegara A. and Sadarman S. (2022). Effects of Fibre-rich Ingredient Levels on Goose Growth Performance, Blood Profile, Foie Gras Quality and its Fatty Acid Profile: A Meta-Analysis. *Journal of Animal and Feed Sciences*, 31(4), 301–309.

Anggraeni A.S., Jayanegara A., Laconi E.B., Kumalasari N.R. and Sofyan A. (2022). Marine by-Products and Insects as a Potential Chitosan Source for Ruminant Feed Additives. *Czech Journal of Animal Science*, 67(8), 295–317.

Balehegn M., Ayantunde A., Amole T., Njarui D., Nkosi B.D., Müller F.L., Meeske R., Tjelele T.J., Malebana I.M., Madibela O.R. and Others. (2022). Forage Conservation in Sub-Saharan Africa: Review of Experiences, Challenges, and Opportunities. *Agronomy Journal*, 114(1), 75–99.

De Morais J.P.G., Júnior R.C., Garcia T.M., Capucho E., Campana M., Gandra J.R., Ghizzi L.G. and Del Valle, T.A. (2021). Chitosan and Microbial Inoculants in Whole-plant Soybean Silage. *The Journal of Agricultural Science*, 159(3–4), 227–235.

Del Valle T.A., Antonio G., De Castro Zilio E.M. da Silva Dias M.S., Gandra J.R., de Castro F.A.B., Campana M. and de Morais J.P.G. (2020). Chitosan Level Effects on Fermentation Profile and Chemical Composition of Sugarcane Silage. *Brazilian Journal of Veterinary Research and Animal Science*, 57(3), e162942–e162942.

Del Valle T.A., Zenatti T.F. Antonio G., Campana M., Gandra J.R., Zilio E.M.C., de Mattos L.F.A., and de Morais J.G.P. (2018). Effect of Chitosan on the Preservation Quality of Sugarcane Silage. *Grass and Forage Science*, 73(3), 630–638.

Gandra J.R., Oliveira E.R., Takiya C.S., Goes R., Paiva P.G., Oliveira K.M.P., Gandra E.R.S., Orbach N.D. and Haraki H.M.C. (2016). Chitosan Improves the Chemical Composition, Microbiological Quality, and Aerobic Stability of Sugarcane Silage. *Animal Feed Science and Technology*, 214, 44–52.

Gandra J.R., Takiya C.S., Del Valle T.A., Oliveira E.R. de Goes R., Gandra E.R.S., Batista J.D.O. and Araki H.M.C. (2018). Soybean Whole-plant Ensiled with Chitosan and Lactic Acid Bacteria: Microorganism Counts, Fermentative Profile, and Total Losses. *Journal of Dairy Science*, 101(9), 7871–7880.

Harahap R.P., Suharti S., Ridla M., Laconi E.B., Nahrowi N., Irawan A., Kondo M., Obitsu T. and Jayanegara A. (2022). Meta-analysis of Dietary Chitosan Effects on Performance, Nutrient Utilization, and Product Characteristics of Ruminants. *Animal Science Journal*, 93(1), e13676.

Jayanegara A., Harahap R.P., Suharti S. and Nahrowi N. (2021). Chitosan as a Feed Additive: Its Modulatory Effect on Methane Emission and Biohydrogenation Under Artificial Rumen System. *IOP Conference Series: Materials Science and Engineering*, 1098(4), 42101.

Jayanegara A., Sujarnoko T.U.P., Ridla M., Kondo M. and Kreuzer M. (2019). Silage Quality as Influenced by Concentration and Type of Tannins Present in the Material Ensiled: A Meta-Analysis. *Journal of Animal Physiology and Animal Nutrition*, 103(2), 456–465.

Jayanegara A., Wina E. and Takahashi J. (2014). Meta-analysis on Methane Mitigating Properties of Saponin-rich Sources in the Rumen: Influence of Addition Levels and Plant Sources. *Asian-Australasian Journal of Animal Sciences*, 27(10), 1426.

Muck R.E., Nadeau E.M.G., McAllister T.A., Contreras-Govea F.E., Santos M.C. and Kung Jr L. (2018). Silage Review: Recent Advances and Future uses of Silage Additives. *Journal of Dairy Science*, 101(5), 3980–4000.

Niderkorn V. and Jayanegara A. (2021). Opportunities Offered by Plant Bioactive Compounds to Improve Silage Quality, Animal Health and Product Quality for Sustainable Ruminant Production: A Review. *Agronomy*, 11(1), 86.

Pereira F.M., Carvalho G.G.P., Magalhães T.S., Júnior, J.E.F., Pinto L.F.B., Mourão G.B., Pires A.J. V, Eiras C.E., Novais-Eiras D., Azevêdo J.A.G. and Others. (2018). Effect of Chitosan on Production Performance of Feedlot Lambs. *The Journal of Agricultural Science*, 156(9), 1138–1144.

Sirakaya S. and Beyzi S.B. (2022). Treatment of Alfalfa Silage with Chitosan at Different Levels to Determine Chemical, Nutritional, Fermentation, and Microbial Parameters. *Journal of Animal and Feed Sciences*, 31 (1), 73–80.

Sauvant D., Schmidely P., Daudin J.-J. and St-Pierre N.R. (2008). Meta-analyses of Experimental Data in Animal Nutrition. *Animal*, 2(8), 1203–1214.

Tufail M.S., Mbuku S., Mutimura M., GuoX., Piltz J. and Others. (2020). *Utilisation of Conserved Forage to Improve Livestock Production on Smallholder Farms in Asia and Africa.*

Developing Modern Livestock Production in Tropical Countries – Adli et al. (eds)
© 2023 The Authors, ISBN 978-1-032-44025-5
Open Access: www.taylorfrancis.com, CC BY-NC-ND 4.0 license

Thiobarbituric Acid Reactive Substances (TBARS) and quality of poultry meat as affected by electron beam irradiation: A meta-analysis study

T. Wahyono, A.M. Firmansyah, A. Febrisiantosa, A.I. Setiyawan, M.F. Karimy,
A.C. Trinugraha & T. Ujilestari
*Research Center for Food Technology and Processing, National Research and Innovation Agency
(BRIN), Gunungkidul, Indonesia*

M.M. Sholikin
Research Center for Animal Husbandry, BRIN, Bogor, Indonesia

A.M. Benita
Research Center for Radiation Process Technology, BRIN, South Jakarta, Indonesia

A. Jayanegara
Faculty of Animal Science, IPB University, Bogor, Indonesia
Animal Feed and Nutrition Modelling (AFENUE) Research Group, Bogor, Indonesia

ABSTRACT: Irradiation is a safe and effective approach for food preservation since it reduces food spoilage and improves food hygiene and shelf life. However, irradiation can decrease food quality by causing lipid oxidation and off-odors/flavors. The thiobarbituric acid-reactive substances (TBARS) assay can be used to evaluate the degree of mal-ondialdehyde produced in meat. The effect of irradiation by the electron beam on TBARS and quality in poultry meat (duck and chicken) was investigated. The source of data in the meta-analysis study was conducted on search engines (Scopus®, and PubMed®), searched with "irradiation", "meat", "chicken" and/or "duck" as keywords. The mixed model methodology was used in the present study. After evaluation, 9 articles and 38 studies were chosen to be included in the database. Electron beam irradiation significantly ($p < 0.05$) increased the amount of TBARS. With regard to meat quality, electron beam irradiation increased the redness of poultry meat ($p < 0.01$) and decreased the total bacteria and coliforms ($p < 0.01$). However, there were no differences among the control and irradiation treatment groups for any of the sensory attributes tested (taste, texture, and flavor). In the present meta-analysis study, it can be concluded that irradiation by electron beam had no effect on meat quality properties. However, irradiation could increase TBARS values.

1 INTRODUCTION

In the 2019–2025 period, the highest increase in chicken meat production was produced by Indonesia (417.22%) (Uzundumlu & Dilli 2023). From 2016 to 2019, the export value of poultry products from Indonesia increases by approximately 96.90% (Livestock and Animal Health Statistics 2020). Meat export policies need to be followed by supporting technology. Meat preservation techniques are required to ensure the safety of exported products. Irradiation is one of the appropriate industrial uses that has demonstrated

DOI: 10.1201/9781003370048-9

effectiveness in inhibiting spoilage and harmful microorganisms in meat and fish products (Rosario *et al.* 2020). In addition to spoilage bacteria, meat products may include parasites and dangerous bacteria that could be eradicated with irradiation (Kanatt *et al.* 2005).

Among various food processing techniques, electron beam (e-beam) food irradiation is a non-thermal approach that uses high-energy electrons to break the DNA of pathogens, hence inhibiting their growth. E-beam is considered safer than gamma irradiation since it is produced using electricity rather than radioactivity (Jo *et al.* 2017). However, irradiation degrades food quality by causing lipid oxidation and developing off-flavors and smells (Rababah *et al.* 2004). The thiobarbituric acid-reactive substances (TBARS) assay can evaluate the degree of malondialdehyde produced in meat (Rababah *et al.* 2006). To our knowledge, there is no study to date attempted to quantitatively summarise the effect of electron beam irradiation on the TBARS value of poultry meat. Furthermore, meat quality also needs to be observed because it is related to consumer acceptance. Accordingly, this meta-analysis study aimed to analyze the effect of irradiation by the electron beam on TBARS and quality in poultry meat (duck and chicken).

2 MATERIAL AND METHODS

2.1 *Data collection*

We collected articles published in Scopus® and PubMed®, selected based on suitability with the keywords ("irradiation", "meat", "chicken" and/or "duck"). Approximately 217 articles were retrieved that outlined studies of irradiation for poultry meat, yet only 40 articles of these published articles showed potential for inclusion based on their title, keywords, and abstracts. After evaluation, 9 articles and 38 studies were selected for inclusion in the database (Table 1). The selected articles confirmed that chicken and duck meat were irradiated with different pre-treatments (no treatment, cooked, smoked, infused with water, green tea extract, grape seed extract, and art-butyl hydroquinone). The irradiation doses were 0, 1, 1.5, 1.8, 2, 3, 4.5, 5, and 7 kGy. The parameters included were (1) TBARS; (2) pH; (3) total volatile base nitrogen (TVBN); (4) the possible extent of the oxidation caused by lipids (POV); (5) microbial loads: total bacteria, and coliform; (6) heme pigment: myoglobin (Mb), metmyoglobin (MMb), and oxymyoglobin (MbO$_2$); (7) Hunter's color: lightness (L*), redness (a*), and yellowness (b*); (8) sensory parameters: appearance, taste, texture, flavor, and overall acceptability. If any data used a different measurement unit, these data were transformed into the same measurement units.

Table 1. Study included in the meta-analysis of electron beam irradiation effects on thiobarbituric acid reactive substances (TBARS) and quality of poultry meat.

No	Reference	Meat Sample	Energy (MeV)	Dosage (kGy)
1	Lewis *et al.* (2002)	Chicken	10	0; 1; and 1.8
2	Rababah *et al.* (2004)	Chicken	No information	0; and 3
3	Rababah *et al.* (2006)	Chicken	10	0; and 3
4	Gomes *et al.* (2006)	Chicken	10	0; 2; 3; and 7
5	Kwon *et al.* (2008)	Chicken	10	0; and 5
6	An *et al.* (2017a)	Duck	10	0; 1.5; 3; and 4.5
7	An et al. (2017b)	Duck	10	0; 1; 3; and 7
8	An *et al.* (2018)	Duck	10	0; 1; 3; and 7
9	Arshad *et al.* (2020)	Duck	10	0; 3; and 7

2.2 Data analysis

Data were analyzed for statistical analyses using a mixed model methodology (St-Pierre 2001; Sauvant 2008). Different studies were treated as random effects, whereas the dosages of electron beam irradiation were treated as fixed effects. Root mean square error (RMSE) and p-value were the model statistics used. The statistical analysis was performed using R software version 4.1.2 developed by R Core Team 12 (2022) and a "lme4" package version 1.1-28. Statistical significance was stated if $p<0.05$. If the p-value ranged between 0.05 and 0.10, there was a tendency to be significant.

3 RESULT AND DISCUSSION

Table 2 presents the effect of electron beam irradiation on TBARS and poultry meat quality. The present meta-analysis revealed that electron beam irradiation increased TBARS value at 0 ($p<0.01$), 14 ($p<0.05$), and 21 ($p<0.05$) days of storage. POV value was elevated due to irradiation treatment ($p<0.01$). Concerning microbial loads, electron beam irradiation

Table 2. Effect of electron beam irradiation on thiobarbituric acid reactive substances (TBARS) and quality of poultry meat.

Response parameter	Unit	N	Intercept	SE Intercept	Slope	SE slope	p-value	RMSE	R^2
			TBARS (d)						
0	mg MDA/kg	82	2.06	0.28	0.23	0.06	0.001	0.75	0.72
7	mg MDA/kg	12	0.82	0.75	0.15	0.09	0.159	0.72	0.65
14	mg MDA/kg	15	1.99	1.64	0.37	0.24	0.029	1.84	0.64
21	mg MDA/kg	16	1.58	1.17	0.44	0.16	0.017	1.25	0.71
pH		15	6.01	0.18	0.03	0.03	0.296	0.19	0.69
TVBN	mg%	7	1.84	1.55	0.21	0.09	0.101	0.44	0.93
POV	meq peroxide/kg	7	0.53	0.31	0.09	0.01	0.001	0.03	0.99
			Microbial loads						
Total bacteria	log CFU/g	18	4.98	1.03	−0.72	0.13	0.001	1.09	0.81
Coliform	log CFU/g	18	1.98	0.47	−0.40	0.14	0.009	1.32	0.01
			Heme pigment						
Mb	%	7	40.8	3.83	0.24	0.24	0.015	1.07	0.93
MMb	%	7	29.3	14.2	0.33	0.33	0.664	1.48	0.99
MbO$_2$	%	7	16.5	6.07	0.22	0.22	0.051	1.01	0.98
			Hunter's color						
L*		22	51.2	3.91	−0.45	0.23	0.071	2.05	0.94
a*		22	7.28	2.07	0.32	0.13	0.025	1.14	0.93
b*		22	8.53	1.63	0.27	0.08	0.005	0.74	0.95
			Sensory parameters						
Appearance		10	7.00	0.39	0.01	0.03	0.939	0.16	0.91
Taste		7	7.08	0.22	−0.04	0.05	0.443	0.26	0.26
Texture		14	5.88	0.82	0.01	0.04	0.815	0.24	0.97
Flavor		10	6.87	0.28	−0.04	0.05	0.496	0.25	0.64
Overall acceptability		10	6.93	0.27	−0.03	0.05	0.524	0.25	0.60

decreased total bacteria and coliforms (p<0.01) in poultry meat. Irradiation treatment reduced the amount of myoglobin (p<0.05) and tended to increase oxymyoglobin (p<0.1). Concerning Hunter color changes, the mean values of a* and b* significantly (p<0.05) increased with the dosage of irradiation. The L* values decreased after irradiation treatment (p<0.1). Generally, electron beam irradiation did not affect all the sensory parameters of meat and TVBN value. Because irradiation is believed to promote lipid oxidation due to free radical production, TBARS analysis was performed to test for any increase in lipid oxidation. In each storage time, as the electron beam irradiation level increased, there was an increase in the TBA values indicating increased oxidation (Lewis *et al.* 2002). The increase in TBARS may have been caused by lipid oxidation, which is initiated by hydroxyl radicals produced by irradiation and carbonyl production, breakdown of peroxides, and interaction with nucleophilic molecules (Arshad *et al.* 2020). Free radicals induce lipid oxidation by altering the unsaturated fatty acids or triglycerides (An *et al.* 2017). Strategies are required to prevent the effects of oxidation after irradiation treatment. Rababah *et al.* (2004; 2006) demonstrated that infusing antioxidants and plant extracts into raw and cooked poultry meat reduced lipid oxidation in both irradiated and unirradiated chicken.

Coliforms and total bacteria count of the poultry meat were decreased and eliminated after irradiation treatment. The contamination caused by dangerous microorganisms originating from animal flesh and unclean handling techniques endangers the health of humans (An *et al.* 2018). . Food irradiation's greatest health benefit is its ability to remove nearly all hazardous bacteria, parasites, and pests to maintain a safe and healthy food supply (Huang *et al.* 2007). The effectiveness of irradiation against pathogens is mostly attributable to the creation of hydrogen peroxide as a result of the production of free radicals during irradiation (Lewis *et al.* 2002). Irradiation is an efficient method for decreasing or eliminating microbial contamination by damaging the bacterial nucleic acid and extending the shelf life of poultry meat (Baptista *et al.* 2014). Gomes and da Silva (2006) reported that mesophilic and psychrotrophic bacteria count decreased with the increase in radiation dosage. In our findings, irradiation treatment had no effect on the sensory parameters, which is consistent with the previous study's findings (An *et al.* 2017a; Arshad *et al.* 2020).

4 CONCLUSION

The results showed that electron beam irradiation has a significant effect on reducing microbial activity in poultry meat. Furthermore, there were no differences between the control and irradiation treatment groups for any of the sensory attributes tested (taste, texture, and flavor). However, irradiation of poultry meat can generate lipid oxidation, as demonstrated by an increase in TBARS value. According to our results, strategies are required to prevent the effects of oxidation after irradiation treatment.

ACKNOWLEDGMENTS

We are grateful for the support of this study by the Research Center for Food Technology and Processing, National Research and the Innovation Agency Republic of Indonesia.

REFERENCES

An K.A., Arshad M.S., Jo Y., Chung N., and Kwon J.H. (2017a). E-beam Irradiation for Improving the Microbiological Quality of Smoked Duck Meat with Minimum Effects on Physicochemical Properties During Storage. *Journal of Food Science*, 82(4), 865–872.

An K.A., Jo Y., Akram K., Suh S.C. and Kwon J.H. (2018). Assessment of Microbial Contaminations in Commercial Frozen Duck Meats and the Application of Electron Beam Irradiation to Improve their Hygienic Quality. *Journal of the Science of Food and Agriculture*, 98(14), 5444–5449.

An K.A., Jo Y., Arshad M.S., Kim G.R. Jo, C. and Kwon J.H. (2017b). Assessment of Microbial and Radioactive Contaminations in Korean Cold Duck Meats and Electron-beam Application for Quality Improvement. *Korean Journal for Food Science of Animal Resources*, 37(2), 297–304.

Arshad M.S., Kwon J., Ahmad R.S., Ameer K., Ahmad S. and Jo Y. (2020). Influence of E-beam Irradiation on Microbiological and Physicochemical Properties and Fatty Acid Profile of Frozen Duck Meat. *Food Science and Nutrition*, 8, 1020–1029.

Baptista R.F., Teixeira C.E., Lemos M., Monteiro L.G., Vital H.C., Mársico E.T., Júnior C.A.C. and Mano S.B. (2014). Effect of High-dose Irradiation on Quality Characteristics of Ready-to-eat Broiler Breast Fillets Stored at Room Temperature. *Poultry Science*, 93(10), 2651–2656.

Gomes C., Da Silva P.F., Castell-Perez M.E. and Moreira R.G. (2006). Quality and Microbial Population of Cornish Game Hen Carcasses as Affected by Electron Beam Irradiation. *Journal of Food Science*, 71(7), E327–E336.

Gomes H.A. and da Silva E.N. (2006). Effects of Ionizing Radiation on Mechanically Deboned Chicken Meat During Frozen Storage. *Journal of Radioanalytical and Nuclear Chemistry*, 270(1), 225–229.

Huang C.L., Wolfe K. and McKissick J. (2007). Consumers' Willingness to Pay for Irradiated Poultry Products. *Journal of International Food and Agribusiness Marketing*, 19(2–3), 77–95.

Jo Y., An K, Arshad M.S. and Kwon J. (2017). Effects of E-beam Irradiation on Amino Acids, Fatty Acids and Volatiles of Smoked Duck Meat During Storage. *Innovative Food Science and Emerging Technologies*, 47, 101–109.

Kanatt S.R., Chander R. and Sharma A. (2005). Effect of Radiation Processing on the Quality of Chilled Meat Products. *Meat Science*, 69, 269–275.

Kwon J.H., Kwon Y., Nam K.C., Lee E.J. and Ahn D.U. (2008). Effect of Electron-beam Irradiation before and After Cooking on the Chemical Properties of Beef, Pork, and Chicken. *Meat Science*, 80(3), 903–909.

Lewis S.J., Vela´squez A., Cuppet S.L. and McKee S.R. 2002. Effect of Electron Beam Irradiation on Poultry Meat Safety and Quality. *Poultry Science*, 81(6), 896–903.

Livestock and Animal Health Statistics. (2020). Ministry of Agriculture Republic Indonesia.

Rababah T., Hettiarachchy N., Horax R., Eswaranandam S., Mauromoustakos A., Dickson J. and Niebuhr S. (2004). Effect of Electron Beam Irradiation and Storage at 5°C on Thiobarbituric Acid Reactive Substances and Carbonyl Contents in Chicken Breast Meat Infused with Antioxidants and Selected Plant Extracts. *Journal of Agricultural and Food Chemistry*, 52, 8236–8241.

Rababah T., Hettiarachchy N.S., Horax R., Cho M.J., Davis B. and Dickson J. (2006). Thiobarbituric Acid Reactive Substances and Volatile Compounds in Chicken Breast Meat Infused with Plant Extracts and Subjected to Electron Beam Irradiation. *Poultry Science*, 85, 1107–1113.

Rosario D.K.A., Rodrigues B.L., Bernardes P.C. and Conte-Junior C.A. (2020). Principles and Applications of Non-thermal Technologies and Alternative Chemical Compounds in Meat and Fish. *Critical Reviews in Food Science and Nutrition*, 61(7), 1163–1183.

Uzundumlu A.S. and Dilli M. (2023). Estimating Chicken Meat Productions of Leader Countries for 2019–2025 years. *Ciência Rural*, 53(2), 1–12.

Sauvant, K.P. *Appeals Mechanism in International Investment Disputes*. New York: Oxford University Press.

Developing Modern Livestock Production in Tropical Countries – Adli et al. (eds)
© 2023 The Authors, ISBN 978-1-032-44025-5
Open Access: www.taylorfrancis.com, CC BY-NC-ND 4.0 license

Quality of chicken liver nuggets to the addition of spinach flour from fat content, p content and ash content

D. Amertaningtyas, F. Mu'tashim & L.R. Chamidah
Faculty of Animal Science, University of Brawijaya, Jl. Veteran, Malang, Indonesia

ABSTRACT: The study was conducted to determine the effect of adding green spinach flour (*Amaranthus tricolor*) to chemical quality in terms of fat content and ash content. The observation materials were chicken liver and spinach flour using a completely randomized design (CRD) with 4 treatments and 4 replications, P0 (0%), P1 (5%), P2 (10%), and P3 (15%). The parameters measured were fat content, protein content, and ash content. Statistical analysis was done using analysis of variance (ANOVA). The addition of spinach flour had no significant effect ($P>0.05$) on the fat content, protein content, and ash content of chicken liver nuggets, and the best treatment in this study was chicken liver nuggets without the addition of spinach flour (P0) with a fat content of 20.07 %, protein content of 12.02%, and ash content of 1.62%. For further research, it is necessary to add spinach flour (*Amaranthus tricolor*) and other vegetable flour to chicken liver nuggets by testing different variables.

Keywords: chicken liver nuggets, spinach flour, fat content, protein activity, ash content.

1 INTRODUCTION

Nuggets are restructured meat products with dough and coating to maintain quality. Chicken nuggets are a popular product among the public, but because of the relatively high price, not all people can consume them. The development of innovation in processed nugget products is increasingly diverse, such as using chicken liver. Broiler liver was chosen because of the taste that is liked by the community and has nutritional content such as 5,43 g/100 g fat, 16,92 g/100 g protein, minerals, and vitamins (Permadi et al. 2012). The innovation of processing chicken liver can be in the form of nuggets so that the shelf life and economic value of chicken liver will increase.

Nugget products generally have the disadvantage of only having a fiber content of 2,16%, which is not sufficient for dietary fiber needs (Permadi et al. 2012). The recommended daily dietary fiber requirement for male adolescents is 35–37 g/day and for female adolescents is 30 g/day (Islami *et al.* 2016). Moreover, the addition of vegetables to nuggets will increase the fiber content because vegetables are a source of dietary fiber which is proven to have an important role in maintaining a healthy body, one of which is spinach (All *et al.* 2018). Green spinach (*Amaranthus tricolor*) is a nutritious vegetable. 100 g of spinach leaves (*Amaranthus tricolor*) contained 39.9 mg of protein, 358 mg of calcium, 2,4 mg of iron, 0,8 mg of zinc, 18 mg of vitamin A, 62 mg of vitamin C, and 8 mg of fiber (Zuryanti et al. 2016). Spinach can be processed into flour to extend its shelf life of spinach and make it easier to mix spinach into various processed foods. One of the efforts to improve the quality of chicken liver nugget products is to treat different additions of spinach flour (*Amaranthus tricolor*) to nuggets in terms of fat, protein, and ash content.

DOI: 10.1201/9781003370048-10
This chapter has been made available under a CC BY NC ND license

Based on the description above, it is important that this study was conducted to determine the effect on the quality of using chicken liver nuggets with the addition of spinach flour (*Amaranthus tricolor*) in terms of fat content, protein content, and ash content.

2 MATERIALS AND METHODS

The research was conducted at the Meat Laboratory of the Animal Products Processing Division, Faculty of Animal Science, Universitas Brawijaya for making nuggets, and at the Laboratory of Food Quality and Safety Testing, Department of Agricultural Product Technology Faculty of Agricultural Technology, Universitas Brawijaya for sample testing. The materials used include chicken liver, green spinach flour (*Amaranthus tricolor*), tapioca flour, eggs, salt, pepper, garlic, bread flour, and cooking oil. The equipment used includes stoves, LPG gas, frying pans, boilers, choppers, basins, knives, cutting boards, digital scales, and rulers. The method used is a laboratory experiment using a completely randomized design (CRD) with 4 treatments and 4 replications. The treatments were T0 (addition of 0% spinach flour), T1 (addition of 5% spinach flour), T2 (addition of 10% spinach flour), and T3 (addition of 15% spinach flour).

3 VARIABLE TEST AND DATA ANALYSIS

3.1 *Variable test*

3.1.1 *Fat content*
The fat content test was determined using Soxhlet extraction (AOAC 2005) using a sample of 2 grams (W1) inserted into filter paper and a fat sleeve, then inserted into a fat flask whose fixed weight was weighed (W2) and connected to a Soxhlet tube. The fat sleeve was inserted into the extractor chamber of the Soxhlet tube and rinsed with fat solvent. The extraction tube was mounted on a Soxhlet distillation apparatus and then heated at 40°C with an electric heater for 6 hours. The fat solvent in the fat flask is distilled until all the fat solvent has evaporated.

3.1.2 *The ash content*
The ash test was carried out by dry ashing (AOAC 2005) by cleaning the porcelain ash dish and drying it in an oven at a temperature of about 105°C for 30 minutes. The porcelain ash dish was then put into a desiccator (30 minutes) and then weighed. A sample of 5 grams was weighed and then put into a porcelain ash dish. The cup was then burned on an electric stove until it was smokeless and put in an ashing furnace at a temperature of 600°C for 7 hours.

3.2 *Data analysis*

The data obtained were analyzed using analysis of variance (ANOVA). Then if there is a difference, it is continued with Duncan's Multiple Range Test (DMRT) (Sudarwati et al. 2019).

4 RESULTS AND DISCUSSION

4.1 *The fat content*

Measurement of fat content was carried out using the Soxhlet extraction method. The value of fat content in broiler liver nuggets with the addition of green spinach flour (*Amaranthus tricolor*) can be seen in Table 1. The value of fat content ranged from 20.27% to 23.57%.

Table 1. The average fat, protein, and ash content on chicken liver nuggets with the addition of green spinach flour (*Amaranthus tricolor*).

Treatments	Fat Content (%)	Protein Content (%)	Ash Content (%)
T0	20,27 ± 1,84	12,02 ± 0,43	1,62 ± 0,27
T1	21,23 ± 1,97	11,53 ± 0,76	1,65 ± 0,14
T2	23,57 ± 1,68	11,20 ± 0,20	1,77 ± 0,17
T3	20,93 ± 1,00	11,21 ± 0,34	1,77 ± 0,15

The results of the analysis showed that the addition of spinach flour (*Amaranthus tricolor*) did not have a significant effect ($P>0.05$) on the fat content of chicken liver nuggets. The highest fat content value was found in the T2 treatment (with the addition of 10% spinach flour) which was 23.57%, while the lowest fat content value was in the T0 treatment (0% spinach flour addition) which was 20.27%.

The fat content of broiler liver nuggets with the addition of green spinach flour (*Amaranthus tricolor*) ranged from 20.27% to 23.57% higher when compared to the study of chicken nuggets with broiler liver substitution (Yuliana et al. 2013) which resulted in fat content with an average of 9.77% to 12.92%. This can be due to differences in the basic materials and supporting materials used in making nuggets. A mixture of meat and broiler liver with a percentage of 10%, 20%, 30%, and 40% of the weight of chicken meat was used (Yuliana N. *et al.* 2013).

The value of fat content is higher when compared to the study of chicken nuggets with the addition of spinach flour conducted (Nisa K.M 2021) which has an average fat content of 3.45%. This is presumably due to differences in testing methods, so the values obtained are also different. The average value of liver nugget fat content in the T0 treatment (the addition of 0% spinach flour) was 20.27%, this result was lower when compared to research conducted (Amertaningtyas *et al.* 2021) the fat content obtained from making steamed chicken liver nuggets that is equal to 27.12%. This can be caused during the processing. The steaming process can also be the cause of the reduced fat content of the nuggets. The fat melts during cooking (Soeparn 2005).

4.2 The protein content

Protein content was measured using the Kjeldahl method. Chicken liver nugget protein with the addition of green spinach flour (*Amaranthus tricolor*) can be seen in Table 1. The results of the analysis of the addition of green spinach flour (*Amaranthus tricolor*) had no significant effect ($P>0.05$) on the protein content of chicken liver nuggets. The use of different amaranth flour (*Amaranthus tricolor*) according to the treatment of T1 (addition of 5% spinach flour), T2 (addition of 10% spinach flour), and T3 (addition of 15% spinach flour) in chicken liver nuggets did not affect protein content because spinach flour was not is a source of protein. The protein content of spinach is 35 g/100 g (Ningsih S. 2005). The protein content in 100 g of green spinach (*Amaranthus tricolor*) is 1.3% (Indraswari D.H. *et al.* 2017). The decrease in protein content was in line with the increase in the concentration of green spinach flour (*Amaranthus tricolor*). The decrease in protein content is influenced by the addition of flour concentration (Meitta A.P. et al. 2014).

4.3 The ash content

The addition of spinach flour had no significant effect ($P>0.05$) on the ash content of chicken liver nuggets. The average value of ash content ranged from 1.62% to 1.77%. The lowest ash content value was found in treatment T0 (with the addition of 0% spinach flour) which was 1.62 and the highest ash content value was found in T3 (with the addition of 15% spinach flour). The research on chicken nuggets with the addition of spinach flour (Nisa K. M 2021) had an ash content of 2.38%. The study of broiler liver nuggets (Amertaningtyas et al. 2021) found that the average value of steamed chicken liver ash content was 2.50%. Chicken liver nuggets use tapioca flour to get an ash content of 3.53% (Hanif M 2021). For fried foods, the high or low ash content depends on the length and temperature of the frying pan. The increase in ash content is thought to be caused by high temperatures so a lot of water content is lost (Sundari D et al. 2015).

5 CONCLUSION

The addition of spinach flour (*Amaranthus tricolor*) with a percentage of 0 to 15% in chicken liver nuggets did not affect the fat content, protein content, and ash content, with 20.27–23.57% of fat content, 11.20–12.02% of protein content, and 1.62–1.77% of ash content. Suggestions from this study need to do further research on adding flour from other types of vegetables to chicken liver nuggets by testing different variables.

ACKNOWLEDGEMENT

Acknowledgments for the Brawijaya University Research and Community Service Institute through Dana Penerimaan Negara Bukan Pajak (PNBP) following the DIPA of Brawijaya University Number: DIPA-: 974.36/UN10.C10/PN/2022 on the Hibah Penelitian Pemula (HPP) scheme.

REFERENCES

Agustina A.S., Choiril H.M. and Rohmat H. (2017). Effect of Boiling on Calcium Levels in Green Spinach (Amaranthus tricolor, L) with Complexometric Method. *Motorik*, 12(24), 75–83.

Amertaningtyas D.A. (2021). Penggunaan Tepung Terigu dan Tepung Tapioka Pada Nugget Hati Ayam dan Nugget Hati Sapi. *Jurnal Ilmu Ternak Universitas Padjadjaran*, 21(2).

Amertaningtyas D., Evanuarini H. and Apriliyani M.W. (2022). Chemical Quality and Amino Acid Profile of Liver Nuggets Using Different Flours. In *IOP Conference Series: Earth and Environmental Science* (Vol. 1020, No. 1, p. 012025). IOP Publishing.

AOAC. (2005). *Official Methods of Analysis. Association of Officials Analysis Chemist*, 14th ed. Assoc. Agric. Chemist, Washington, D.C.

BSN. (2014). SNI.01-6683-2014. Nugget Ayam. Badan Standarisasi Nasional. Jakarta.

Gobel M., Fahmi F. and Pakaya I. (2018). Mutu Kimia dan Organoleptik Nugget Ikan Tuna dengan Penambahan Berbagai Kombinasi Tepung Wortel. *Jurnal Agroindustri Halal*, 4(1), 053–059.

Hamidiyah A. (2018, October). Composition of Chicken Liver Nugget to Organoleptic and Hemoglobin Levels in the Efforts to Prevent Adolescent Female Anemia. In *International Conference on Sustainable Health Promotion* (pp. 114–118).

Hanif M. (2021). *Protein Content, Ash Content, and Iron Content of Chicken Liver and Beef Liver Nuggets using Wheat Flour and Tapioca Flour*. Thesis. Fakultas Peternakan. Universitas Brawijaya. Malang.

Hanifah N.I.D. and Dieny F.F. (2016). *Hubungan Total Asupan serat, Serat Larut Air (Soluble), dan Serat Tidak Larut Air (Insoluble) Dengan Kejadian Sindrom Metabolik Pada Remaja Obesitas* (Doctoral Dissertation, Diponegoro University).

Hermanaputri D.I., Ningtyias, F.W. and Rohmawati N. (2017). Pengaruh Penambahan Bayam *[Amaranthus Tricolor]* Pada "Nugget" Kaki Naga Lele *[Clarias Gariepinus]* Terhadap Kadar Zat Besi, Protein, Dan Air. *Nutrition and Food Research*, 40(1), 9–16.

Meitta A.P., Rosyidi D. and Widyastuti E.S. (2013). Pengaruh Penambahan Pati Biji Durian Terhadap Kualitas Kimia dan Organoleptik Nugget Ayam. *Jurnal Ilmu-Ilmu Peternakan (Indonesian Journal of Animal Science)*, 23(3), 17–26.

Ningsih S. (2005). *The Effect of Spinach Flour Substitution on the Making of Steamed Sponge Cake on the Taste and fe Levels.* Thesis. Faculty of Public Health. Universitas Sumatera Utara. Medan.

Nisa K.M. (2021). Effect of Addition of Spinach Flour *(Amaranthus Tricolor)* on the Chemical Quality of Chicken Nuggets. Thesis. Fakultas Peternakan. Universitas Brawijaya. Malang.

Permadi S. N., Mulyani S., and Hintono A. (2012). Kadar Serat, Sifat Organoleptik, dan Rendemen Nugget Ayam Yang Disubstitusi Dengan Jamur Tiram Putih *(Plerotus ostreatus)*. *Jurnal Aplikasi Teknologi Pangan*, 1(4).

Soeparno. (2005). *Ilmu dan Teknologi Daging.* Indonesia: Gadjah Mada University Press.

Sudarwati H., Natsir M.H. and Nurgiartiningsih V.A. (2019). *Statistika dan Rancangan Percobaan: Penerapan dalam Bidang Peternakan.* Universitas Brawijaya Press.

Sundari D., Almasyhuri A. and Lamid A. (2015). Pengaruh Proses Pemasakan Terhadap Komposisi Zat Gizi Bahan Pangan Sumber Protein. *Media Litbangkes*, 25(4), 235–242.

Wijayanti D.A., Hintono A. and Pramono Y.B. (2013). Kadar Protein dan Keempukan Nugget Ayam Dengan Berbagai Level Substitusi Hati Ayam Broiler. *Animal Agriculture Journal*, 2(1), 295–300.

Yuliana N., Pramono Y.B. and Hintono A. (2013). Kadar Lemak, Kekenyalan dan Cita Rasa Nugget Ayam Yang Disubstitusi Dengan Hati Ayam Broiler. *Animal Agriculture Journal*, 2(1), 301–308.

Zuryanti D., Rahayu A. and Rochman N. (2016). Pertumbuhan, Produksi dan Kualitas Bayam (Amaranthus Tricolor L.) Pada Berbagai Dosis Pupuk Kandang Ayam dan Kalium Niitrat (KNO3). *Jurnal Agronida*, 2(2).

Developing Modern Livestock Production in Tropical Countries – Adli et al. (eds)

The proportion of fetal sex using double dose artificial insemination of sexed semen in Holstein Friesian crossbred cows

A.P.A. Yekti, N. Hulaida, G. Ciptadi & T. Susilawati*
Faculty of Animal Science, Universitas Brawijaya, Malang, Indonesia

S. Rahayu
Faculty of Mathematics and Natural Sciences, Universitas Brawijaya, Jl. Veteran, Malang, Indonesia

ABSTRACT: Artificial insemination (AI) using sexed semen is the technology applied to obtain the sex offspring as expected. However, the concentration of sexed frozen semen has lower number than non-sexed frozen semen. This study aimed to evaluate the proportion of fetal sex resulting from artificial insemination using frozen semen with unsexed and double-dose sexed semen on Holstein Friesian Crossbred. A total of 100 Holstein Friesian crossbred dairy housed on farmers' farms in the Pujon sub-district, Malang district. The cows were divided into two treatments consisting of 50 cows, including AI with unsexed semen (T1) and sexed semen (T2). The semen used was frozen semen with X-chromosomes bearing sperm that were separated using the Percoll density gradient centrifugation method. The fetal sex was observed using ultrasonography (USG) 50–90 days after insemination. The parameters observed were pregnancy rate (PR), percentage of fetal sex, and proportion of sperm. The results showed that the pregnancy rate of T1 was 50% and T2 was 52%, respectively. In addition, the female fetal of T1 was 77.78%, while T2 was 81.25%. Furthermore, the X and Y sperm proportions in frozen semen sexed X-bearing chromosomes were 77.9% and 22.1%, respectively. At the same time, the proportion of spermatozoa X and Y in non-sexed semen was 49.7% and 50.3%, respectively. To sum up, the proportion of female fetal by artificial insemination using sexed semen is higher than unsexed semen, with 81.25% and 77.78%, respectively.

Keywords: Artificial Insemination, Percoll gradient, double dose, sex ratio, Holstein Friesian

1 INTRODUCTION

The value of artificial insemination (AI) technology can be improved by using sexed semen to obtain the sex of offspring as expected. The sex calf is determined by the presence of X and Y chromosomes, each of which differs in size, shape, weight, density, charge, motility, motility, phytochemicals on its surface (Prakash 2014), and DNA content (Rahman & Pang 2019). The Percoll density gradient centrifugation sexing method (PDGC) is a method that produces sexed semen with low cost and effectiveness in the separation process. The principle of the sexing method using Percoll centrifugation is the density difference between X and Y-bearing spermatozoa. The density of X-bearing spermatozoa is higher than Y-bearing spermatozoa causing X spermatozoa to reach the lower fraction faster, while Y spermatozoa will remain in the upper fraction (Kusumawati *et al.* 2019). The sexing process reduces the

---

*Corresponding Author: tsusilawati@ub.ac.id

DOI: 10.1201/9781003370048-11

concentration of spermatozoa because there is a long process starting from separation through gradient levels, centrifugation, dilution, and freezing. The previous studies showed that the concentration of PDGC sexing results in frozen Limousin Y semen was 12.125 ± 4.19 million/straw (Mahfud *et al.* 2019) which does not meet the SNI standard of 25 million/straw. The decrease in spermatozoa concentration can reduce the success of AI. Therefore, it is necessary to increase the concentration of sperm by using double-dose AI. Double-dose artificial insemination can significantly increase the conception and pregnancy rate (Kuswati *et al.* 2022; Yekti *et al.* 2022). In addition, ultrasonography (USG) can detect the pregnancy and sex of the conceptus earlier (Quintela *et al.* 2011). This research aims to evaluate the proportion of fetal sex resulting from artificial insemination using frozen semen with unsexed and double-dose sexed semen on Holstein Friesian Crossbred by using USG.

2 MATERIALS AND METHODS

A total of 50 acceptors were obtained from Holstein Friesian crossbred with the following criteria: having a normal reproduction system and a body conditioning score (BCS) of 2.5–4. Deposition of sperm was in position 4 or corpus uteri. The sexing method used was Percoll Density Gradient Centrifugation (Susilawati 2014). The unsexed and sexed semen was produced by the artificial insemination center in Singosari, Malang. The treatments were divided into cows inseminated by unsexed semen 25 acceptors (T1) and cows inseminated by double dose sexed semen 25 acceptors (T2). According to Kumar *et al.* (2017), X spermatozoa are larger than average and Y spermatozoa are smaller than average. Double-dose insemination was performed twice, the first 2 hours after the onset of estrous and the second 8 hours after the onset of estrous (Yekti *et al.* 2022). The fetal sex was observed by using USG mindray-50 to observe the genital tubercle development (Quintela *et al.* 2011). In addition, the proportion of sperm was calculated by measuring the head size using the Olympus cellSens Dimension software. The parameters observed include the pregnancy rate (PR), the percentage of fetal sex, and the proportion of spermatozoa. Prior to the statistical analysis, the data were observed using the chi-square test.

3 RESULTS AND DISCUSSION

3.1 *Pregnancy rate*

Two months after insemination, USG was used to evaluate the pregnancy in cows. The pregnancy rate can be used to evaluate the success of AI. The pregnancy rate value shows the number of pregnant acceptors in the AI acceptor group after pregnancy examination using rectal palpation or USG method (Jainudeen & Hafez 2000).

Table 1 shows that the pregnancy rate of AI using sexed frozen semen with double doses of AI is higher than the unsexed single dose AI. The pregnancy rate for cows in unsexed semen was 50%, while in sexed semen, it is 52%. Process sexing can damage the sperm cell membrane, reducing spermatozoa's ability to fertilize the egg (Kusumawati *et al.* 2017; Susilawati *et al.* 2017). In addition, the concentration produced in sexed semen is much lower

Table 1. Pregnancy rate on AI with unsexed and sexed semen.

Frozen semen	Number of cows (n)	Pregnantt (n)	PR (%)
Unsexed single dose (T1)	50	25	50.00
Sexed double dose (T2)	50	26	52.00

than in unsexed semen. The double-dose AI method produces a higher pregnancy rate than unsexed AI. Several factors, including silent heat, the age of cows, and false estrus detection by farmers, can cause a low pregnancy rate value. The accuracy of estrus detection will increase the percentage of pregnancy in cows because the perfect timing of AI in the estrus phase will result in a high chance of fertilization. Farmers' lack of knowledge in estrus detection can result in AI implementation delays, resulting in AI failure (Garmo *et al.* 2008). Moreover, inseminator skills also play a role in the success of AI, including the thawing method (Nisa *et al.* 2022). In this study, using warm water at a temperature of 37°C for 30 seconds followed the national standard Indonesian.

3.2 *Sex ratio of fetal sex in unsexed and sexed frozen semen*

The sex ratio between treatments, both in unsexed and sexed semen, was observed using ultrasound. Fetal sex in cattle can be observed by looking at the genital tubercle of the fetus. The genital tubercle in males can be found near the tail of the umbilical cord, while in females, it is under the tail (Quintela *et al.* 2011). In this study, the semen used was sexed semen spermatozoa X-bearing, expecting to produce more female calves. The percentage of fetal sex unsexed and sexed semen with double doses is listed in Table 2.

Table 2. The sperm proportion and sex ratio of male and female calves.

| | Unsexed (T1) | | | Sexed (T2) | | |
| | Sperm proportion Mean (%) | Sex | | Sperm proportion Mean (%) | Sex | |
Sex		n	Percentage (%)		n	Percentage (%)
X sperm/Female	49.7	14	77.78	77.9	13	81.25
Y sperm/Male	50.3	4	22.22	22.1	3	18.75
Total	100	18	100	100	16	100

The results showed that the sex percentage of the female fetus in unsexed semen was 77.78%. Meanwhile, on a double dose, sexed semen was 81.25%. It is shown that AI using double doses of sexed semen had a higher percentage of females than AI using unsexed semen. Furthermore, the sperm proportion of spermatozoa X and Y in unsexed semen was found to be 49.7% and 50.3%, respectively, which is categorized as an average proportion of unsexed semen. In addition, the proportion of spermatozoa X in sexed semen was 77.9% higher than spermatozoa Y, 22.1%. The accuracy of semen sexing can be seen based on the proportion of X and Y spermatozoa after the sexing process. Several studies have stated that the Percoll density gradient centrifugation can separate the X and Y spermatozoa ratio with high separation. The top layer produces Y spermatozoa as much as 72%. In comparison, the lower layer produces X spermatozoa 77.5% compared to non-sexing, which has a proportion of X and Y spermatozoa, respectively, 50.4% and 49.6% (Kusumawati *et al.* 2019). Yekti *et al.* (2019) reported the proportion of X and Y spermatozoa after sexing in the upper fraction was around 80.79% compared to non-sexing, which only had 52.77% Y spermatozoa. Silva *et al.* (2017) stated that the success rate of the PDGC method varies from 86% to 94%. The sex ratio of female and male fetuses in AI using unsexed semen was 77.78% and 22.22%, respectively. This result shows different values with the proportion of X and Y spermatozoa on straw. In contrast, Yekti *et al.* (2019) stated that unsexed semen had a spermatozoa percentage of 47.23% and produced 45.83% of the female calf. Meanwhile, the Y spermatozoa had a percentage of 52.77% and 54.17% of the male calf. The analysis using Chi-square test for sex accuracy showed a significant difference ($P<0.05$) between the proportion of spermatozoa in unsexed semen and the fetal sex. In this research, the AI deposition of semen was in corpus uteri or position 4, which can increase the chance of the X spermatozoa fertilizing the egg and resulting in more female calves (Susilawati 2014). The timing of AI can also affect the success of pregnancy. The proportion of female calf births in their off-spring increased with early AI in the first 18 hours from the onset of estrus (Martinez *et al.* 2004).

4 CONCLUSION

In conclusion, the sex ratio of fetuses from AI using frozen sexed semen X chromosome-bearing has a higher percentage than AI using non-sexed semen. Either female or male fetuses from AI using non-sexed semen had a percentage of 72.89% and 27.11%, while for sexed semen, it is 82.93% and 17.07%, respectively. Furthermore, the proportions of X and Y spermatozoa in unsexed frozen semen were 49.7% and 50.3%. In contrast, for sexing frozen semen, the percentages were 77.9% and 22.1%.

ACKNOWLEDGEMENT

The author would like to thank the Directorate General of Higher Education, The Ministry of Education, Culture, Research and Technology, which provides funding through the Doctor Dissertation Research scheme 2022.

REFERENCES

Garmo R.T., Refsdal A.O., Karlberg K., Ropstad E., Waldmann A., Beckers J.F. Reksen O. (2008). Pregnancy Incidence in Norwegian Red Cows Using Nonreturn to Estrus, Rectal Palpation, Pregnancy-Associated Glycoproteins, and Progesterone. *Journal of Dairy Science*, 91, 3025–3033.

Jainudeen M.R. & Hafez E.S.E. 2000. *Cattle and Buffalo in Reproduction in Farm Animals*. USA, Blackwell Publishing.

Kumar N., Gebrekidan B., Gebrewahd T.T. Hadush B. (2017). Sexed Semen Technology in Cattle. *Indian Journal Animal Health*, 56, 157–168.

Kusumawati E.D., Isnaini N., Yekti A.P.A., Luthfi M., Affandhy L., Pamungkas D., Kuswati, Ridhowi A., Sudarwati H., Rahadi S., Rahayu S., Susilawati T. (2019). The Motility and Ratio of X and Y Sperm Filial Ongole Cattle Using Different Sexed Semen Methods. *American Journal of Animal And Veterinary Sciences*, 14, 111–114.

Kusumawati E.D., Isnaini N., Yekti A.P.A., Luthfi M., Affandhy L., Pamungkas D., Kuswati, Ridhowi A., Sudarwati H., Susilawati T., Rahayu S. (2017). The Quality of Sexed Semen on Filial Ongole Bull Using Percoll Density Gradient Centrifugation Method *Asian Journal of Microbiololgy Biotechology Envinroment Science*, 19, 189–199.

Kuswati, Septian W.A., Rasyad K., Prafitri R., Huda A.N., Yekti A.P.A., Susilawati T. (2022). The Increase Of Madura Cows Reproduction Performance With Double-Dose Method of Artificial Insemination. *American Journal of Animal and Veterinary Sciences*, 17, 198–202.

Mahfud A., Isnaini N., Yekti A.P.A., Kuswati K., Susilawati T. (2019). Kualitas Spermatozoa Post Thawing Semen Beku Sperma Y Hasil Sexing Pada Sapi Limousin. *Ternak Tropika Journal of Tropical Animal Production*, 20, 1–7.

Martinez F., Kaabi M., Martinez-Pastor F., Alvarez M., Anel E., Boixo J.C., De Paz P., Anel L. 2004. Effect of the Interval Between Estrus Onset and Artificial Insemination on Sex Ratio and Fertility in Cattle: A Field Study. *Theriogenology*, 62, 1264–70.

Nisa D.C., Rachmawati A., Susilawati T., Yekti A.P.A. (2022). The Quality of Frozen Semen with Different Thawing Duration and Temperature on Simmental Bull. *Jurnal Ilmu-Ilmu Peternakan*, 32, 108–117.

Prakash M.A. (2014). Sexing of Spermatozoa in Farm Animals: A Mini Review. *Advances In Animal and Veterinary Sciences*, 2, 226–232.

Quintela L.A., Becerra J.J., Perez-Marin C.C., Barrio M., Cainzos J., Prieto A., Diaz C. Herradon P.G. (2011). Fetal Gender Determination by First-Trimester Ultrasound in Dairy Cows Under Routine Herd Management in Northwest Spain. *Animal Reproduction Science*, 125, 13–19.

Rahman M.S., Pang M.G. (2019). New Biological Insights on X And Y Chromosome-Bearing Spermatozoa. *Front Cellular Development Biology*, 7, 388.

Silva J.C.F., Moura M.T., Basto S.R.L., Oliveira L.R.S., Caldas E.L.C., Filho M.L.S., Oliveira M.A.L. (2017). Use of Percoll Density Centrifugation for Sperm Sexing in Small Ruminants. *Global Journal of Science Frontier Research: D Agriculture And Veterinary*, 17, 2017, 55–59.

Susilawati T. (2014). *Sexing Spermatozoa*, Malang, UB Press.

Susilawati T., Kusumawati E.D., Isnaini N., Yekti A.P.A., Sudarwati H., Ridhowi A. (2017). Effect of Sexing Process Using Percoll Density Gradient Centrifugation and Frozen on Motility and Damage to Spermatozoa Membrane Of Filial Ongole. *Advances In Health Sciences Research (Ahsr), 1st International Conference In One Health (Icoh 2017)*, 5, 5.

Yekti A.P.A., Bustari W.O., Kuswati, Huda A.N., Satria A.T., Susilawati T. 2019. Male Calf Proportion Of Artificial Insemination Results By Using Sexed Sperm With Double Dose on Ongole Crosbred Cows. *Iop Conferences Series: Earth Environmental Sciences, 387, 012029.*

Yekti A.P.A., Prafitri R., Kuswati, Huda A.N., Kusmartono K., Susilawati T. (2022). The Success of Double Dose Artificial Insemination at Different Times in Ongole Crossbred Cattle. *American Journal of Animal And Veterinary Sciences*, 17, 26–30.

Developing Modern Livestock Production in Tropical Countries – Adli et al. (eds)
© 2023 The Authors, ISBN 978-1-032-44025-5
Open Access: www.taylorfrancis.com, CC BY-NC-ND 4.0 license

Comparison of morphology and morphometry of ovaries and uterine horns of two breeds of rabbits after being induced superovulation using FSH and bovine pituitary extracts

S. Wahyuni, T.N. Siregar & H. Hafizuddin*
Universitas Syiah Kuala, Aceh, Indonesia

ABSTRACT: The administration of BPE will increase the steroid hormone concentration, followed by an increase in the morphology and morphometry of the reproductive organs, especially the ovaries and uterine horns. This study aims to determine the potency of BPE as an alternative preparation for induced superovulation based on the morphological and morphometric observations of the ovaries and uterine horns of two breeds of rabbits, namely local rabbits (LR) and New Zealand White (NZW) rabbits. Morphometrically, the length and width of the rabbit ovaries induced by FSH and BPE in both groups of rabbits showed no significant difference (P>0.05) and also with control rabbits. Furthermore, the length of the uterine horns was also not different between induced superovulation groups and control rabbits (P>0.05). Based on the morphology and morphometry observations on the ovaries and uterine horns, it can be concluded that BPE has the potential as an alternative preparation for superovulation in different breeds of rabbits and other female species.

Keywords: morphology and morphometry, ovaries, superovulation, uterine horn

1 INTRODUCTION

Herbal superovulation is a method used to increase, develop, and mature the ovarian follicles that contain oocytes. The superovulation method can be used to increase the number of ovulated ova in an estrous cycle. Furthermore, superovulation is applied to increase reproductive capabilities by obtaining offspring with better genetic quality. In rabbits, superovulation is considered a method to study the development of reproductive technology and further research in other animal species (Garnier *et al.* 1988). In the field of research, especially in reproductive studies, rabbits are widely used as laboratory animals because of their favorable reproductive characteristics and low breeding costs (Saratsi *et al.* 2002).

The hormone used in the superovulation method is the gonadotropin hormone. In performing superovulation, gonadotropin hormones are used to increase the stimulation of follicular growth. The hormone commonly used is FSH. In addition to FSH, another hormone that has a similar action to FSH is PMSG (Dianti *et al.* 2011). Superovulation treatment with PMSG induction often shows unsatisfactory results, while previous studies have shown that FSH is very effective in producing a high number of embryos per animal (Techakumphu *et al.* 2002). Several recent studies have demonstrated that pituitary extract can be used as an alternative hormone to increase livestock productivity (Amiruddin *et al.* 2014; Iskandar & Setiaji 2018; Outang *et al.* 2017; Suriansyah *et al.* 2013; Zulkarnain *et al.* 2015). However, the information regarding the use of pituitary extracts for the purpose of superovulation is still limited (Arum *et al.* 2013).

---

*Corresponding Author: hafizuddin_umar@unsyiah.ac.id

DOI: 10.1201/9781003370048-12
This chapter has been made available under a CC BY NC ND license

2 MATERIALS AND METHODS

2.1 *Animals*

The experimental animals used in this study were nine local rabbits (LR) and NZW rabbits and also male LR and NZW. All rabbits used were 1.5–2 years old and weighed 2–3 kg. All rabbits were in good health condition, not pregnant, have given birth, and were not disabled. The experimental rabbits were obtained from a rabbit farm located in Aceh Tamiang, Aceh Province.

2.2 *Preparation of BPE*

This study used cattle's pituitary glands that were collected from a slaughterhouse. The pituitary samples that have been obtained were kept in a cool box and immediately taken to the laboratory. The pituitary gland extraction was carried out based on the method applied by Isnaini *et al.* (1994) cited by Sayuti *et al.* (2022). In this study, nine local rabbits (LR) and NZW rabbits were used as animal models. The criteria for rabbits used were rabbits that have given birth before and weigh between 2 and 3 kg. In this study, we also used two male rabbits each from the LR and NZW breeds. Before treatment, all rabbits were adapted for 30 days in separate cages. Anatomical observations were carried out by observing the shape (morphology) of the ovaries and uterus of LR and NZW rabbits from all treatment groups. The ovarian and uterine organs were then documented (photographed) using a digital camera. Measurements of ovaries and uterine horns were carried out on the right and left of both organs including length and width in centimeters (cm). In the part of the uterine horn that forms the curve, length measurements were made using a thread following the curve of organs. Next, the thread was stretched on the surface of the ruler in cm. The morphological data of rabbit ovaries and uterine horns are presented in the form of images. The morphometric data were analyzed using a two-way analysis of variance (ANOVA).

3 RESULTS AND DISCUSSION

3.1 *Morphology of ovaries and uterine horns*

Based on the results of the observation of the ovarian morphology of the two rabbit breeds induced by superovulation with FSH and BPE, the ovaries were very different from the ovaries of the two control rabbit breeds (Figure 1).

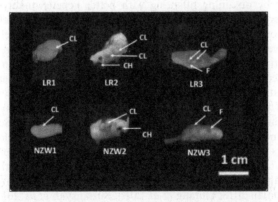

Figure 1. The morphology of ovaries in local rabbit (LR) and New Zealand White (NZW) rabbit after being induced superovulation. The LR control (LR1), LR injected by follicle-stimulating hormone/FSH (LR2), and bovine pituitary extract/BPE (LR3); NZW control (NZW1), NZW injected by FSH (NZW2), and NZW injected by BPE (NZW3). The presence of corpus luteum (CL), corpus hemorrhagic (CH), and follicle (F) is found on the surface of ovaries.

3.2 *Morphometric of ovaries and uterine hoens*

The morphometric measurements (length and width) of the ovaries and uterine horns are presented in Table 1. Morphometrically, the length and width of the ovaries in LR2, NZW2, LR3, and NZW3 rabbits were not significantly different from those of LR1 and NZW1 rabbits (P>0.05). The length and width of the uterine horn in the two treatment groups were also not significantly different from the length and width of the uterine horn in the control group (P>0.05).

Table 1. Morphometry (mean ± SD) of ovaries and uterine horns of the local and NZW rabbits after being induced superovulation using FSH and BPE.

| | Superovulation Treatment | | | | | |
| | Control | | FSH | | BPE | |
Organ	Right	Left	Right	Left	Right	Left
Ovaries Length (cm)						
– Local rabbit	1.20 ± 0.26	1.26 ± 0.32	1.60 ± 0.26	1.66 ± 0.41	1.43 ± 0.25	1.43 ± 0.15
– NZW	1.46 ± 0.40	1.40 ± 0.40	1.10 ± 0.45	1.10 ± 0.20	1.30 ± 0.10	1.20 ± 0.26
Width (cm)						
– Local rabbit	0.66 ± 0.11	0.56 ± 0.15	0.70 ± 0.10	0.56 ± 0.05	0.66 ± 0.05	0.83 ± 0.25
– NZW	0.53 ± 0.25	0.56 ± 0.25	0.50 ± 0.20	0.50 ± 0.10	0.56 ± 0.05	0.63 ± 0.05
Uterine Horns						
Length (cm)						
– Local rabbit	3.66 ± 0.28	4.10 ± 0.26	9.46 ± 5.22	7.76 ± 2.98	4.56 ± 2.07	4.86 ± 1.67
– NZW	7.56 ± 1.55	6.96 ± 1.00	8.60 ± 2.22	8.33 ± 1.78	4.86 ± 1.55	4.56 ± 1.59
Width (cm)						
– Local rabbit	0.86 ± 0.15	0.83 ± 0.15	0.73 ± 0,05	0.76 ± 0.05	0.80 ± 0.10	0.76 ± 0.11
– NZW	0.70 ± 0.30	0.70 ± 0.30	0.50 ± 0,26	0.46 ± 0.25	0.76 ± 0.05	0.73 ± 0.11

Based on Table 1, the morphometric data in terms of ovary length and width were not significantly different between the two rabbit breeds induced by superovulation using FSH and BPE compared to the two control groups. This indicates that the rabbits used in this study did not have the same weight and age even though both rabbit breeds were adults. Hernandez *et al.* (2010) stated that body weight in female rabbits has more influence on the anatomy and function as well as the maturity level of the reproductive organs. The effect of body weight on reproductive organs can be determined based on the differences in morphology and histology of the reproductive tract in female NZW rabbits. NZW rabbits with a body weight of about 2 kg and not induced by superovulation had the mean right and left ovary lengths of 1.12 ± 0.09 and 0.98 ± 0.10 cm, respectively, and the length of the right and left uterine horns was 8.56 ± 0.78 and 7.82 ± 0.81 cm. The ovarian size of NZW rabbits and local control rabbits in this study with a body weight range of 2–3 kg was almost the same as the data reported by Hernandez *et al.* (2010), while the uterine horns of control NZW rabbits were shorter.

4 CONCLUSION

Based on the morphology and morphometry observation on the ovaries and uterine horns, it can be concluded that BPE has the potential as an alternative preparation for superovulation in different breeds of rabbits.

REFERENCES

Amiruddin Siregar T.N., Hamdan, Azhari, Jalaluddin, Zulkifli and Rahman A,A, (2014). The Effect of Pituitary Extract Administration to Increase the Productivity of Layer on Final Period of Production. *Jurnal Kedokteran Hewan*, 8, 80–84.

Arum W.P., Siregar T.N. and Melia J. (2013). The Effect of Bovine Pituitary Extract on Superovulatory Response of Aceh Cattle. *Journal Medicine Veteriner*, 7(2), 71–74.

Dianti D., Udin and Jaswandi. (2011). Pengaruh Penambahan *Follicle Stimulating Hormone* (fsh) dan *Pregnant Mare's Serum Gonadotropin* (pmsg) Dalam Sel Granulosa Terhadap Konsentrasi Progesteron Pada Tingkat Maturase Oosit. *Journal Peternakan Indonesia*, 13(1), 1–6.

Garnier V., Renard J.P. and Menezo Y. (1988). Vianility and Freezing Ability of Rabbit Embryos Collected in the Vagina After Prostaglandin Treatment. *Japan Journal Physiology*, 38(4), 585–589.

Hernández J.A, Sánchez J.S. and Pérez-Martínez M. (2010). Morphometric Characteristics of Female Reproductive Organs of New Zealand Rabbits with Different Body Weight in Peripuberal Period of Transition. *Veterinary México*, 41(3), 211–218.

Iskandar F. and Setiaji C.A. (2018). Peningkatan Kesuburan Menggunakan Ekstrak Hipofisa Pada Kambing Kaligesing Betina Yang Birahinya Diserempakkan Dengan Progesterone Acetate. *Surya Agritama*, 7, 122–138.

Outang T.M.T, Nalley W.M. and Hine T.M. (2017). Utilization of Cattle Hypophysis Extract to Improve Reproductive of Postpartum Sows. *Journal Veterinary*, 18, 383–392.

Saratsi A., Tsiligianni T.H., Besenfelder U., Anastasiadis A., Vainas E. and Brem G. (2002). Induction of Multiple Ovulation in Rabbits Using PMSG and hCG. *Journal Hellenic Veterinary Medicine Society*, 53, 228–236.

Sayuti A., Hamdan H., Jannah M., Safriadi S., Nasri T. and Siregar T.N. (2022). Superovulation Induction with Bovine Pituitary Extract in Local Rabbits. *Punjab University Journal of Zoology*, 37(1), 29–34.

Subchan F.A., Handarini R. and Siswanti S.W. (2016). Perbedaan Waktu Penyuntikan Hormon FSH Terhadap Respon Superovulasi Sapi Angus. *Jurnal Peternakan Nusantara*, 2(1), 34–42.

Suriansyah M., Kamil T. and Bugar H. (2013). Effectiveness and Efficiency of the Pituitary Gland Extract for Spawning of Climbing Perch Fish (*Anabas testudineus* Bloch). *Jurnal Ilmu Hewani Tropika*, 2,46–51

Techakumphu M., Numchaisrika P., Suktrakun V., Phanitkitcharoen S., Kaewnanuer A. and Suwajanakorn S. (2002). Superovulation Responses in Rabbits to Different Does of Follicle Stimulating Hormone. *Thailand Journal Veterinary Medicine*, 32(2), 53–58.

Zulkarnain, Sutiyono and Setiatin E.T. (2015). The Use of Goat Hypothalamic Extract to Optimize Fertility of Female Kejobong Goats. *Journal Veterinary*, 16, 343–350.

The potential of biomass of sweet sorghum (sorghum bicolor L. Moench) planted with different planting systems in acid dry land of lampung

R.D. Tambunan
Research Center for Animal Husbandry, Research Organization for Agriculture and Food, National Research and Innovation Agency, Cibinong, West Java, Indonesia

N.D. Suretno
Research Center for Sustainable Production System and Life Cycle Assessment, Research Organization for Energy and Manufacture, National Research and Innovation Agency, Tangerang Selatan, Banten, Indonesia

ABSTRACT: This research was conducted at Natar Agricultural Science Park, Lampung Province, from April to August 2021. Sweet sorghum (Sorghum bicolor L. Moench) variety used in this study was Bioguma 1 Agritan. The seeds were planted with two different planting systems (zigzag and linear). The treatments were arranged in a Randomized Block Design with three replications. Data collected were analyzed statistically using ANOVA with Minitab 20 software. When the F-test for the treatment was significant ($P \leq 0.05$), treatments were compared using the Tukey test with a significance value of 5%. The results showed that at maturity, sorghum planted using a linear system was significantly taller ($P<0.05$) than the zigzag (275.93 cm vs. 264.57 cm). However, they have a similar fresh weight and panicle weight per plant compared to their counterparts ($P>0.05$). Biomass production of the zigzag (56.00 tons/ha/season) was significantly higher ($P<0.05$) than the linear's (31.95 tons/ha/season), which may accommodate approximately 3–5 cattle per year.

1 INTRODUCTION

The main factor determining the success of the livestock industry is the provision of feed, such as forage and concentrate. However, the availability of forage for animal feed is increasingly narrowed due to limited land caused by the shift of function from native pasture to horticulture and crop fields or settlements (Baba et al. 2019), resulting in a shortage of herbage production. Sweet sorghum (Sorghum bicolor L Moench) is considered to be able to provide a solution to limited land. It can live on marginal or barren lands that do not compete with productive land for food crop production (Capriyati & Tohari 2014; Ristiani et al. 2021). It has wide adaptability and is tolerant to drought stress and high temperatures (Barcelos et al. 2016; Borghi et al. 2013), with high resistance to saline-alkaline soils (Vasilakoglou et al. 2011). Additionally, from the agronomic perspective, it is more environmentally friendly than corn due to its relatively low requirement for nitrogen (Barbanti et al. 2006) and water (Vasilakoglou et al. 2011). Under conditions of limited water supply, sweet sorghum still produces well (Capriyati & Tohari 2014).

Many studies have been conducted on the biomass potential of sorghum planted using the conventional (linear) planting system (Capriyati & Tohari 2014; Dinata 2017; Hajar et al.

2019; Suwarti et al. 2017; Syuryawati et al. 2017). However, there has been no research on sorghum biomass potential using the zigzag method. Therefore, this study aims to determine the potential biomass of sweet sorghum planted with different planting systems on the acid-dry land of Lampung Province.

2 MATERIAL AND METHODS

This research was conducted at Natar Agricultural Science Park, Lampung Province, Indonesia ($-5°19'30''$, $105°10'29''$, 126 m above sea level) from April to August 2021. The sweet sorghum (Sorghum bicolor L. Moench) variety cultivated in this study was Bioguma 1 Agritan, planted on 1 April 2021 with two different planting systems (zigzag and con-ventional/linear) arranged in a Randomized Block Design with three replications. The zigzag planting system in the study used 75 cm × 25 cm × 25 cm spacing, while the conventional planting system was 75 cm × 25 cm (Figure 1). The number of seeds per planting hole was 2–3 seeds. Based on the Schmith Firguson's classification, the climate around the research location was categorized as B type, with an average rainfall of 1,786 mm/year. Cow manure applied at the beginning of land tillage was 2.5 tons/ha, and dolomite was 150 kg/ha. Chemical fertilizers, consisting of 200 kg/ha NPK 16:16:16, 150 kg/ha urea, and 50 kg/ha SP-36, were applied a few days after planting (DAP). Urea and NPK were employed twice, viz. 35% of the doses simultaneously with SP-36 were given at 7 DAP, while the remaining fertilizers were at 30 DAP.

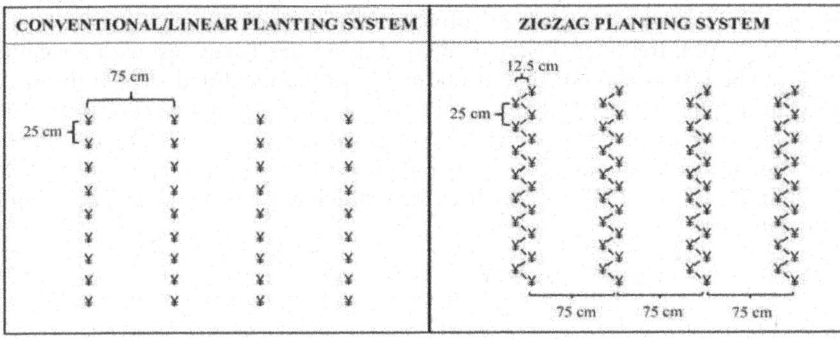

Figure 1.   The zigzag and the linear (conventional) planting systems.

Sweet sorghum from both planting systems was harvested at 105 DAP. The samples of each treatment were taken from five plots. The plot size was 3 m × 4 m. The parameters observed were the number of plants per plot, the height of the plant, fresh weight per plant, panicle weight per plant, total biomass production, and chemical composition of sorghum per treatment. The total biomass production is the weight of leaves and stems per plant multiplied by the number of plants per hectare. The data were analyzed statistically using ANOVA with Minitab 20 software. When the F-test for the treatment was significant ($P \leq 0.05$), treatments were compared using Tukey's test with a significance value of 5%.

3 RESULTS AND DISCUSSION

This research aimed to provide information regarding the potential of biomass of sweet sorghum planted with different planting systems. Table 1 showed that at maturity, sweet

Table 1. The mean harvest performance of sweet sorghum grown with zigzag and linear planting systems.

Planting system	Plant population/ ha	The number of plants/plot	Plant height (cm)	Fresh weight per plant (g)	Panicle weight per plant (g)	Calculated total biomass production/ ha (ton)
Linear	53,333	96.80[a]	275.93[a]	599.00[a]	78.38[a]	31.95[b]
Zigzag	93,333	127.60[a]	264.57[b]	600.05[a]	72.58[a]	56.00[a]

Note: Different letters in the superscript in the same column indicate that values are significantly different by Tukey's test ($P < 0.05$).

sorghum planted using a linear planting system was significantly ($P<0.05$) taller than the zigzag planting system (275.93 cm vs. 264.57 cm). However, it has a significantly lower total biomass production/ha ($P<0.05$) than the zigzag pattern (31.95 tons/ha vs. 56.00 tons/ha). The linear pattern also has a slightly higher panicle's weight per plant than the zigzag (78.38 g vs. 72.58 g), even though the difference was not significant ($P>0.05$). These results indicate that morphologically, the higher the plant density, the smaller the size of individual plants. Low plant density will produce larger individual plants because they will get a better-growing space and adequate nutrients. Hidayat et al. (2018) stated that plants with an ideal growing area would receive better conditions for growth, such as sufficient sunlight, nutrients, and water.

Sorghum biomass can be used as an alternative for animal feed, especially for cattle, because of its nutritive values that are similar to Elephant grass (Irawan & Sutrisna 2011) and comparable to corn (Zea mays L.). Based on the proximate analysis at the Laboratory of Agricultural Product Technology, Politeknik Negeri Lampung (2021), sorghum planted using a zigzag pattern had higher crude protein (CP) and carbohydrates than those on conventional planting systems. On the other hand, sorghum planted using a linear planting system had higher crude fiber and crude fat than their counterparts (Table 2). The CP content of sorghum leaves and stems in the current study was higher than that reported by Yuliatun and Triantarti (2021). The CP of sorghum in their study was 4.82% dry weight. The difference in CP content in both studies was caused by the variety. Yuliatun and Triantarti (2021) used the B6 variety, while this study used Bioguma 1 Agritan. Several studies reported that CP concentrations are affected by the genetic characteristics of the selected variety, the plant environment, and the maturity stage of the plants at harvest (Qu et al. 2014).

Table 2. Chemical composition of sweet sorghum (mixed of leaves and stems) grown with zigzag and linear planting system.

Planting system	Water content (%)		% dry weight			
		Ash	Crude fiber	Crude protein	Crude fat	Carbohydrate
Linear	76.84	7.57	43.19	10.45	4.06	34.73
Zigzag	78.97	2.17	39.76	12.52	3.34	42.21

Source: Laboratory of Agricultural Product Technology, Politeknik Negeri Lampung (2021).

4 CONCLUSION

The present study demonstrated that the zigzag planting system produced higher sorghum biomass than the linear system. This biomass may accommodate approximately 3 5 cattle per year. The high nutritional value of sweet sorghum makes it suitable to be used as an alternative to animal feed. Sweet sorghum is also grown well in the acid-dry land of Lampung Province.

ACKNOWLEDGEMENTS

The authors wish to acknowledge Dr. Slameto, Ade Sopandi, and Sunaryo for technical support; Indonesia Cerdas Desa (ICD) East Lampung Regency for the fund; and Lampung Assessment Institute for Agricultural Technology for research facilities during the study.

REFERENCES

Agung G.A.M.S., Sardiana I.K., Diara I.W., and Nurjaya G.M.O. (2013). Adaptation, Biomass and Ethanol Yields of Sweet Sorghum (Sorghum bicolor L. Moench) Varieties at Dryland Farming Areas of Jimbaran Bali, Indonesia. *Journal of Biology, Agriculture and Healthcare*, 3(17), 111–115.

Andrzejewski B., Eggleston G. and Powell R. (2013). Pilot Plant Clarification of Sweet Sorghum Juice and Evaporation of Raw and Clarified Juices. *Industrial Crops and Products*, 49, 648–658.

Baba S., Dagong M.I.A., Sohrah S., and Utamy R.F. (2019). Factors Affecting the Adoption of Agricultural by-products as Feed by Beef Cattle Farmers in Maros Regency of South Sulawesi, Indonesia. *Tropical Animal Science Journal*, 42(1), 76–80.

Barbanti L., Grandi S., Vecchi A., and Venturi G. (2006). Sweet and Fibre Sorghum (Sorghum bicolor (L.) Moench), Energy Crops in the Frame of Environmental Protection From Excessive Nitrogen Loads. *European Journal of Agronomy*, 25(1), 30–39.

Barcelos C.A., Maeda R.N., Santa Anna L.M.M., and Pereira Jr, N. (2016). Sweet Sorghum as a Whole-crop Feedstock for Ethanol Production. *Biomass and Bioenergy*, 94, 46–56.

Borghi E.C.A.C., Crusciol C.A.C., Nascente A.S., Sousa V.V., Martins P.O., Mateus G.P., and Costa C. (2013). Sorghum Grain Yield, Forage Biomass Production and Revenue as Affected by Intercropping Time. *European Journal of Agronomy*, 51, 130–139.

Capriyati R., and Tohari D.K. (2014). Pengaruh Jarak Tanam Dalam Tumpangsari Sorgum Manis (Sorghum bicolor L. Moench) dan Dua Habitus Wijen (Sesamum indicum L.) Terhadap Pertumbuhan dan Hasil. *Vegetalika*, 3(3), 49–62.

Dinata A.A.N.B.S. *Produktivitas Biomassa Sorgum Batang Manis Yang Memperoleh Biourin Sebagai Sumber Pakan Hijauan Untuk Ternak Sapi.*

Gunawan S., St Aisyah S., and Hafsan H. (2017). Sorgum Untuk Indonesia Swasembada Pangan (Sebuah Review). In *Prosiding Seminar Nasional Biologi* (Vol. 3, No. 1).

Hajar H., Abdullah L., and Diapari D. (2019). Produksi dan Kandungan Nutrien Beberapa Varietas Sorgum Hybrid dengan Jarak Tanam Berbeda sebagai Sumber Pakan. *Jurnal Ilmu Nutrisi Dan Teknologi Pakan*, 17(1), 1–5.

Hidayat K.F., Sunyoto S., and Saputro A.D. (2018, August). Pengaruh Kerapatan Tanaman dan Varietas Sorgum Terhadap Pertumbuhan dan Produksi Biomassa Sorgum Pada Sistem Tumpangsari Sorgum Dengan Ubikayu. In *Prosiding Seminar Nasional Fakultas Pertanian UNS* (Vol. 2, No. 1, pp. A-336).

Indonesian Agency for Agricultural Research and Development. (2019). *Description of Sweet Sorghum Bioguma 1 Agritan Variety*. (in Indonesian.)

Irawan B., and Sutrisna N. (2011). Prospek Pengembangan Sorgum di Jawa Barat Mendukung Diversifikasi Pangan. In *Forum Penelitian Agro Ekonomi* (Vol. 29, No. 2, pp. 99–113).

Khalilian M.E., Habibi D., Golzardi F., Aghayari F., and Khazaei A. (2022). Effect of Maturity Stage on Yield, Morphological Characteristics, and Feed Value of Sorghum [Sorghum bicolor (L.) Moench] Cultivars. *Cereal Research Communications*, 1–10.

Qu H., Liu X.B., Dong C.F., Lu X.Y., and Shen Y.X. (2014). Field Performance and Nutritive Value of Sweet Sorghum in Eastern China. *Field Crops Research*, 157, 84–88.

Ristiani D.N., Hadi M.S., Kukuh S., and Pramono E. (2021). Biomass and Yield of Five Genotypes Sorghum (Sorghum bicolor [L.] Moench) in Dry Land Tanjung Bintang South Lampung. *Inovasi Pembangunan–Jurnal Kelitbangan*, 9(1), 71–85.

Sulistyowati Y., Nurhasanah A.N., Widyajayantie D., Astuti D., Rachmat A., Pantouw C.F., and Nugroho S. (2022). Seleksi dan Evaluasi Sorgum Mutan Generasi M2 Hasil Radiasi Sinar Gamma untuk Peningkatan Karakter Biomassa. *Jurnal Penelitian Pertanian Terapan*, 22(2), 138–145.

Suwarti S., Efendi R., and Pabendon M. (2017). Populasi Optimum Sorgum Manis Sebagai Hijauan Pakan Ternak Dengan Pengaturan Populasi Tanaman. In *Prosiding Seminar Nasional Teknologi Peternakan dan Veteriner* (Vol. 2017, pp. 540–548).

Lalu M.S., and Pabendon M.B. Peningkatan Produksi Brangkasan Sorgum Mendukung Ketersediaan Pakan dan Peningkatan Pendapatan Petani. *Prosiding Seminar Nasional Teknologi Peternakan dan Veteriner*.

Vasilakoglou I., Dhima K., Karagiannidis N., and Gatsis T. (2011). Sweet Sorghum Productivity for Biofuels Under Increased Soil Salinity and Reduced Irrigation. *Field Crops Research*, 120(1), 38–46.

Yu J., Zhang T., Zhong J., Zhang X., and Tan T. (2012). Biorefinery of Sweet Sorghum Stem. *Biotechnology Advances*, 30(4), 811–816.

Yuliatun S., and Triantarti T. (2021). Kualitas dan Nilai Nutrisi Silase Daun Sorgum Manis Untuk Pakan Ternak. *Indonesian Sugar Research Journal*, 1(2), 78–88.

Developing Modern Livestock Production in Tropical Countries – Adli et al. (eds)
© 2023 The Authors, ISBN 978-1-032-44025-5
Open Access: www.taylorfrancis.com, CC BY-NC-ND 4.0 license

Effect of plant regulators on fiber fraction content of Mangrove leave (*Rhizopora apiculata*) as animal feed

G. Yanti*, N. Jamarun, Suyitman, B. Satria, R.W.W. Sari & Z. Ikhlas
Faculty of Animal Science, Andalas University, Padang City, West Sumatra, Indonesia

ABSTRACT: Carbohydrates are a form of carbon storage resulting from photosynthesis, which consists of crude fiber and fiber fraction, which is stored by plants in the form of leaves, branches, and twigs. The yield of plant biomass can be increased by defoliation and giving plant regulators in the vegetative phase. Exogenous cytokinin application has been reported to stimulate the growth and development of lateral shoots. Aims the study was to see the effect of plant regulators on the fiber fraction and lignin content of the leaves of Mangrove (*Rhizopora apiculata*) as forage for animal feed. This study used a Randomized Block Design (RBD) with 5 treatments and 4 replications, which consists of T1: control, T2: BAP, T3: TDZ, T4: JM, and T5: AK. The results of the study show that the lowest NDF and ADF content found in the T5 treatment were 38.53% and 28.23%. This value was significantly different ($P<0.05\%$) with the control treatment, T2, T3, and T4. The lowest lignin content was found in the T4 treatment (9.32%) and the highest in the control treatment (T1) (13.01%). The lignin content of T4 was significantly different ($P>0.05\%$) with T2, T3, and T5 treatments. The conclusion is plant regulators reduced the content of ADF, NDF, and lignin in *Rhizopora apiculata* leaves. Giving Plant Regulator slows down the aging process so that it reduces the lignin content.

Keywords: Plant regulators, Rhizopora apiculata, fiber fraction

1 INTRODUCTION

One of the mangrove plants that are widely found in the mangrove ecosystem is the type *Rhizopora apiculata* which is included in the Rhizophoraceae family. This mangrove is one of the most important species in the mangrove ecosystem. According to Sari *et al.* (2021) *R. apiculata* has a very hard, fast-growing mangrove wood, breath roots, and types of opocyte leaves. In its development, *R. apiculata* was used as food and feed ingredients. According to Sari (2021), *R. apiculata* contains 5.76% crude protein, 16.83% crude fiber, 3.07% crude fat, 48.62% Acid Detergent Fiber (ADF), and 54.51% neutral detergent fiber (NDF). In terms of nutritional content, mangrove leaves have the potential to be used as feed forage.

The mangrove plants need the right technology to maintain their survival if make to feed forages. The quality and production of forage are influenced by the type of plant, the age of the plant, and the place of production (climate and soil fertility). Forage harvesting is affected by the season, cutting age, and cutting interval. Pruning (defoliation) will increase the plant's ability to promote growth. Taiz and Zeiger (2002) explained that plants will continue to experience cell division, cell lengthening, and cell differentiation during the vegetative phase so that there is an increase in leaf and twig biomass. Pruning was intended to stimulate new shoots so that it is able to produce more shoots and biomass. The biomass

---

*Corresponding Author. gusriyanti594@gmail.com

DOI: 10.1201/9781003370048-14
This chapter has been made available under a CC BY NC ND license

could be increased in yield by defoliation and administration of plant growth regulators (PGr) in the immature plant phase. Branch formation and bud growth in plants could be spurred by cytokinin hormones that play a role in the activation of cell division (George et al. 2008). Cytokinin hormone was an adenine-derived compound that was useful for stimulating the formation of buds, affecting cell metabolism, and stimulating dormant cells (Karjadi & Buchori 2008).

Trimmed plants will increase the fixation of carbon in the air. The main product of carbon fixation is the formation of carbohydrates consisting of starch and fructans. Carbohydrates are the main benchmark in determining the quality of forage in addition to the content of proteins, fats, and minerals. In fermentative digestion in the rumen with the help of enzymes produced by rumen microbes, carbohydrates are hydrolyzed into volatile fatty acids (VFA), ammonia (NH_3), CO_2, and methane gas (CH_4). The main purpose of this study was to increase the amount of mangrove forage production by pruning and applying growth regulators.

2 MATERIALS AND METHODS

At the beginning of the study, mangrove plants that were the subject of the study were pruned 15 cm long from the leaflets to equalize the condition of the plant. The growth regulators used are types of cytokinins that come from various sources. The treatment consisted of T1:Control, T2:Benzyl amino purines, T3:Thiadozuron, T4:Young Corn Extract, and T5:Young Coconut Water. Benzyl amino purines and thiadozuron are given with a concentration of 60 ppm, while young corn and coconut water with a concentration of 50%.

During the observation period, plants sprayed growth regulators 1 time per 2 weeks. Spraying is carried out at 08 Am. The treatment is given until the age of 16 weeks. After collecting, the leaf samples are placed at room temperature for 24 hours and dried in a 60°C oven for 3 hours. The sample is finely ground until it passes through a 1 mm sieve, then the sample is stored for testing. The results were analyzed using the Randomize Complete Block method with IBM SPSS Statistics 26.0 Version (IBM corp., NY, USA).

3 RESULTS AND DISCUSSION

The content of NDF, ADF, and Lignin of mangrove leaves (*Rhizopora apiculata*) which are given the practice of various types of growth regulators is presented in Table 1. Van Soest et al. (1991) divide forage into two fractions, namely cell contents and cell walls. The contents of the cell consist of protein fractions, non-structural carbohydrates, minerals, and fats that are easily soluble in neutral detergent solvents. Cell walls that are insoluble in neutral detergent solvents (NDF) are divided into fractions based on their solubility in acid

Table 1. The content of NDF, ADF, and lignin leaves of *Rhizopora apiculata* treated with various types of ZPT.

Parameters (%)	Treatment				
	T1	T2	T3	T4	T5
Dry matter	32.74[b]	31.44[b]	31.24[b]	32.09[b]	35.05[a]
NDF	38.43[b]	38.11[b]	37.23[a]	38.71[b]	38.53[b]
ADF	29.84[bc]	28.47[a]	29.06[ab]	30.80[c]	28.23[a]
Lignin	13.01[c]	10.87[b]	9.98[bc]	9.32[a]	11.04[b]

Description: different superscripts on the same line show noticeable differences (P<0.05)

detergent solvents. The soluble fraction consists of hemicellulose and cell wall proteins, while the insoluble ones are selulosa, lignin, lignocellulose, and silica called acid detergent fiber (ADF).

The ADF describes the indigestible part of the forage. Feed ingredients with a lower NDF content have a higher quality than ingredients with a high NDF content. The results showed that the difference in the type of PGr given had a significant effect ($p<0.05$) on the content of NDF, ADF, and lignin of *Rhizopora apiculata* leaves. The content of NDF and ADF varies with each treatment. PGr removal does not necessarily decrease the NDF and ADF content of *Rhizopora apiculata* leaves. The varying fiber fraction content in each treatment is estimated to be due to the accumulation of organic carbon produced. The application of PGr to rhizopora apiculata plants is able to increase dry matter. The highest dry matter in the T5 (coconut water) treatment is thought to be because coconut water contains not only cytokinins but also gibberellin. Cytokinins play a role in chlorophyll synthesis and leaf expansion resulting from cell enlargement. According to Naor *et al.* (2005), cytokinin and gibberellin compounds increase plant physiological activity and affect protein synthesis, increase sugar content, and chlorophyll in plants.

4 CONCLUSION

The results of the study show that the lowest NDF and ADF content found in the T5 treatment were 38.53% and 28.23%. The lowest lignin content was found in the T4 treatment (9.32%) and the highest in the control treatment (T1) (13.01%).

REFERENCES

Anjarsari I.R.D., Hamdani J.S., Suherman C., Nurmala T., Khomaeni H.S. & Rahadi V.P. (2021). Studi Pemangkasan dan Aplikasi Sitokinin-Giberelin pada Tanaman Teh (Camellia Sinensis (L) O. Kuntze) Produktif Klon GMB 7. *Jurnal Agronomi Indonesia (Indonesian Journal of Agronomy)*, 49(1), 89–96.

George E.F., Hall M.A. & De Klerk G.J. (2008). *Plant Propagation by Tissue Culture*, 3rd Edition. The Netherland, The Back Ground Springer.

Goering H.K.(1970). *Forage Fiber Analyses (Apparatus, Reagents, Procedures, and Some Applications)* (No. 379). US Agricultural Research Service.

Herdiawan I., Abdullah L. & Sopandi D. (2014). Status Nutrisi Hijauan Indigofera Zollingeriana pada Berbagai Taraf Perlakuan Stres Kekeringan dan Interval Pemangkasan. *JITV*, 19(2), 91–103.

Karjadi A.K. & Buchory A. (2008). Pengaruh Auksin dan Sitokinin terhadap Pertumbuhan dan Perkembangan Jaringan Meristem Kentang Kultivar Granola. *Journal of Horticulture*, 18(4), 380–384

Liu Q., Luo L. & Zheng L. (2018). Lignins: Biosintesis and Biologycal Function in Plants. *International Journal of Moleculer Science*, 19, 335.

Naor V., Kigel J. & Ziv M. (2004, April). The Effect of Gibberellin and Cytokinin on Floral Development in Zantedeschia spp. In Vivo and In Vitro. In *IX International Symposium on Flower Bulbs 673* (pp. 255–263).

Oba M. & Allen M.S. (1999). Evaluation of the Importance of the Digestibility of Neutral Detergent Fiber from Forage: Effects on Dry Matter Intake and Milk Yield of Dairy Cows. *Journal of Dairy Science*, 82(3), 589–596.

Sari R.W.W., Jamarun N., Pazla R., Yanti G. & Ikhlas Z. (2022, April). Nutritional Analysis of Mangrove Leaves (Rhizophora apiculata) Soaking with Lime Water for Ruminants Feed. In *IOP Conference Series: Earth and Environmental Science* (Vol. 1020, No. 1, p. 012010). IOP Publishing.

Taiz L. and Zeiger E. (2002) *Plant Physiology*, 3rd Edition, Sinauer Associates, Inc. Publishers, Sunderland, MA, USA.

Van Soest P.V., Robertson J.B. & Lewis B.A. (1991). Methods for Dietary Fiber, Neutral Detergent Fiber and Nonstarch Polysaccharides in Relation to Animal Nutrition. *Journal of Dairy Science*, 74(10), 3583–3597.

Wu W., Du K., Kang X. & Wei H. (2021). The Diverse Roles of Cytokinins in Regulating Leaf Development. *Horticulture Research*, 8.

Developing Modern Livestock Production in Tropical Countries – Adli et al. (eds)

Histopathological changes of the endometrium of white rats (*Rattus norvegicus*) infected with *Escherichia coli*

T. Armansyah, T.N. Siregar, Hafizuddin, Nazaruddin, C.A.A. Shakina,
B. Panjaitan & A. Sutriana
Faculty of Veterinary Medicine, Universitas Syiah Kuala, Banda Aceh, Aceh, Indonesia

Suhartono
Department Biology, Faculty of MIPA, Universitas Syiah Kuala, Banda Aceh, Aceh, Indonesia

ABSTRACT: The purpose of this study was to determine the histopathological change of endometrium of white rats infected with different concentration of *E. coli*. For that purpose, 9 white rats were randomly divided into 3 treatment groups consisted of 3 rats each. The rats in control group (P0) was inoculated with NaCl solution, while the rats in group I (PI) and group II were inoculated with *E. coli* at concentration of 1.0×10^5 CFU/ml and 1.5×10^8 CFU/ml, respectively. The rats were sacrificed 36 hours post inoculation to evaluate the histophatological change in endometrium. Data were analyzed using the Kruskal-Wallis non-parametric test and continued with the Mann-Whitney U test. The results showed that the level of necrosis and proliferation of endometrial epithelial cells were significantly higher ($P<0.05$) in groups PI and PII as compared to group P0. It could be concluded that the higher the concentration of inoculated *E. coli*, the higher the damage to the endometrium in terms of the decrease in lumen size, the level of necrosis and proliferation of endometrial epithelial cells.

Keywords: endometrium, histopathological, proliferation, rat

1 INTRODUCTION

Endometritis is an inflammation in the endometrium caused by bacterial infection and can be classified into acute endometritis and chronic endometritis (Barański *et al.* 2012; Sendana *et al.* 2019). Cows affected by endometritis can have a negative impact on farmers, causing economic losses due to decreased reproductive performance. There are several non-specific microorganisms that can cause endometritis in cattle due to poor cage sanitation such as *Streptococcus*, *Staphylococcus*, *Escherichia coli*, and *Corynebacterium pyogenes* (Sinaga *et al.* 2021). Rafika *et al.* (2020) reported that most of Gram-negative bacteria found in cattle were *E. coli* (30.00%) due to contamination of the reproductive tract by feces containing *E. coli*. The use of mice as animal models for endometritis case in cattle will facilitate the understanding of disease pathogenesis in cattle. Previous studies have reported that intravaginal inoculation of *E. coli* in mice at a dose of 1.5×10^6 could induce acute endometritis with an infection rate of 66.7% (Dar *et al.* 2016). However, the reports regarding histopathological changes in the endometrium of white mice infected with *E. coli* that induce endometritis are still limited. Therefore, this study aims to evaluate the histopathological changes of white rat endometrium infected with *E. coli* with a concentration of 1.5×10^5 CFU/ml and 1.5×10^8 CFU/ml in experimental animals. The data can be used as a basis for determining the degree of pathogenicity of bacteria causing endometritis in cattle.

DOI: 10.1201/9781003370048-15

2 METHODS

This research was designed using completely randomized design (CRD) with 3 treatments and 3 replications. The samples used in each experimental group were 3 female white rats, thus the total rats used were 9 female white rats aged 3–4 months and weighed 160–200 grams. During adaptation, the rats were given a standard T29-4 ration, and their body weight and activity were continuously monitored. After 2 weeks acclimatization, the rats were conditioned to be in the luteal phase by injecting hormone progesterone (potahormon) subcutaneously for 5 days at a dose of 16 mg/kg. The rats were then divided into 3 treatment groups and bacteria were inoculated into their uterine horn. Control group (P0) was inoculated with 50 μl NaCl solution as a negative control, group I (PI) was inoculated with 50 μl of *E. coli* per rat with a concentration of 1.0×10^5 CFU/ml (Demirel *et al.* 2019), and group II (PII) was inoculated with 50 μl of *E. coli* per rat with a concentration of 1.5×10^8 CFU/ml. The rat uterus was taken 36 hours post *E. coli* inoculation. Prior to uterus collection, the rats were sacrificed by cervical dislocation. Then surgery was performed to remove the uterine organs. Uterine organ samples were fixed in 10% NBF solution to prevent tissue damage or decay due to the influence of bacteria or autolysis (Duwiri *et al.* 2019). Histopathological preparation and examination were conducted using Kiernan method (1990), which was made in several stages: fixation, dehydration, clearing, infiltration, embedding, sectioning, staining, and microscopic examination. The staining process was carried out using hematoxylin–eosin (HE) and the observations were made under a light microscope. Parameters assessed were histopathological features of necrosis and proliferation of epithelial cells, and swelling of the endometrium (assessed by the wide and narrowed lumen). Histological preparations were observed through 5 fields of view and scored based on the categories according to Duwiri *et al.* (2019). Necrosis was given a score of 0 if there was no necrosis, a score of 1 if there was focal necrosis (mild), a score of 2 if there was multifocal necrosis (moderate), and a score of 3 if there was diffuse (severe). The data were analyzed using Kruskal-Wallis non-parametric test followed by Mann-Whitney U test (Steel & Torrie 1991).

3 RESULTS AND DISCUSSION

Image of cell necrosis in groups P0, PI, and PII is presented in Figure 1. In group P0, the whole uterus from the three replicates of white rat samples in normal conditions with a regular arrangement of ciliated columnar epithelium, and no necrosis or cell proliferation was found. In groups PI and PII, mild to severe necrosis was found which was characterized by lost blood supply during cell swelling and protein denaturation and organ damage during the stages of necrosis, namely psychosis, karyorhexis, and karyolitic. However, there were no inflammatory cells found in group PI. In group PII, the necrosis was more severe, the endometrial epithelium was lysed and inflammatory cells (lymphocytes and neutrophils) and fibroblasts appeared.

The results of Mann Whitney analysis showed that cell necrosis and cell proliferation significantly increase (P<0.05) in rats infected with *E. coli* (group P1 and PII) compared to

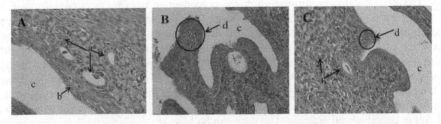

Figure 1.   Epithelial cell proliferation of white rat endometrium in group PO (A), group P1(B), and group P2 (C). a. uterine glands, b. epithelial cell, c. lumen, d. epithelial cell proliferation. (HE:400X).

the rats in control group (P0). The difference in the concentration of the inoculated bacteria (1.0×10^5 CFU/ml and 1.5×10^8 CFU/ml) also had a significant effect ($P<0.05$) on the increase of necrosis. However, the number of cell proliferation between group infected with bacteria at a dose of 1.0×10^5 CFU/ml was not significantly different ($P>0.05$) compared to the group infected with bacteria at a dose of 1.5×10^8 CFU/ml. Cell proliferation activity is influenced by the expression of oncogenes, tumor suppressor genes as well as repair genes, and apoptosis genes. The activity of these various genes causes uncontrolled proliferation (Watuguly & Samsuria 2018). The average scores for necrosis and epithelial cell proliferation in the white rat uterus in groups P0, P1, and PII are presented in Table 1.

Table 1. Average score of necrosis and epithelial cell proliferation in the endometrium of white rats inoculated with different concentrations of *E. coli*.

Parameter	Treatment		
	P0	PI	PII
Necrosis	0.00 ± 0.00^a	1.66 ± 0.58^a	3.00 ± 0.00^b
Epithelial cell proliferation	0.00 ± 00^a	2.33 ± 0.58^b	1.33 ± 0.58^b

[a,b]Different superscripts in the same row show significant differences between treatment groups ($P<0.05$)

4 CONCLUSION

Induction of endometritis using *E. coli* caused histopathological changes in the form of narrowing of the lumen, increased necrosis and epithelial cells proliferation in the endometrium of white rats. However, the difference in the concentration of *E. coli* used to induce endometritis in white rats only affected the rate of necrosis cell.

REFERENCES

Barański W. Podhalicz-Dziegielewska M. Zduńczyk S. and Janowski T. (2012). The Diagnosis and Prevalence of Subclinical Endometritis in Cows Evaluated by Different Cytologic Thresholds. *Theriogenology*, 78(9), 1939–1947.

Dar S.H., Qureshi S., Palanivelu M., Muthu S., Mehrotra S., Jan M.H., Chaudhary G.R., Kumar H., Saravanan R. and Narayanan K. 2016. Evaluating a Murine Model of Endometritis using Uterine Isolates of Escherichia Coli from Postpartum Buffalo. *Iranian Journal of Veterinary Research*, 17(3), 171–176.

Demirel M.A., Han S., Tokmak A., Ercan Gokay N., Uludag M.O., Yildirir Ustun T. and Cicek A.F. (2019). Therapeutic Effects of Resveratrol in Escherichia Coli-induced Rat Endometritis Model. *Naunyn-Schmiedeberg's Archives of Pharmacology*, 392(12), 1577–1589.

Duwiri C.V., Samsuri S. and Berata I.K. (2019). Perubahan Histopatologi Ovarium Pada Tikus Putih (*Rattus norvegicus*) Akibat Pemberian Ragi Tape. *Indonesia Medicus Veterinus*, 8(3), 338–346.

Kiernan J.A. (1990). *Histological and Histochemical Methods: Theory and Practice*. England: Pergamon Press.

Rafika I., Thasmi C.N., Herrialfian H., Rosmaidar R. and Hafizuddin H. (2020). Isolasi dan Identifikasi Bakteri Gram Negatif Pada Uterus Sapi Aceh Yang Mengalami Repeat Breeding. *Jurnal Agripet*, 20(2), 187–192.

Sendana L., Wandia I.N. and Dada IKA. (2019). Laporan Kasus: Penanganan Bedah Terhadap Kejadian Endometritis Pada Kucing Lokal. *Indonesia Medicus Veterinus*, 8(5), 572–582.

Sinaga E., Karja N.W.K. and Amrozi A. (2021). Nanokitosan Efektif Menekan Jumlah Bakteri Gram Negatif Dan Gram Positif Penyebab Endometritis Pada Sapi Friesian Holstein Secara in Vitro. *Jurnal Veteriner*, 22 (2), 198–206.

Steel R.G.D. and Torrie J.H. (1991). *Prinsip dan Prosedur Statistika*. Indonesia: Gramedia Pustaka Utama.

Watuguly T.W. and Samsuria I.K. (2018). *Aspek Dasar Molekular Proliferasi dan Apoptosis*. Indonesia: Alfabeta.

Developing Modern Livestock Production in Tropical Countries – Adli et al. (eds)

The effect of carrot extract addition (*Daucus carota* L.) into the diluent of tris aminomethan egg yolk on the quality of Boer goat's frozen semen

M.N. Ihsan, C.N.A. Simbolon, H. Pratiwi & S. Wahjuningsih*
Universitas Brawijaya, Malang, Indonesia

ABSTRACT: Artificial insemination is one of the reproductive biotechnology methods used to improve the genetic quality of livestock. Some factors affect the success of artificial insemination, including the quality of the frozen semen. This research examined the effects of carrot extract addition in egg yolk diluent tris aminomethane on the quality of frozen semen of Boer goats. Fresh semen was collected from 5 male Boer goats aged 5–7 years, with minimum mass sperm motility of ++ and individual motility of at least 70%. The semen was diluted using tris aminomethane egg yolk added with different concentrations of carrot extract. In this experimental research, 4 treatments with 5 replications and a laboratory experiment using a completely randomized design (CRD) were carried out. The treatments in this study were P0:0% carrot extract + 80% tris aminomethane + 20% egg yolk, P1:1% carrot extract + 80% tris aminomethane + 20% egg yolk, P2: 2% carrot extract + 80% tris aminomethane + 20% egg yolk, P3: 3% carrot extract + 80% tris aminomethane + 20% egg yolk. The addition of carrot extract in egg yolk tris aminomethane had a significant effect ($P<0.05$) on sperm individual motility and viability. To sum up, the addition of 1% carrot extract had better results than other treatments.

Keywords: Boer, carrot, egg yolk. semen

1   INTRODUCTION

Boer goats are superior meat goats originating from South Africa. Boer goats are superior as they grow weight faster, have excellent reproduction, have strong resistance to digestive tract parasites, are adaptive to different environments, and their meat quality is good. The Indonesian Directorate General of Livestock and Animal Health (2021) reported decreases in national goat meat production from 72,852 tons in 2019 to 61,711 tons in 2020 and 61,724 tons in 2021. This declining goat meat production can be addressed by increasing the goat population and improving genetic quality through artificial insemination. Artificial insemination is one of the reproductive technologies that can increase livestock populations and improve the genetic quality of livestock. The artificial insemination process goes through several stages, starting from superior male semen collection, semen assessment, cement dilution, cement freezing, and artificial insemination outcome assessment. The success of artificial insemination is influenced by several factors, including the quality of frozen semen used. The freezing process of semen can cause cold shock in spermatozoa and damage its plasma membrane due to lipid peroxidation reactions by free radicals produced during the metabolic process, thereby reducing the quality of semen. Spermatozoa membrane damage

---

*Corresponding Author: yuning@ub.ac.id

DOI: 10.1201/9781003370048-16

can be minimized by adding antioxidants to the diluent. Carrots (*Daucus carota* L.) contain antioxidant compounds such as vitamin C and β-carotene. β-carotene in carrots acts as an antioxidant compound that breaks the chain of lipid peroxidation reactions. Barek et al. (2020) found the addition of carrot juice (*Daucus carota* L.) in citrated egg yolk (S-KT) had a positive effect on the quality of liquid semen of Bligon goats. Vitamin C and β-carotene contained in carrots act as antioxidants that minimize the number of spermatozoa that die due to free radicals. It is necessary to conduct research on the quality of Boer goat spermatozoa with the addition of carrot extract (*Daucus carota* L.) in egg yolk tris amino-methane diluent stored in a container at $-196°C$. The carrot extract can supply antioxidants to maintain the quality of Boer goat semen during freezing.

2 MATERIALS AND METHODS

Semen samples were collected from 4 healthy bucks, aged 5 to 7 years old with a body weight of 65 to 80 kg, using an artificial vagina. Semen was collected three times a week. The standard quality of sample semen was the individual motility which should be $\geq 70\%$ (Purdy et al. 2021). Fresh semen was diluted in tris aminomethane egg yolk as a base diluent with a 1:10 ratio. The sample of semen was divided into four treatments: T0: (Tris Aminomethan Egg Yolk + 0% Carrot Extract), T1: (Tris Aminomethan Egg Yolk + 1% Carrot Extract), T2: (Tris Aminomethan Egg Yolk + 2% Carrot Extract), T3: (Tris Aminomethan Egg Yolk + 3% Carrot Extract). The diluted semen was put in a 0.25 ml straw at 4°C using an automatic filling and sealing machine. After that, the straw was put in a goblet and placed on the surface of liquid nitrogen for 9 minutes before being plunged into liquid temperature $-196°C$ and stored at least 24 hours prior to the analysis. Thawing was conducted by dipping the straw into the waterbath at a temperature of 37°C for 30 seconds (Pedrosa et al. 2021). Sperm motility was examined using a light microscope at 400X magnification, while sperm viability was observed by placing a drop of cement on a warm glass slide to be added with one drop of dual staining eosin negrosin. The solution was then mixed gently and observed under the microscope at 400 × magnification. Unlike the healthy sperm, the dead sperm would absorb the stain. A total of 200 sperm were examined in each sample. A completely randomized design with 5 replicates of each treatment was employed in this research using Microsoft excel. The data on semen quality traits were analyzed in Analysis of Variance (ANOVA) followed by Duncan Multiple Range Tests (DMRT) to determine the differences among the treatments, with statistical significance set at $P<0.05$.

3 RESULTS AND DISCUSSIONS

The results of the experiment done in this research are presented in Tables 1 and 2. How carrot extract worked as an antioxidant on tris aminomethane egg yolk diluent before freezing and post-thawing semen quality was examined. An average score of the spermatozoa motility and viability for each carrot extract concentration was measured, showing scores of 79 ± 5.48 and 87.73 + 1.05, respectively, in fresh semen. Carrot extract concentrations of 1%, 2%, and 3% were found suitable and showed a positive effect on spermatozoa motility and viability before freezing. The addition of carrot extract at the concentrations of 1% and 2% increased the motility before freezing of 75 ± 3.5% and 73 ± 2.7%, showing a significantly higher value (P<0.05) than the control treatment (70 ± 3.5%). Similarly, the addition of carrot extract at the concentrations of 1% and 2% also increased the viability percentage count of 81.26 ± 2.0% and 79.69 ± 1.0% respectively, showing a significantly higher result (P<0.05), higher than the control treatment (74.33 ± 1.4%). Carrot extract concentrations of 1% and 2% were found suitable and positively affected the post-thawing motility. The addition of carrot extract at the concentrations

Table 1. Effects of different carrot extract concentrations on before freezing semen quality.

Parameters (%)	Fresh Semen	Semen Quality Before Freezing (%)			
		0% carrot extract	1% carrot extract	2% carrot extract	3% carrot extract
Sperm Motility	79 ± 5.48	70 ± 3.5[a]	75 ± 3.5[b]	73 ± 2.7[b]	67 ± 4.5[a]
Sperm Viability	87.73 + 1.05	74.33 ± 1.4[a]	81.26 ± 2.0[b]	79.69 ± 1.0[b]	75.53 ± 1.1[a]

Different superscripts within rows indicate significant differences at P<0.05

Table 2. Effects of different carrot extract concentrations on post-thawed semen quality.

Parameters (%)	Fresh Semen	Semen Quality Post Thawing (%)			
		0% carrot extract	1% carrot extract	2% carrot extract	3% carrot extract
Sperm Motility	79 ± 5.48	3939 ± 2.2[a]	48 ± 2.7[b]	45 ± 3.5[b]	36 ± 4.2[a]
Sperm Viability	87.73 + 1.05	58.42 ± 2.7[a]	65.03 ± 1.4[b]	62.11 ± 1.0[b]	59.78 ± 3.1[a]

Different superscripts within rows indicate significant differences at P<0.05.

of 1% and 2% increased the post-thawing motility of 48 ± 2.7% and 45 ± 3.5%, respectively, whose values were significantly (P<0,05) higher than the control treatment (39 ± 2.2%). Carrot extract at concentrations of 1% and 2% also increased the viability percentage count 65.03 ± 1.4% and 62.11 ± 1.0%, respectively, which are significantly (P<0.05) higher than the control treatment (58.42 ± 2.7%). Whereas the addition of carrot extract at a concentration of 3% did not have any significant effect before freezing and post-thawing parameters.

Spermatozoa are highly sensitive to lipid peroxidation resulting from the oxidation of membrane lipids by superoxide, hydrogen peroxide, and hydroxyl radicals. Spontaneous lipid peroxidation of the spermatozoa membranes destroys the structure of the lipid matrix. Reactive oxygen species ultimately lead to the impairment of sperm functions, such as sperm motility, functional membrane integrity, leakage of intracellular enzymes, and damage to the sperm DNA through oxidative stress (Gangwar et al. 2015). Oxidative stress is a physiological state of spermatozoa triggered by ROS during cryopreservation and is associated with cellular disorders (Ahmed et al. 2020). The continuous production of ROS as a result of sperm metabolism can result in increased numbers of immature sperm cells. Furthermore, semen freezing-thawing processes often result in lesser concentrations of antioxidants in the sperm and seminal plasma, resulting in sperm oxidative stress (Eidan 2016).

At a concentration of 1%, carrot extract showed an optimal antioxidant effect compared to 2% carrot extract. However, at a concentration of 3%, the addition of carrot extract decreased sperm motility and lower viability compared to the 2% concentration. Excessive addition of antioxidants will affect the rate of oxidation even causing antioxidants to become pro-oxidants. The change from antioxidants to pro-oxidants or free radicals causes more unsaturated fatty acids produced which can accelerate and expand the occurrence of lipid peroxidation due to damaged sperm plasma membrane following the loss of essential unsaturated fatty acids that make up the membrane (Wahjuningsih & Ihsan 2018). The results of the lipid peroxide radical chain reaction can only be stopped by antioxidants that can break the chain reaction. Antioxidants maintain the spermatozoa during cryopreservation by reducing, eliminating, or suppressing free radical reactions (Zidni et al. 2022). At this stage, β-carotene in carrots is a fat-soluble antioxidant that inhibits lipid peroxidation and increases the activity of various antioxidants that can bind to free radicals during the reduction of molecular oxygen. In addition, carrots also contain Vitamin C which can capture free radical activity, prevent chain reactions, and reduce the peroxidative damage that can affect the viability and fertility of spermatozoa. The mechanism of carotenoids as antioxidants in neutralizing free radicals is by donating one of their electrons to free radicals (unstable molecules) to make them become stable molecules.

4 CONCLUSIONS

The addition of (*Daucus carota* L.) at a concentration of 1% in tris aminomethane egg yolk diluent can maintain the motility and viability of frozen goat spermatozoa.

ACKNOWLEDGMENTS

The authors thank the faculty of animal husbandry for providing funds for this research, through public funds DPA (Budget Realization Document) PTNBH (Legal State-Owned Universitas Brawijawa), Number: DPA-FPt-251101/2022, Dated January 4, 2022.

REFERENCES

Ahmed H., Jahan S., Ullah H., Ullah F., and Salman M.M. (2020). The Addition of Resveratrol in Tris Citric Acid Extender Ameliorates Post-thaw Quality Parameters, Antioxidant Enzymes Levels, and Fertilizing Capability of Buffalo (Bubalus bubalis) Bull Spermatozoa. *Theriogenology*, 152, 106–113.

Barek M.E., Hine T.M., Nalley W.M., and Belli H.L. (2020). The Effect of Carrot Juice Supplementation in Citrate-egg yolk Extender on Spermatozoa Quality of Bligon Goat. *Jurnal Nukleus Peternakan*, 7(2), 109–117.

Direktorat Jenderal Peternakan dan Kesehatan Hewan. (2021). *Statistik Peternakan dan Kesehatan Hewan.* Jakarta

Eidan S.M. (2016). Effect on Post-cryopreserved Semen Characteristics of Holstein Bulls of Adding Combinations of Vitamin C and Either Catalase or Reduced Glutathione to Tris Extender. *Animal Reproduction Science*, 167, 1–7.

Gangwar C., Kharche S.D., Ranjan R., Kumar S., Goel A.K., Jindal S.K., and Agarwal S.K. (2015). Effect of Vitamin C Supplementation on Freezability of Barbari Buck Semen. *Small Ruminant Research*, 129, 104–107.

Pedrosa A.C., Torres M.A., Alkmin D.V., Pinzon J.E., Martins S.M.M.K., da Silveira J.C., and de Andrade A.F.C. (2021). Spermatozoa and Seminal Plasma Small Extracellular Vesicles miRNAs as Biomarkers of Boar Semen Cryotolerance. *Theriogenology*, 174, 60–72.

Purdy P.H., Graham J.K., and Azevedo H.C. (2021). Evaluation of Boar and Bull Sperm Capacitation and the Acrosome Reaction Using Flow Cytometry. *Animal Reproduction Science*, 106846.

Wahjuningsih S. and Ihsan M.N. (2018). Supplementation of α Tocopherol on Plasma Membrane Integrity of Goat Sperm After Freezing. *Journal of Innovation and Applied Technology*, 4(1), 580–584.

Zidni I., Lee H.B., Yoon J.H., Park J.Y., Oh Y.D., Jang H.S., and Lim H.K. (2022). Effect of Antioxidants in Cryopreservation Media on Spotted Halibut (Verasfer variegatus) Sperm Quality During Cryopreservation. *Aquaculture*, 738351.

Developing Modern Livestock Production in Tropical Countries – Adli et al. (eds)

Blood metabolite status of peanut goats given basalt ration of sugar cane (*Saccharum officinarum*) and Titonia (*Tithonia diversifolia*) fermentation and addition of peel flour and avocado seeds in concentrate

Z. Ikhlas*
Postgraduate Student of Animal Science Faculty, Andalas University, Padang City, West Sumatra, Indonesia

N. Jamarun, Arief & R. Pazla
Lecturer of Animal Science Faculty, Andalas University, Padang City, West Sumatra, Indonesia

R. Welan
Nutrition Dept. Faculty of Medicine Andalas University, Padang City, West Sumatra, Indonesia

G. Yanti & R.W.W. Sari
Doctoral Student of Animal Science Faculty, Andalas University, Padang City, West Sumatra, Indonesia

ABSTRACT: The fermented sugarcane shoots is intended as a source of energy and fermented Titonia as a forage protein source in goat nut rations. Avocado waste aims to enrich the ration with vitamins and minerals in order to optimize rumen bioprocess. The aim of this study was to obtain a good performance of Kacang goats through appropriate ration formulation based on fermented forage (sugarcane shoots and Titonia) with avocado waste. This formulation is expected to minimize the use of concentrate in the ration. This study used 16 male peanut goats aged 1 year which were divided into 4 groups based on body weight. The concentrate consists of rice bran, corn, palm kernel cake, salt, and minerals. The design used was a randomized block design with 4 ration treatments and 4 weight groups of goats as replicates, namely: (T0 = Sugarcane Tops 35% + Titonia 5% + 0% Avocadodo Waste + 60% Concentrate, T1 = Sugarcane Tops 35% + Titonia 9.5% + Avocado 0.5% + Concentrate 55%, T2 = Sugarcane Tops 35% + Titonia 14% + Avocado 1% + Concentrate 50%, P3 = Sugarcane Tops 35% + Titonia 18.5% + Avocado 1.5% + Concentrate 45%). The parameters measured included blood metabolites (cholesterol, high-density lipoprotein (HDL), Low-density lipoprotein (LDL)). The results showed that the P3 treatment gave the best blood metabolites. The cholesterol value was 88.70 mg/dl which normally ranged between 64, 60, and 136.40 mg/dl, HDL with a value of 53.36 (mg/dl) which normally ranges from 22.5–55.67 (mg/dl), and LDL with a value of 29.17 (mg/dl) which normally ranges from 77.32 (mg/dl).

Keywords: peanut goat, Titonia, sugarcane shoots, avocado waste, fermentation, cholesterol

1 INTRODUCTION

Forage plays an important role as a source of fiber used by microorganisms for fermentation in the rumen. Currently, the problems that often occur in the development of ruminant

---

*Corresponding Author: zaitulikhlas98@gmail.com

DOI: 10.1201/9781003370048-17

livestock business are the low productivity of forage in the dry season and the price of protein source feed ingredients which are quite expensive. One solution that is sufficient to overcome this problem is to look for alternative forages with continuous availability and high nutritional levels, both from forages that have not been utilized properly as animal feed or agricultural waste. Agricultural wastes that can be used as feed ingredients include sugarcane shoots and Titonia.

Peanut goat is one of the germplasm of Indonesian ruminant livestock that is kept by many people because it has advantages such as having the adaptability to a barren land with limited feed availability, and resistance to disease (Tunnisa 2013). Rusfidra (2007) stated that the advantages of the Kacang goat are that it has very good production rates and produces quality meat. Biologically, goats are quite productive and easy to develop and are able to produce in unfavorable environments (Sutama 2005). Dwatmadji *et al.* (2008) stated that the peanut goat-rearing system is relatively easy and does not require large costs. Behind these advantages, peanut goat also has a weakness, namely peanut goat meat has high cholesterol levels. Goat meat tends to have high cholesterol levels with an average value of 70 mg/100 g (Sitepoe 1992). Arum *et al.* (2009) stated that goat meat is a familiar thing in the community, but excessive consumption can increase the risk of blockage of blood vessels which will lead to heart disease and stroke. This is caused by the high cholesterol content in goat fat, which is 3.2 mg/g. Cholesterol is an important element in the body that is needed to regulate chemical processes in the form of body metabolism as a building material for cell walls, making bile acids to emulsify fats. Blood cholesterol is bounded by a lipoprotein, which consists of chylomicrons, namely very low-density lipoprotein (VLDL), LDL, and HDL. Excess cholesterol can cause the deposition of LDL-cholesterol on the walls of blood vessels, resulting in the narrowing and hardening of blood vessels known as atherosclerosis (the process of plaque formation in blood vessels). Lee *et al.* (2005) stated that high amounts of cholesterol can cause atherosclerosis which will eventually have an impact on coronary heart disease. Therefore, it is necessary to make efforts to reduce cholesterol by adding skin flour and avocado seeds to goat rations. Avocado leaves and fruit contain saponins, alkaloids, flavonoids, polyphenols, and quercetin while avocado seeds are known to contain flavonoids, tannins, quinones, polyphenols, triterpenoids, saponins, monoterpenoids, and sesquiterpenoids (Rostini 2017). Among these substances, flavonoids are the most effective substances in reducing LDL cholesterol levels in the blood because flavonoids work to increase HDL cholesterol (Nurwahyunani 2006).

2 MATERIALS AND METHODS

2.1 *Study area*

This research was conducted in July–October 2021, in Andalas University Faculty of Animal Husbandry goat stable Padang, West Sumatra Indonesia.

2.2 *Forage materials and nutrition analysis*

In this research, the method used is Group Design (RAK) using 4 treatments and 4 replications. The treatments used in the study are as follows:

P0: Titonia 5% + Sugarcane Tops 35% + Avocado 0% + Concentrate 60%
P1: Titonia 10% + Sugarcane Tops 34.5% + Avocado 0.5% + Concentrate 55%
P2: Titonia 15% + Sugarcane Tops 34% + Avocado 1% + Concentrate 50%
P3: Titonia 20% + Sugarcane Tops 33.5% + Avocado 1.5% + Concentrate 45%

The livestock used in this study were 16 male peanuts, aged 1 year and weighing 10–12 kg, goats from Toke goat breeders in bypass, Padang. The cages used were individual skeleton cages measuring pxlt (1 × 0.7 × 1.5 m) of iron equipped with a place to eat and drink, 16 pieces each. The materials used in this study were sugarcane shoots, Titonia, white rot mold (Pleurotus ostreatus), Lactobacillus bulgaricus, Potato Dextrose Agar (PDA) medium, aquades, avocado waste, palm kernel cake, rice bran, broken corn, salt, minerals, goat peanuts, ad libitum drinking water, H2SO4, selenium, and materials for chemical analysis. The materials used in this study were sugarcane shoots, Titonia, white rot mold (Pleurotus ostreatus), Lactobacillus bulgaricus, Potato Dextrose Agar (PDA) medium, aquades, avocado waste, palm kernel cake, rice bran, broken corn, salt, minerals, goat peanuts, ad libitum drinking water, H2SO4, selenium, and materials for chemical analysis.

2.3 *Statistical analysis*

All the data obtained were described descriptively.

3 RESULTS AND DISCUSSION

The content of the blood profile with the provision of rations according to the treatment given to peanut goats is presented in Table 1. The blood profile consists of cholesterol, LDL-cholesterol, and HDL-cholesterol. Cholesterol in the body binds to a type of protein to form lipoproteins. These lipoproteins are divided into LDL) and HDL (Soehardi 2004). LDL or bad cholesterol is a type of cholesterol that has a fairly bad impact on the body if its levels are too high. It is known that LDL has atherogenic properties (easily attached to the inner walls of blood vessels and reduces the formation of LDL receptors). HDL is often called the "good" cholesterol because it is a lipoprotein that transports lipids from the periphery to the liver. HDL is synthesized and secreted mainly by the liver and to a lesser extent in the intestinal epithelium during fat absorption from the intestine.

Table 1. The effect of giving rations to the blood profit of Kacang goats.

Parameter (mg/dl)	T0	T1	T2	T3
Blood Cholesterol	111,80	101,86	96,57	88.70
Blood HDL-Cholesterol	39.08	39.80	51.60	53.36
Blood LDL-Cholesterol	62.55	42.59	39.04	29.17

Note: P0: Titonia 5% + Sugarcane Tops 35% + Avocado 0% + Concentrate 60%
P1: Titonia 10% + Sugarcane Tops 34.5% + Avocado 0.5% + Concentrate 55%
P2: Titonia 15% + Sugarcane Tops 34% + Avocado 1% + Concentrate 50%
P3: Titonia 20% + Sugarcane Tops 33.5% + Avocado 1.5% + Concentrate 45%
Description: different superscripts on the same line show noticeable differences ($P<0.05$)

Analyzing the different blood profiles aims to see if the blood profiles produced in offering rations provide optimal results to Kacang goats. In the analysis of blood cholesterol, the lowest was found in the P3 treatment with a blood cholesterol content of 88.70%. The lower the blood cholesterol value obtained, the better the quality of the peanut goat. According to Gurvey (2003), cholesterol is an intermediate material for the formation of a number of important components such as vitamin D (to form and maintain healthy bones), forming hormones (estrogen and testosterone), and bile acids (for digestive function). Therefore, as long as cholesterol levels are still within normal limits, there is no need to worry because cholesterol has various important functions. In the P3 treatment, the blood cholesterol content value was classified as normal, namely 88.70. Rostini (2016) stated that the normal range of cholesterol in goats is between 64.6 and 136.4.

4 CONCLUSION

The results showed that the P3 treatment gave the most optimal results than the other treatments for each blood profit parameter, consisting of blood cholesterol with a value of 88.79 mg/dl, HDL with a value of 53.36 (mg/dl), and LDL with a value of 29.17 (mg/dl) against Kacang goat.

ACKNOWLEDGMENT

This study was supported by a research institution and community service at Andalas University, Indonesia (Grant No: 011/E5/PG.02.00.PT/2022)

REFERENCES

Arum R. & Müller W. (Eds.). (2009). *The Reemergence of Self-Employment: A Comparative Study of Self-employment Dynamics and Social Inequality*. Princeton University Press.

Dwatmadji D. & Efrianto E. (2008). Scrotal Circumference dan Hubungannya Dengan Ukuran Tubuh Kambing Kacang Pada Sistem Pemeliharaan Yang Berbeda. *Jurnal Sain Peternakan Indonesia* Vol, 3(1).

Guryev O., Carvalho R.A., Usanov S. Gilep A. & Estabrook R.W. (2003). A Pathway for the Metabolism of Vitamin D3: Unique Hydroxylated Metabolites Formed During Catalysis with Cytochrome P450scc (CYP11A1). *Proceedings of the National Academy of Sciences*, 100(25), 14754–14759.

Haque R.A., Iqbal M.A., Budagumpi, S., Khadeer Ahamed M.B., Abdul Majid A.M. & Hasanudin N. (2013). Binuclear meta-xylyl-linked Ag (I)-N-Heterocyclic Carbene Complexes of N-alkyl/aryl-alkyl-substituted Bis-benzimidazolium Salts: Synthesis, Crystal Structures and In Vitro Anticancer Studies. *Applied Organometallic Chemistry*, 27(4), 214–223.

Kostaman T. & Sutama I.K. (2005). Laju Pertumbuhan Kambing Anak Hasil Persilangan Antara kambing Boer Dengan Peranakan Etawah Pada Priode Pra- sapih. *JITV*, 10(2), 106–112.

Lee G.A., Rao M.N. & Grunfeld C. (2005). The Effects of HIV Protease Inhibitors on Carbohydrate and Lipid Metabolism. *Current HIV/AIDS Reports*, 2(1), 39–50.

Nurwahyunani A. (2006). Efek Ekstrak daun Sambung Nyawa Terhadap Kadar Kolesterol Ldl dan Kolesterol Hdl Darah Tikus Diabetik Akibat Induksi Streptozotocin. *Universitas Negri Semarang, Semarang. (Disertasi)*.

Prayitno R.S. & Heni N. (2021). Pengaruh Pemberian Limbah Daun Bawang Merah (Allium Ascalonicum L.) Sebagai Hijauan Alternatif Terhadap Profil Lemak Darah Domba. *Jurnal Peternakan*, 18(1), 19–24.

Rostini T. & Zakir I. (2017). Performans Produksi, Jumlah Nematoda Usus, dan Profil Metabolik Darah Kambing Yang Diberi Pakan Hijauan Rawa Kalimantan. *Jurnal Vet*, 18(3), 469–477.

Rostini T., Ni'mah G.K. & Sosilawati S. (2016). Pengaruh Pemberian Pupuk Bokashi Yang Berbeda Terhadap Kandungan Protein dan Serat Kasar Rumput Gajah (Pennisetum Purpureum). *Ziraa'ah Majalah Ilmiah Pertanian*, 41(1), 118–126.

Rusfidra A. 2007. Studies on the Cock Crowing Bioacoustics Ballenger *"Local Chicken Singer"* from West Sumatra.

Sitepoe M. (1992). *Kolesterol Fobia: Keterkaitannya Dengan Penyakit Jantung*. Penerbit PT Gramedia Pustaka Utama.

Soehardi S. (2004). *Memelihara Kesehatan Jasmani Melalui Makanan*. Bandung: ITB.

Tunnisa R. (2013). Keragaman Gen IGF-1 Pada Populasi Kambing Kacang di Kabupaten Jeneponto. *Skripsi. Universitas Hasanuddin. Makasar*.

Developing Modern Livestock Production in Tropical Countries – Adli et al. (eds)
© 2023 The Authors, ISBN 978-1-032-44025-5
Open Access: www.taylorfrancis.com, CC BY-NC-ND 4.0 license

Application of *Eupencillium javanicum* BS4 enzyme powder in Palm Kernel Meal feed for layer chicken

T. Haryati*, A.P. Sinurat & A. Herliatika
Research Center of Animal Husbandry, Research Organization for Agriculture and Food, National Research Innovation Agency of the Republic of Indonesia (BRIN), Cibinong Sciences Center, Cibinong, Bogor, Indonesia

ABSTRACT: Palm Kernel Meal (PKM) is a waste product from the palm oil industry which has potential energy and protein content for animal feed ingredients. However, the use of PKM is limited due to its high crude fiber content and low nutrient digestibility. The β-Mannanase liquid enzyme produced from *Eupenicillium javanicum* BS4, a mesophyll fungus isolated from royal palm seeds (*Roystone regia*), has been used to increase nutrient availability and reduce the mannan content in PKM. In this experiment, we compared the effectiveness of free liquid enzyme and pollard-immobilized enzyme in the performance of the layer chicken. First, the recovery of immobilized enzyme in different ratio of enzyme and pollard was measured (1:1, 1:2, and 1:3 w/v), and we concluded that the 1:1 ratio has the highest recovery activity (75%). That recovery value showed not all enzymes added expressed the activity in vitro. Five treatments were assigned randomly to four contiguous cages in each of four rows in a randomized complete block design: (i) positive control (commercial), negative control, liquid enzyme treatment, pollard immobilized enzyme added at 20ml/kg PKM and 26.7ml/kg PKM, respectively. The result showed that pollard immobilized enzyme treatment (20ml/Kg PKM) has the lowest feed conversion ratio (4.16), liquid enzyme treatment has 4.80 FCR, and pollard-immobilized enzyme (26.7ml/Kg PKM) has the highest FCR (8.72). Feed consumption and egg quality did not differ significantly among the treatments. We concluded that the most efficient feed is the one that was added with pollard immobilized enzyme 20ml/kg PKM.

Keywords: Palm Kernel Meal, mannannase-enzymes, laying hen

1 INTRODUCTION

Chicken eggs are a relatively cheap source of protein compared to beef or chicken and are widely consumed by Indonesian people. Chicken eggs are mainly supplied from chicken farms that use imported feed ingredients such as corn and soybean meal (Aziz et al. 2021). This condition causes quite high fluctuations in the price of these feed ingredients. The solution to overcome the increase in imported feed prices is to use local raw materials we have not used optimally as feed ingredients. One of the local raw materials that we can use is palm kernel cake (PKC).

PKC is a biomass waste from the oil palm plantation industry that can be used as an alternative feed source because of its high potential for protein content (Sharmila et al. 2014). However, PKC cannot be added directly to animal feed, especially chickens. There are still shell fragments due to the imperfect palm kernel oil extraction process which can cause shell contamination. The shell is sharp and can damage the intestinal wall of young birds.

The addition of β-mannanase enzyme can increase the ileal digestibility energy of broilers aged 28 days (Latham et al. 2018). Adding PKC in poultry feed can also function as mannan

---

*Corresponding Author: tharyati2017@gmail.com

DOI: 10.1201/9781003370048-18

oligosaccharides (MOS) or prebiotics (Osorio et al. 2022). The prebiotics is degraded by gut microbiota and produces short-chain fatty acids as degradation products (Davari et al. 2019), which helps to reduce gut pathogens.

In a previous study conducted by Balitnak, the β-mannanase enzyme was used in liquid form (Sinurat 1999). In this study, immobilization of the β-mannanase enzyme was carried out in pollard powder, which aims to prevent the enzyme from being damaged easily and to facilitate its handling in the field. The cations contained in pollard powder also have a function as a coenzyme and can increase enzyme activity (Purwadaria et al. 2003).

This study aimed to compare the performance of chickens fed with PKM content treated with immobilized β-mannanase enzyme and free enzyme treatment in liquid form.

2 MATERIALS AND METHODS

The production of the β-mannanase enzyme was carried out using the submerged culture method. 50 ml of Mandels medium and 3% coconut cake were added into a 250 ml Erlenmeyer flask. It was inoculated with E. javanicum BS4, after which it was incubated for 5 days in an incubator shaker at 150rpm at room temperature (300C).

After five days, the cultures in Erlenmeyer flasks were collected, then centrifuged at 4800 g for 10 minutes at 70°C. The filtrate containing the mannanase enzyme was added with ammonium sulfate salt to precipitate the protein (mannanase enzyme). Then the filtrate was stored in the refrigerator overnight. The filtrate was then centrifuged at 4800 g for 10 minutes at 70°C. Then the precipitate was dissolved with 0.1M Na-acetate buffer pH 5.8 and stored the enzyme with a concentration of 10×.

The immobilized enzyme was obtained by mixing the ground pollard powder and liquid enzyme (1:1; 1:2 and 1:3 w/v) and dried at 40°C. The activity of the mannanase enzyme was measured using the saccharification method on the PKM substrate.

A completely randomized experimental design for laying hens was carried out with five treatments with a total of 80 laying hens aged 19 weeks. Treatment 1 was a positive control (commercial feed); Treatment 2 was a negative control, feed containing 20% PKC without enzyme addition; Treatment 3 was feed containing 20% PKC with the addition of liquid β-mannanase enzyme as much as 20ml/kg PKC; Treatment 4 was feed containing 20% PKC with the addition of β-mannanase enzyme as much as 20ml/kg PKC immobilized in polar with a ratio of 1:1 (v/w); Treatment 5 was feed containing 20% PKC with the addition of β-mannanase enzyme with the same expression activity as the liquid enzyme (iso expression) immobilized with pollard (table 1). The duration of the feeding trial was ten weeks. Egg

Table 1. The composition of the feed in the experiment.

Parameter	Negative Control	Liq Enzyme 20ml/kg PKC	Pow Enzyme 20ml/kg PKC (%)	Pow Enzyme 26.7ml/kg PKC
Corn meal	40	40	40	40
Palm Kernel Cake	20	20	20	20
Soybean Meal 44%	16.25	16.06	16.06	16.06
Calcium Carbonate	8.58	8.59	8.59	8.59
Meat Bone Meal	5.17	5.07	5.07	5.07
Hominy feed	4.77	6.1	6.1	6.1
Olein Oil	2.54	1.47	1.47	1.47
Corn Gluten Flour	2	2	2	2
Salt/ NaCl	0.2	0.2	0.2	0.2
Methionine	0.12	0.12	0.12	0.12

collection starts from week 5 to week 10. The observed variables were the number of eggs produced, egg weight, feed consumption, feed-to-egg conversion, and egg quality.

3 RESULTS AND DISCUSSION

In the liquid enzyme saccharification test, the enzyme activity obtained was 9.72 units/ml at 1000× dilution. In vitro test results showed that the recovery of enzyme activity was 75.67% at 1:1 composition and 55.58% at 1:2 composition and 35.86% at 1:3 composition. Subsequent experiments using a 1:1 composition and a recovery value of 75% were taken into account to determine isoexpression. The best result was 75.67% at the ratio (1:1 w/v). This shows that in vitro values, not all enzymes can be separated from pollard. This is because pollard contains 10% crude fiber and contains mannan, causing an association between the β-mannanase enzyme and its substrate (Purwadaria et al. 2003). The value of 75% was taken into account to determine the isoexpression treatment.

The feeding trial started when the hens were 19 weeks old, and the firstegg was laid at 23 weeks old, in the production variable (% Hen-Day), the enzyme addition treatment with the highest yield was the addition of 20ml/kg PKC enzyme powder (46.58%), followed by 20ml/kg PKC (46.43%) liquid enzyme and isoexpression powder enzyme (37.5%) (table 2). When compared with the positive control, the treatment of 20ml/Kg PKC liquid enzyme and 20ml/Kg PKC enzyme powder showed lower results (2.94% and 2.79%). The isoexpression powder enzyme treatment showed the lowest egg production (11.87%). Based on statistical analysis, all treatments did not show a significant difference, although the difference for the isoexpression treatment was quite large.

Table 2. Effect of addition of liquid enzymes, powder enzymes, and isoexpression powder enzymes treatment on the performance of laying hens from week 23 to 28.

Parameter	Production (%HD)	Consumption (g/cage)	Egg weight (g/cage)	FCR (feed (g)/ egg (g)	Mortality %
Positive Control	49.37	2615.41b	814.10	4.60	6.25
20% PKC – Enzyme	46.87	2801.61a	783.10	6.75	6,25
20% PKC + Liq enzyme 20ml/kg PKC	46.43	2718.75ab	720.20	4.80	0,00
20% PKC + Pow enzyme 20ml/kg PKC	46.58	2705.83ab	741.10	4.16	6,25
20% PKC + Pow enzyme isoexpression	37.50	2747.29ab	610.20	8.72	0,00

Different superscripts in the same column show significant differences (P<0.05)

The level of consumption affects the FCR variable, where the 20ml/kg PKC liquid enzyme treatment and 20ml/kg PKC enzyme powder have a better value than the negative control treatment. The best FCR values were obtained from treatment with 20ml/kg BIS enzyme powder (4.16), followed by positive control (4.60), liquid enzyme 20ml/kg PKC (4.80), negative control (6.75), and isoexpression powder enzyme (8.72).

Egg quality parameters such as yolk color and weight, Haugh unit, shell weight, and shell thickness did not show significant differences between treatments (table 3). In egg quality parameters, there was no significant difference between treatments. This indicates that the addition of PKC does not have a negative effect on the quality of eggs produced by livestock. The report of Herliatika et al. (2021) research shows the results that the inclusion of 10% of

Table 3. Effect of treatment with the addition of liquid enzymes, powder enzymes, and isoexpression powder enzymes on the quality of chicken eggs from week 26.

Parameter	Yolk (index)	Weight (g)	HU Test	Shell Weight (g)	Thick shell Upper	(index)
Positive Control	8.00	13.81	102.62	6.12	0.46	0.42
20% PKC – Enzyme	8.47	14.25	107.16	5.95	0.42	0.42
20% PKC + Liq enzyme 20ml/kg PKC	8.68	14.18	100.59	5.94	0.45	0.44
20% PKC + Pow enzyme 20ml/kg PKC	8.72	13.95	105.30	5.86	0.41	0.43
20% PKC + Pow enzyme isoexpression	8.62	13.93	106.93	5.59	0.44	0.39

the PKC had no significant effect on feed consumption, hen-day, egg weight, FCR, HU, and eggshell thickness; however, decreased egg yolk score of 13.46% was noticed.

4 CONCLUSION

It can be concluded that the best enzyme treatment for improving the performance of laying hens is enzyme powder 20 ml/Kg PKC.

REFERENCES

Aziz M.N., Loh A.C., Foo H.L., and Chung E.L.T. (2021). Is Palm Kernel Cake a Suitable Alternative Feed Ingredient for Poultry? *Animals*, 11(2), 338.

Davari D.D., Negahdaripour M., Karimzadeh I., Seifan M., Mohkam M., Masoumi S.J., Berenjian A., and Ghasemi Y. (2019). Prebiotics: Definition, Types, Sources, Mechanisms, and Clinical Applications. *Food*, 8 (3), 92.

Gomez-Osorio L.M., Nielsen J.U., Martens H.J., & Wimmer R. (2022). Upgrading the Nutritional Value of PKC Using a Bacillus Subtilis Derived Monocomponent β-Mannanase. *Molecules*, 27(2), 563.

Herliatika A., Sinurat A.P., Haryati T., & Subeni I. (2022, April). Effect of Palm Kernel Cake (PKC) Inclusion and Multi-Enzyme Supplementation on Layer Performances. In *6th International Seminar of Animal Nutrition and Feed Science (ISANFS 2021)* (pp. 55–60). Atlantis Press.

Karimi K., and Zhandi M. (2015). The Effect of β-mannanase and β-glucanase on Small Intestine Morphology in Male Broilers Fed Diets Containing Various Levels of Metabolizable Energy. *Journal of Applied Animal Research*, 43(3), 324–329.

Latham R.E., Williams M.P., Walters H.G., Carter B., and Lee J.T. (2018). Efficacy of β-mannanase on Broiler Growth Performance and Energy Utilization in the Presence on Increasing Dietary Galactomannan. *Poultry Science*, 97(2), 549–556.

Purwadaria T., Ketaren P.P., Sinurat A.P., and Sutikno I. (2003). Identification and Evaluation of Fiber Hydrolytic Enzymes in the Extract of Termites (Glyptotermes montanus) for Poultry Feed Application. *Indonesia Journal of Agricultural Science*, 4(2), 40–47.

Sharmila Alimon A., Azhar A.R., Noor K., and Samsudin H.M. (2014). Improving Nutritional Values of Palm Kernel Cake (PKC) as Poultry Feeds: A Review. *Malaysian Society of Animal Production*, 17(1), 1–18.

Sinurat A.P. (1999). Recent Development on Poultry Nutrition and Feed Technology and Suggestions for Topics of Researches. *Indonesian Agricultural Research & Development Journal*, 21(3), 37–45.

Sinurat A.P., Purwadaria T., and Haryati T. (2016). Effectivity of BS4 Enzyme Complex on the Performance of Laying Hens Fed with Different Ingredients. *Indonesian Journal of Animal and Veterinary Sciences*, 21(1), 1–8.

Developing Modern Livestock Production in Tropical Countries – Adli et al. (eds)
© 2023 The Authors, ISBN 978-1-032-44025-5
Open Access: www.taylorfrancis.com, CC BY-NC-ND 4.0 license

Evaluation of additional chestnut tannins in complete feed silage on pH post incubation and product rumen fermentation in vitro

Sadarman*, Dewi Febrina & D. Mastin
Department of Animal Science, Sultan Syarif Kasim State Islamic University, Pekanbaru, Indonesia

R. P. Harahap
Study Program of Animal Science, Faculty of Agriculture, Tanjungpura University, Pontianak, Indonesia
Animal Feed and Nutrition Modelling (AFENUE) Research Group, Faculty of Animal Science, IPB University, Bogor, Indonesia

N. Qomariyah
Research Center for Animal Husbandry, Research Organization for Agriculture and Food, National Research and Innovation Agency (BRIN), Cibinong Sciences Center, Cibinong, Bogor, Indonesia
Animal Feed and Nutrition Modelling (AFENUE) Research Group, Faculty of Animal Science, IPB University, Bogor, Indonesia

D.N. Adli
Faculty of Animal Science, Universitas Brawijaya, Malang, Indonesia

R.A. Nurfitriani
Department of Animal Science, Politeknik Negeri Jember, East Java
Animal Feed and Nutrition Modelling (AFENUE) Research Group, Faculty of Animal Science, IPB University, Bogor, Indonesia

A. Jayanegara
Department of Nutrition and Feed Technology, Faculty of Animal Science, IPB University, Bogor, Indonesia
Animal Feed and Nutrition Modelling (AFENUE) Research Group, Faculty of Animal Science, IPB University, Bogor, Indonesia

ABSTRACT: This study aimed to evaluate the effect of adding chestnut tannins to complete feed silage in vitro. A completely randomized design with 5 treatments and 5 replications was used in the manufacture of complete feed silage. The treatment in question is T1 = Complete Feed. Furthermore, for T2, T3, T4, and T5 each added chestnut tannins (% DM) 0.50; 1; 1.50; and 2%, then ensiled for 30 days, dried, and floured to a size of 1 mm, then tested in vitro. The parameters measured were post-incubation rumen pH and rumen fermentation products (ammonia and total VFA). The data obtained were analyzed based on analysis of variance and if there was a significant effect between treatments, then Duncan's test was continued at a 5% level. The results of this study showed that the use of chestnut tannins as a silage additive to synthesize complete feed had a significant effect ($P<0.05$) on ammonia with an average value ranging from 15.2 to 17.1 mM. Overall ammonia concentration in each treatment was still within normal limits, i.e., 6–21 mmol/l. Post-incubation rumen pH and total VFA were not affected by chestnut tannins, but the values of these two variables were still within normal limits. The conclusion of this study is that the addition of 0.50% DM chestnut tannins in complete feed silage can stabilize the pH of post-incubation rumen fluid and rumen fermentation products in vitro.

Keywords: ammonia, chestnut tannins, complete feed, in vitro, pH, silage, total VFA

---

*Corresponding Author: sadarman@uin-suska.ac.id

DOI: 10.1201/9781003370048-19
This chapter has been made available under a CC BY NC ND license

1 INTRODUCTION

Completed feed is a mixture of various kinds of feed ingredients that are given to livestock according to their needs. The manufacture of complete feed aims to utilize agro-industrial waste that is quickly damaged into a mixture of feed ingredients that meet specific nutrient needs and can improve feed efficiency. Efforts that can be made to enhance complete feed digestibility are through the manufacture of silage that can strengthen its palatability (Kondo et al. 2016). Silage is fermented or pickling feed produced from chopped plants, animal feed forage, agricultural waste, and so on, with a certain level of water content then stored in an airtight silo (Kondo et al. 2016). The process of making silage (ensilage) can run optimally if additives are added, both stimulant and inhibition such as tannins which can minimize protein damage during ensilage (Siddiqui et al. 2022a; Siddiqui et al. 2022b). This study aims to determine the effect of the addition of chestnut tannins on complete feed silage on in vitro fermentation of the rumen, including the pH of the post-incubation rumen fluid, NH_3, and total VFA.

2 MATERIALS AND METHODS

Complete feed silage treatment refers to Kondo et al. (2016), that is, complete feed consisting of 30 kg of field grass, palm fronds 17 kg, 25 kg of palm kernel meal that has been chopped, and 15 kg of tofu dregs that have been squeezed, aerated in advance, after which the dry matter is evaluated. The feed will be completely weighed according to the capacity of the silo contents used, which is 1.50 kg of laboratory scale. Complete feed is put in containers, added molasses, salt, urea, $CaCO_3$, and chestnut tannins, are stirred until evenly distributed, next put into a silo. The silo is tightly closed so that the conditions inside are anaerobic; then, the silo is stored in a place that is not exposed to sunlight for 30 days. Next, it is dried and then mashed with a sieve size of 1 mm.

2.1 Treatment

The treatment of the addition of tannins as silage additives refers to the results of the study by Sadarman et al. (2020). The in vitro incubation consisted of five treatments with five replications by following a randomized block design Petrie and Watson (2013). Treatments consisted of: P1 = complete feed (control), P2 = P1 + chestnut tannins 0.50% DM (2.63 g), P3 = P1 + chestnut tannins 1% DM (5.25 g), P4 = P1 + chestnut tannins 1.50% DM (7.88 g), and P5 = P1 + chestnut tannins 2% DM (10.5 g).

2.2 Parameters measured

Parameters measured in the in vitro evaluation were pH, NH_3, and total VFA. Data were tested using analysis of variance (ANOVA) (Petrie and Watson 2013), and if there was a significant difference at $P<0.05$, then continued with Duncan's multiple range test.

3 RESULTS AND DISCUSSION

3.1 pH rumen

The pH of the rumen is the degree of acidity of the rumen of the cattle (McDonald et al. 2012). The pH value of the rumen can determine the condition of the rumen that will affect the growth of rumen microbes and rumen fermentation products. Data on the effect of adding chestnut tannins 0.50–2% DM on the rumen pH in vitro can be seen in Table 1.

Table 1.   Effect of treatment on post-incubation rumen pH in vitro.

Treatment	pH
P1	6.71 ± 0,12
P2	6.67 ± 0,30
P3	6.78 ± 0,15
P4	6.75 ± 0,13
P5	6.73 ± 0,10

Note: P1 = complete feed (control), P2 = P1 + chestnut tannins 0.50% DM (2.63 g), P3 = P1 + chestnut tannins 1% DM (5.25 g), P4 = P1 + chestnut tannins 1.50% DM (7.88 g), and P5 = P1 + chestnut tannins 2% DM (10.5 g)

The results of the analysis of the variety of addition of chestnut tannins 0.50–2% DM did not significantly affect (P>0.05) the pH of the rumen after incubation of complete feed silage. The addition of a CT of 0.50% DM resulted in the pH of the rumen being relatively the same as the control. Chestnut tannins added as much as 0.50–2% DM still produce a rumen pH in the normal range of 6.67–6.78. This condition shows that a complete feed has been degraded so that microbes producing digestive enzymes can live and breed in it. According to McDonald et al. (2012), the rumen is a suitable environment for the growth and propagation or proliferation of microbes, which is supported by the availability of substrates, so that the microbes can produce digestive enzymes, which can be directly utilized by the landlady, namely ruminants such as buffaloes, cows, goats, sheep, and other ruminants. According to Dryden (2021), fermentation of organic matter by various rumen microbes can cause pH changes in the rumen ecosystem, this condition can determine the growth of specific microbial species so that it can affect the type and quantity of fermentation products produced. Kellems and Church (2009) explain that the fermentation of carbohydrates will produce organic acids that can lower the pH of acids during the rumen fermentation. McDonald et al. (2012) added that protein fermentation or nonprotein nitrogen will release excess $N-NH_3$, which is immediately joined by protons, this activity can increase the pH of the base.

3.2   *Ammonia content*

Ammonia is a chemical compound that has an essential contribution to the presence of nutrients in the rumen, and the final product of protein degradation in the rumen, so the high or low production of ammonia indicates the degree of damage to the feed inside the rumen.

The variety analysis results showed that adding chestnut tannins up to 2% DM in complete feed silage had a very noticeable effect on ammonia production (P<0.01) in vitro. Based on Duncan's test, ammonia concentration at P2 (17.1 mM) is different from P3 (15.9 mM), P4 (16.7 mM), and P5 (15.6 mM) (table 2). Ammonia production in P3 is the same as in P5 but different from P4. Ammonia concentrations at P1 (15.2 mM) were lower than all treatments, while the highest ammonia production in this study resulted in P2. The average ammonia concentration in this study ranged from 15.2–17.1 mM. Ammonia concentration in each treatment is still within normal limits, which is 6–21 mmol /l (McDonald et al. 2012) and 5–25 mmol/l (Wu 2017). Menci et al. (2021) said that the addition of extracts of both types of tannins (condensed, hydrolyzed) to frozen-dried dried vetch (*Vicia sativa* L.) grasses with different doses can decrease ammonia production in vitro. According to Xie et al. (2021), the feeding of tannin-rich sorghum to castrated young bulls does not affect ammonia production.

Table 2. Effect of per behavior on product ammonia rumen in vitro.

Treatment	NH_3 (mM)
P1	$15.2^a \pm 24.9$
P2	$17.1^d \pm 27.9$
P3	$15.9^b \pm 25.9$
P4	$16.7^c \pm 27.3$
P5	$15.6^b \pm 25.4$

a-d means in the same column with varying superscript differ significantly ($P<0.05$); P1 = complete feed (control), P2 = P1 + chestnut tannins 0.50% DM (2.63 g), P3 = P1 + chestnut tannins 1% DM (5.25 g), P4 = P1 + chestnut tannins 1.50% DM (7.88 g), and P5 = P1 + chestnut tannins 2% DM (10.5 g)

4 CONCLUSION

The use of 0.50% DM chestnut tannins as a complete feed silage additive made from tofu pulp, palm kernel meal, field grass, and palm fronds can maintain the pH of post-incubation rumen fluid to close to normal, can reduce ammonia concentrations, and does not affect the total VFA value.

REFERENCES

Dryden G.M. (2021). *Fundamentals of Applied Animal Nutrition*. England: CABI Press.

Jayanegara A., Goel G., Makkar H. and Becker K. (2015). Divergence Between Purified Hydrolysable and Condensed Tannin Effects on Methane Emission, Rumen Fermentation and Microbial Population in vitro. *Animal Feed Science Technology*, 209, 60–68.

Jayanegara A., Sujarnoko T.U.P., Ridla M., Kondo M., and Kreuzer M. (2019). Silage Quality as Influenced by Concentration and Type of Tannins Present in the Material Ensiled: A Meta-Analysis. *Journal of Animal Physiology and Animal Nutrition*, 103(2), 456–465.

Kellems R., and Church D. (2009). *Livestock Feeds and Feeding*. England: Pearson Press.

Kondo M., Shimizu K., Jayanegara A., Mishima T., Matsui H., Karita S., Goto M. and Fujihara T. (2016). Changes in Nutrient Composition and in Vitro Ruminal Fermentation of Total Mixed Ration Silage Stored at Different Temperatures and Periods. *Journal Science Food Agriculture*, 96(4), 1175–1180.

Kondo M., Hirano Y., Ikai N. Kita K., Jayanegara A., and Yokota H. (2014). Assessment of Anti-nutritive Activity of Tannins in Tea by-products Based on in vitro Rumen Fermentation. *Asian-Australasian Journal Animal Science*, 27, 1571–1576.

McDonald P., Greenhalgh J.F.D., Morgan C.A., Edwards R., Sinclair L. and Wilkinson R. (2012). *Animal Nutrition* 7th Edition. England: Prentice Hall, Harlow.

McNabb W.C., Waghorn G.C., Peters J.S. and Barry T.N. (1996). The Effect of Condensed Tannins in Lotus Pedunculatus on the Solubilization and Degradation of Ribulose-1,5-Bisphosphate Carboxylase (EC 4.1.1.39/Rubisco) Protein in the Rumen and the Sites of Rubisco Digestion. *British Journal Nutrition*, 76, 535–549.

Menci R., Coppa M., Torrent A., Natalello A., Valenti B., Luciano G., Priolo A. and Niderkorn V. (2021). Effects of Two Tannin Extracts at Different Doses in Interaction with a Green or Dry Forage Substrate on *in vitro* Rumen Fermentation and Biohydrogenation. *Animal Feed Science and Technology*, 278, 114977.

Mendez C.R., Plascencia A., Torrentera N. and Zinn R.A. (2017). Effect of Level and Source of Supplemental Tannin on Growth Performance of Steers During the Late Finishing Phase. *Journal of Applied Animal Research*, 45, (1), 199–203.

Petrie A., and P. Watson. 2013. *Statistics for Veterinary and Animal Science*. London (UK): John Wiley and Sons, Ltd.

Sadarman S., Ridla M. and Nahrowi. (2020). Evaluation of Ensiled Soy Sauce by-product Combined with Several Additives as an Animal Feed. *Veterinary World*, 13, (5), 940–946.

Santoso B., Widayati T.W. and Hariadi B.T. (2020). Improvement of Fermentation and the in vitro Digestibility Characteristics of Agricultural Waste-based Complete Feed Silage with Cellulase Enzyme Treatment. *Advances in Animal and Veterinary Sciences*, 8, (8), 873–881.

Siddiqui S.A., Asif Z., Murid M., Fernando I., Adli D.N., Blinov A.V., Golik A.B., Nugraha W.S., Ibrahim S.A. and Jafari S.M., (2022a). Consumer Social and Psychological Factors Influencing the Use of Genetically Modified Foods—A Review. *Sustainability*, 14(23), 15884.

Siddiqui S.A., Alvi T., Sameen A., Khan S., Blinov A.V., Nagdalian A.A., Mehdizadeh M., Adli D.N. and Onwezen M., (2022b). Consumer Acceptance of Alternative Proteins: A Systematic Review of Current Alternative Protein Sources and Interventions Adapted to Increase Their Acceptability. *Sustainability*, 14 (22), 15370.

Theodorou M., and Brooks A. (1990). *Evaluation of A New Laboratory Procedure for Estimating the Fermentation Kinetics of Tropical Feeds*. Annual Report. Meidenhead (GB): AFRC Inst.

Wu G. (2017). *Principles of Animal Nutrition*. New York, NY: Taylor & Francis Group, LLC.

Xie B., Yang X., Yang L., Wen X. and Zhao G. (2021). Adding Polyethylene Glycol to Steer Ration Containing Sorghum Tannins Increases Crude Protein Digestibility and Shifts Nitrogen Excretion From Feces to Urine. *Animal Nutrition*, 7, (3), 779–786.

Developing Modern Livestock Production in Tropical Countries – Adli et al. (eds)
© 2023 The Authors, ISBN 978-1-032-44025-5
Open Access: www.taylorfrancis.com, CC BY-NC-ND 4.0 license

Edamame isoflavones and omega-3 source supplementation to quail (*Coturnix coturnix japonica*): Effect on egg production and physical quality

R.T. Hertamawati, R. Rahmasari & M.M.D. Utami
Animal Husbandry Department, Politeknik Negeri Jember, East Java, Indonesia

M.A. Bagaskara
Postgraduate Biology Reproduction, Veterinary Medicine Faculty, Airlangga University, Surabaya, Indonesia

ABSTRACT: In the present study, we investigated the effects of dietary edamame iso-flavones (eISF) and fish oil lemuru (*Sardinella lemuru*) (MIL) supplementation on Japanese quail (*Coturnix coturnix japonica*) egg production and physical egg quality. Birds (n = 140; 14 wk old) were randomly assigned to 1 of 5 groups consisting of 28 birds (4 replicates of 7) and were fed a basal diet or the basal diet supplemented with either 0.5% or 1% of eISF and 2% or 4% of MIL. The experimental period lasted 16 wk old with a 16L:8D lighting schedule. Dietary eISF supplementation and fish oil lemuru did not affect feed intake, egg production, egg weight, and shell thickness on the other hand they improved feed efficiency to a greater extent than the other levels (1% eISF and 4 % MIL). However, egg yolk color was increased (P < 0.0001) at the highest level eISF 1% and 4% supplementation. It can be concluded that the present study indicated that supplementing with dietary eISF and fish oil lemuru improved egg yolk color but did not affect egg production.

Keywords: edamame, egg, is flavones, omega-3, quail

1 INTRODUCTION

The incidence of stunting in Indonesia is higher than in other countries in Southeast Asia (Sutarto *et al.* 2018) thus demanding special attention. One of the food ingredients in an effort to prevent stunting cases by fulfilling the nutrition of pregnant women and toddlers with nutritious food is quail eggs. Despite quail eggs being a nutrient-rich food (Shibi *et al.* 2016), consumption of quail eggs is still limited due to public stigma about the high cholesterol levels in quail eggs (Hertamawati *et al.* 2021). High cholesterol is suspected to be the cause of cardiovascular disease, high blood pressure, and obesity; therefore, there is a need for a solution to overcome these obstacles, namely by feeding manipulation.

Feeding manipulation can produce eggs that are low in cholesterol, rich in good fatty acids such as Omega-3, and rich in antioxidants and other nutrients. Isoflavone compounds contained in edamame soybeans have functions such as antioxidants, and they can be accumulated in animal products (Jiang *et al.* 2007) for the production of functional foods for humans. Another significant aspect of feeding manipulation is the enrichment of eggs with omega-3 from lemuru fish, which has been proven by Febrianto and Puspitasari (2015) and Arini *et al.* (2017). The content of omega-3 fish oil is 58,418 mg/g (Rusmana & Natawiharja 2008). Lemuru fish oil has the advantage of being a source of healthy fatty acids (omega-3) in the form of a fairly high content of EPA and DHA (Iriyanti *et al.* 2012).

DOI: 10.1201/9781003370048-20

81

Research on feed enrichment with a combination of isoflavones and lemuru fish oil is still limited so the objectives of this study were to evaluate the effectiveness of dietary edamame isoflavones (eISF) and fish oil lemuru (*Sardinella lemuru*) (MIL) supplementation on Japanese quail (*Coturnix coturnix japonica*) egg production and physical egg quality.

2 MATERIAL AND METHOD

2.1 *Experimental diets*

Two hundred Japanese quail (8 wk old; *Coturnix coturnix japonica*), provided by a commercial company Peksi Yoyakarta, Central Java, were used in accordance with animal welfare regulations at the State Polytechnic of Jember, East Java, Indonesia. After a 7-d adaptation period, the birds were randomly assigned to 5 groups, 40 birds each as 4 replicates.

The treatment feed was P0: control feed (without eISF and MIL); R1: feed containing 2% MIL and 0.5% eISF addition; R2: the feed contains 2% MIL and the addition of eISF 1%; R3: the feed contains 4% MIL and the addition of eISF 0.5%; and R4: feed contains 4% MIL and 1% eISF addition. The diets were prepared by self-mixing. Quails in the laying phase, 85 days old, were fed dietary 20% crude protein and 2800–3000 kcal/kg.

Table 1. Feed formulation and nutrient contents of diet treatments.

	Treatments				
Ingredient	R0	R1	R2	R3	R4
	.... (%)				
Corn	43	45	45	45	45
Rice brand	8	6.5	6.5	6	6
Soybean meal	30	27.9	27.9	28	28
Fish meal	4	5	5	4.9	4.9
Meat bone meal	5	6	6	6	6
Oil	3.9	1.5	1.5	0	0
Lemuru fish oil	0	2	2	4	4
CaCO3	6	6	6	6	6
Premix	0.1	0.1	0.1	0.1	0.1
Additive edamame	0	0.5	1	0.5	1
Total	100	100	100	100	100
Nutrients content[1]					
Energy metabolism (kcal/kg)	2813.4	2823.96	2823.96	2861.24	2861.24
Crude protein (%)	20.72	20.76	20.76	20.70	20.70
Crude fiber (%)	3.02	2.8	2.8	2.78	2.78
Crude fat (%)	6.44	6.16	6.16	6.67	6.67
Ca (%)	3.11	3.3	3.3	2.67	2.67
P available (%)	0.57	0.6	0.6	0.39	0.39

Note: [1]Count from feed formulation.

2.2 *Edamame concentrate isoflavones preparation*

The edamame concentrate isoflavone (eISF) was prepared using the following (Utami & Hertamawati 2020) procedures. The material used is low-grade edamame from PT Mitra Tani 27 Jember. Edamame were sun-dried until the water content was 10% and the procedure of making eISF was used to begin the extracting procedure, which involves macerating it with hexane and then macerating it with methanol.

2.3 *Procedure, performance, and egg quality variables*

Laying quails were divided into 5 groups, each treatment was subjected to four replications. The quail hens were given 25 g of feed per bird each day, and they were fed in the morning and afternoon. Drinking water was given ad-libitum. Edamame isoflavone concentrate (eISF) and lemuru fish oil (MIL) in the ration activity test were carried out in feed supplementary for 14 days. Each group was observed for laying performance (feed intake, egg weight and average hen day production, and feed egg ratio) and physical egg quality (yolk and albumen index, yolk color, and thickness eggshell).

2.4 *Data analysis*

The data obtained were tabulated using excel and analyzed using SPSS ver. 26 Completely Random Design (CRD). Any significant or very significant effect of treatments was followed by Duncan's multiple range test.

3 RESULT AND DISCUSSION

3.1 *Egg production*

Data on production performance are shown in Table 2. The feed intake during the study ranged from 20.11 grams/day to 23.73 grams/day. The results of the analysis of variance showed that the administration of edamame concentrate isoflavones (eISF) and fish oil (MIL) to the level of 1% and 4% reduced feed consumption ($p < 0.05$). The decrease in feed intake is thought to be due to a decrease in feed palatability with increasing fish oil administration. A decrease in feed consumption due to the addition of fish oil by up to 4% was also reported by Istiqomah *et al.* (2017).

The average egg production ranged from 78.30% to 85.019%. The results of the analysis of variance showed that the administration of eISF and fish oil had no significant effect on quail egg production ($p > 0.05$), as well as on egg weight and feed efficiency. The addition of eISF and fish oil proved not to affect the egg formation process so that it did not affect egg production (Sestilawarti & Mirzah 2013).

Table 2. The average egg quail production performance.

Parameter	Dietary Treatment				
	R0	R1	R2	R3	R4
Feed intake (g/bird)	23.73 ± 0.96^b	23.06 ± 1.04^b	23.23 ± 1.24^b	22.66 ± 0.56^b	20.11 ± 2.45^a
Egg weight (g)	10.69 ± 0.23^{ns}	10.82 ± 0.14^{ns}	10.79 ± 0.24^{ns}	10.66 ± 0.15^{ns}	10.51 ± 0.44^{ns}
Hen day production (%)	79.79 ± 6.61^{ns}	85.01 ± 4.11^{ns}	78.79 ± 6.61^{ns}	80.59 ± 7.41^{ns}	78.30 ± 8.83^{ns}
Feed egg ratio	2.22 ± 0.12^{ns}	2.13 ± 0.11^{ns}	2.15 ± 0.16^{ns}	2.13 ± 0.05^{ns}	1.92 ± 0.29^{ns}

[a,b]Different superscripts on the same row show a significant difference ($P < 0.05$).
[ns]Non-significant difference ($P > 0.05$).

3.2 Physicalegg production

The data on physical egg production are shown in Table 3. The results of the analysis of variance showed that the administration of edamame concentrate isoflavones (eISF) and fish oil (MIL) to the level of 1% and 4% increased yolk color (p<0.05). The increase in egg yolk color was due to the presence of lemuru fish oil in the feed, as reported by Darmawan et al. (2017), giving lemuru fish oil up to 2% can increase the yolk color in ducks. The intensity of yolk color is influenced by the presence and role of xanthophyll, a pigment that could be transferred from the feed. Egg yolk color is a quality indicator that can be altered by manipulating a hen's diet.

Table 3. The average physical egg quail production.

Parameter	Dietary Treatment				
	R0	R1	R2	R3	R4
Yolk index	1.15 ± 0.18	1.02 ± 0.25	1.14 ± 0.19	1.11 ± 0.08	1.09 ± 0.02
Albumen index	0.29 ± 0.04	0.36 ± 0.05	0.28 ± 0.04	0.33 ± 0.08	0.27 ± 0.02
Shell thickness	0.16 ± 0.03	0.19 ± 0.05	0.10 ± 0.07	0.16 ± 0.01	0.16 ± 0.06
Yolk color	5.75 ± 0.96^a	7.00 ± 0.82^b	7.50 ± 1.00^b	6.75 ± 0.50^{ab}	7.25 ± 0.50^b

[a,b]Different superscript on the same row shows a significant difference (P<0.05).
[ns]Non-significant difference (P>0.05).

The results of the analysis of variance showed that the administration of eISF and fish oil had no significant effect on the yolk and albumen index (p>0.05), as well as the eggshell thickness. The results of the present study were different from those reported by Sahin et al. (2007) who found that providing isoflavones in quails' diet will increase the eggshell thickness.

4 CONCLUSION

The present study indicates that supplementing with dietary eISF and fish oil lemuru decreased feed intake and improved egg yolk color but did not affect egg production.

ACKNOWLEDGEMENT

We gratefully acknowledge the funding of this research from the Directorate General of Vocational Education, The Ministry of Education, Culture, Research, and Technology through the Research on Leading Products of Vocational Higher Education 2022.

REFERENCES

Arini N.M.J., Sumiati and Mutia R. (2017). Evaluation of Feeding Indigofera Zollingeriana Leaf Meal and Sardinella Lemuru Fish Oil on Lipids Metabolism of Local Ducks. *Journal of the Indonesian Tropical Animal Agriculture*, 42(3), 194–201.

Darmawan A., Sumiati S. and Hermana W. (2017). The Effect of Dietary Vitamin e and Zinc Levels on Performance and Lipid Oxidation in Fresh and Stored Eggs of Laying Ducks. *Buletin Peternakan*, 41(2), 169.

Febrianto A.D.W.I. and Puspitasari R. (2015). Efek Suplementasi Minyak Ikan Lemuru dan L-Karnitin Dalam Rasum Komersial Terhadap Produksi dan Kualitas Telur Burung Puyuh (Coturnix coturnix japonica). *Bioteknologi*, 12(1), 1–7.

Hertamawati R.T., Nusantoro S. and Rahmasari R. (2021). Actions of Edamame Soybean Isoflavones in an Avian Model: The Japanese Quail (Cortunix-cortunix japónica). *IOP Conference Series: Earth and Environmental Science*, 672(1), 012043.

Iriyanti N., Tugiyanti E. and Yuwono E. (2012). Lipid Biosynthesis in Blood and Egg of Local Hen fed with Feed Containing Menhaden Fish Oil as Source of Omega-3 Fatty Acids. *Animal Production*, 14(60), 6–12.

Istiqomah S., Lamid M., and Pursetyo K.T. (2017). Potensi Penambahan Minyak Ikan Lemuru Pada Pakan Komersial Terhadap Kandungan Asam Lemak Omega-3 dan Omega-6 Daging Belut Sawah (Monopterus albus). *Jurnal Ilmiah Perikanan Dan Kelautan*, 9(1), 37.

Jiang Z.Y., Jiang S.Q., Lin Y.C., Xi P.B., Yu D.Q., and Wu T.X. (2007). Effects of Soybean Isoflavone on Growth Performance, Meat Quality, and Antioxidation in Male Broilers. *Poultry Science*, 86(7), 1356–1362.

Rusmana D., and Natawiharja D. (2008). The Effect of Giving Ration Containing Sardinella Oil and Vitamin E on Fat and Cholesterol of Meat in Broiler Chicken. *Jurnal Ilmu Ternak*, 8(1), 19–24. (In Indonesian.)

Sahin N., Onderci M., Balci T.A., Cikim G., Sahin K., and Kucuk O. (2007). The Effect of Soy Isoflavones on Egg Quality and Bone Mineralisation During the Late Laying Period of Quail. *British Poultry Science*, 48(3), 363–369.

Shibi T.K., Jagatheesan R.P., Reetha L.T., and Rajendran D. (2016). Nutrient Composition of Quail Eggs. *International Journal of Science, Environment and Technology*, 5(3)(June), 1293–1295.

Sutarto, Mayasari D. and Indriyani R. (2018). Stunting, Faktor Resiko dan Pencegahannya. *J. Agromedicine*, 5, 243–243.

Utami M.M.D., and Hertamawati R.T. (2020). Dietary Edamame Soybean Isoflavon Concentrate on Improving Carcass Quality of Broilers. *IOP Conference Series: Earth and Environmental Science*, 411(1).

Developing Modern Livestock Production in Tropical Countries – Adli et al. (eds)

Development of black pepper essential oil nanoemulsion using whey protein isolate as a natural emulsifier

Safitri
Master Student, Animal Product Department, University of Brawijaya, Malang, Indonesia

A. Manab* & K.U. Al Awwaly
Lectures, Animal Product Department, University of Brawijaya, Malang, Indonesia

A. Febrisiantosa
Research Centre for Food Technology and Processes, National Research and Innovation Agency (BRIN), Daerah Istimewa Yogyakarta, Indonesia

ABSTRACT: An oil-in-water (O/W) Black Pepper (*Piper nigrum*) essential oil (BPEO) nanoemulsion was made with a biopolymer combination. This study focuses on the effect of whey protein isolate (WPI) as an emulsifier to influence physical characteristics. The oil phase was made from BPEO and corn oil (30:70), and the aqueous phase was made from the modification of glucomannan liquid. The effect of WPI was investigated at different ratios ($T_0 = 0\%$, $T_1 = 2\%$, $T_2 = 4\%$, $T_3 = 6\%$). The experiment was conducted with a completely randomized design (CRD) by using four treatments and three replications, then continued with the Duncan multiple range test (DMRT). The physical character was observed by diameter droplet, polydispersity index, zeta potential, percent transmittance, and optical microscope. Based on its physical character, nanoemulsion can be developed from BPEO, modified glucomannan, WPI, and adding WPI 2% can protect the BPEO's bioactive compound during storage.

Keywords: nanoemulsion, black pepper essential oil, whey protein isolate, antioxidant, antibacterial

1 INTRODUCTION

Black pepper essential oils (*Piper nigrum*) are an excellent source of natural antioxidant and antibacterial molecules because of the bioactive compounds such as terpene and mono-terpene (Wang *et al.* 2020). These bioactive components should be protected when interacting with another food component because those bio-actives are unstable in character, have high volatility, proneness to environmental conditions (i.e., UV, temperature), and hydrophobicity behaviors (Rehman *et al.* 2021). Oil-in-water (O/W) nanoemulsion is one of the methods to encapsulate the EO's bioactive (Farshi *et al.* 2019). Natural emulsifiers become the best alternative to create products with "consumer-friendly" labels, due to the trend to use biopolymers such as proteins or polysaccharides for the preparation of nano-emulsions is increasing (Farshi *et al.* 2019). Whey proteins have function as a natural emulsifier because they have hydrophobic and hydrophilic properties. The utilization of whey proteins (WPI, WPC, and β-lactoglobulin) as emulsifying nano agents has received much attention (Adjonu *et al.* 2014). Assadpour *et al.* (2016) succeeded in optimizing folic

---

*Corresponding Author: manabfpt@ub.ac.id

DOI: 10.1201/9781003370048-21

acid in nanoemulsions and encapsulation of maltodextrin and whey protein. The research of Zhao et al. (2018) also showed the success of using whey protein isolate (WPI) in lutein encapsulation in the form of nanoemulsions. The combination of protein and polysaccharide successfully formed a polyelectrolyte complex, so the nanoemulsion was more stable (Farshi et al. 2019). Modified glucomannan can be used as a stabilizer (Manab et al. 2016). This study was conducted to evaluate the effect of using WPI as a stabilizer with black pepper essential oil and modified glucomannan in the nanoemulsion on physical characters.

2 MATERIALS AND METHODS

The research methodology was a laboratory experiment using a completely randomized design (CRD) with four different treatments containing whey protein isolate (T_0: 0% WPI, T_1: 2% WPI, T_2: 4% WPI, T_3: 6% WPI) (w/v) and using three replicates for every treatment. Analysis of variance (ANOVA) was applied to all data, compared the means of separate replicates using the Duncan's multiple range test. All statistical tests were performed using SAS 9.4 (SAS Institute Inc. 2013). The differences at $P < 0.05$ were considered to be significant.

The nanoemulsion was conducted based on Farshi et al. (2019), who mixed BPEO as the primary oil and corn oil as the carrier oil with a ratio of 1:3. The biopolymer was made from glucomannan as a stabilizer and WPI as an emulsifier. Glucomannan was modified with a combination of lactic acid and microwave irradiation (Manab et al. 2016). 3% wt konjac glucomannan flour was dissolved in 100 ml of distilled water with 4% lactic acid, and then stirred for 15 minutes. The solutions were heated in the microwave for 10 minutes and centrifuged at 5000 rpm for 10 min at 25°C to separate the sediment. The ratio of the oil phase to the aqueous phase was set at 10:90. The first coarse emulsion was made using an Ultra Turrax homogenizer (IKA T25 digital, 20,000 rpm for 3 min) then using ultra-sonication (Lawson®, 20 kHz, 400W for 15 minutes). The emulsifier was prepared by dissolving WPI (2–6% wt) in 100 mL of distilled water and then added to modified glucomannan at ±70°C for 15 min. The droplet diameter (DD), zeta potential (ZP), and polydispersity index (PDI) which is used as a measure of the breadth of the molecular weight distribution were measured using dynamic light scattering (Microtrac, MRB, USA). The samples were diluted 250 folds in twice-distilled water (Farshi et al. 2019). After 7 days, the transmittance was measured using a UV-Vis spectrophotometer (500 nm) with 0.1 ml of nanoemulsion added to 100 ml of distilled water (Senapati et al. 2016). The creaming index measurement using 10 ml of the emulsion was transferred and kept in a test tube and stored for 7 days at room temperature and calculated with the formula $CI = (H_L/H_E) \times 100\%$, in which H_E is the overall height of emulsions and H_L is the total height of the layer of the cream (Mohammed et al. 2020).

3 RESULTS AND DISCUSSIONS

The most important ingredient in nanoemulsion is the emulsifier. Proteins and poly-saccharides have advantages as natural ingredients rather than artificial emulsifiers, but the manufacture of emulsions with these materials must use high energy (McClements & Rao 2011). The development of nanoemulsion in this research combined ultraturrax and ultra-sonication to reduce the size of the droplets to nanometric scales (da Silva et al. 2022). The ultrasonic method uses high-intensity ultrasonic waves to disturb the oil and the water phase so both phases will break up and it will become small droplets (McClements & Rao 2011).

The variance analysis shows that different ratios of whey protein have no significant effects ($p > 0.05$) on DD and ZP, as shown in Figure 1. The data show that all of the treatments produce particles in nano size less than 500 nm. Kotta et al. (2015) explained that the

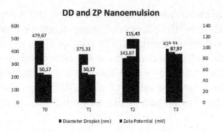

Figure 1. Diameter droplet (nm) and zeta potential (mV) nanoemulsion BPEO.

Table 1. Physical character of black pepper essential oil nanoemulsion.

Parameters	T_0	T_1	T_2	T_3	SEM
PDI	0.06	0.15	0.29	0.01	0.0
Creaming index (%)	20.27[a]	0[b]	0[b]	0[b]	0.09
Percent transmittance (%)	94.83[a]	92.40[a]	84.77[b]	85.23[b]	14.32

*Different superscripts mean significant differences.

size range of nanoemulsion is varied, some consider 200 nm as the upper limit, and some others as 500 nm. All of the treatment indicates around 0.01–0.29, which means that the nanoemulsion has a very homogeneous particle distribution (Agustinisari and Harimurti, 2022). The value of ZP is greater than 30 mV or less than −30 mV (Schreiner et al. 2020) and defined as the strength of electrical repulsion between particles to prevent aggregation (Mohammed et al. 2020). The ultrasonication might lead to the nano formation between oil and stabilizer, but the emulsion could not maintain the formation without an emulsifier.

The variance analysis shows that different ratios of whey protein give a highly significant effect (p<0.01) on the creaming index and give a significant effect (p<0.05) on percent transmittance after 7 days of storage as shown in Table 1. Meanwhile, T_1, T_2, and T_3 indicated stability over the storage time without creaming, and this result showed that WPI has an important role in the oil coating process because WPI is an amphiphilic molecule, and the surface has both polar and non-polar groups. Those surfaces have the ability to reduce the interfacial tension at the oil-water interface (Lam & Nickerson 2013). This result is similar to Mohammed et al. (2020), who explained that enough emulsifiers can adequately encapsulate the droplets of oil. This result is similar to Campelo et al. (2017) who investigated on kinetic stability of lime essential oil emulsion using gum arabic (GA) and WPI. Campelo et al. (2017) successfully preserved the emulsion stability over a period of 4 h during the spray drying process. Mohammed et al. (2020) also studied about creaming index of Nigella sativa essential oil with 10% WPI and resulting in no formation of cream after 7-day storage at 25°C.

T_1 has perfect physical character without creaming and shows transparent or clear transmittance values until 7 days of storage. It could be estimated that the emulsion droplets still reached nanometers after storage. Li et al. (2018) explained that WPI could influence the physical character because the emulsifier molecules are accessible to cover oil-water interface surfaces during the formation of nanoemulsions. T_2 and T_3 indicate that the formation was changing after storage (Mohammed et al. 2020). After the coating is enough, the WPI molecule will accumulate and aggregate on the surface of nanodroplets. It makes the nano formation thicker and increases the percent transmittance (Hosseinnia et al. 2017). The interesting phenomena were T_0 which still has a percent transmittance of more than 90% but have a creaming index of 20,27%. It might be because of the different densities of the oil phase and the aqueous phase but the character of each phase is still on the nanometric scale and the raw material is still at transparency appearance. When the transmittance test is conducted, both phases are mixed because creaming is a reversible process, meaning that the redispersion of a creamed emulsion can be done but is not stable (McSweeney & McNamara 2021).

4 CONCLUSION

Based on its physical character, nanoemulsion can be developed from BPEO, modified glucomannan, and WPI, and adding WPI 2% can protect the BPEO's bioactive compound during storage.

ACKNOWLEDGMENT

This research was supported by BRIN through BARISTA (Bantuan Riset dan Talenta) Programme 2022.

REFERENCES

Adjonu R., Doran G., Torley P. and Agboola S. (2014). Formation of Whey Protein Isolate Hydrolysate Stabilized Nanoemulsion. *Food Hydrocolloids*, 41, 169–177.

Agustinisari I. and Harimurti N. (2022). Production of Clove Oil Nanoemulsion Using Whey Protein-maltodextrin Conjugates and Chitosan. *IOP Conference Series: Earth and Environmental Science*, *1024*(1), 012057.

Assadpour E., Maghsoudlou Y., Jafari S.M., Ghorbani M. and Aalami M. (2016). Optimization of Folic Acid Nano-emulsification and Encapsulation by Maltodextrin-Whey Protein Double Emulsions. *International Journal of Biological Macromolecules*, 86, 197–207.

Campelo P.H., Junqueira L.A., Resende J.V., Zacarias R.D., Fernandes R.V.B., Botrel D.A., and Borges S.V. (2017). Stability of lime Essential Oil Emulsion Prepared Using Biopolymers and Ultrasound Treatment. *International Journal of Food Properties*, 20(1), 564–579.

Da Silva B.D., Do Rosário D.K., Weitz D.A. and Conte-Junior C.A. (2022). Essential Oil Nanoemulsions: Properties, Development, and Application in Meat and Meat Products. *Trends in Food Science & Technology*, 121, 1–13.

Farshi P., Tabibiazar M., Ghorbani M., Mohammadifar M., Amirkhiz M.B. and Hamishehkar H., (2019). Whey Protein Isolate-guar Gum Stabilized Cumin Seed Oil Nanoemulsion. *Food Bioscience*, 28(2019): 49–56.

Hosseinnia M., Khaledabad M.A. and Almasi H. (2017). Optimization of *Ziziphora Clinopodiodes* Essential Oil Microencapsulation by Whey Protein Isolate and Pectin: A Comparative Study. *International Journal of Biological Macromolecules*, 101, 958–966.

Kotta S., Khan A.W., Ansari S.H., Sharma R.K. and Ali J. (2015). Formulation of Nanoemulsion: A Comparison Between Phase Inversion Composition Method and High-Pressure Homogenization Method, *Drug Delivery*, 22(4), 455–466.

Lam R.S. and Nickerson, M.T. (2013). Food Proteins: A Review on Their Emulsifying Properties using a Structure-function Approach. *Food Chemistry*, 141(2), 975–984.

Li Y., Jin H., Sun X., Sun J., Liu C., Liu C. and Xu J. (2018). Physicochemical Properties and Storage Stability of Food Protein-stabilized Nanoemulsions. *Nanomaterials*, 9(1), 25.

Manab A., Purnomo H., Widjarnarko B.S., Radiati L.E. (2016). Modification of Porang (*Amorphophallus Oncophyllus*) Flour by Acid and Thermal Process Using Conventional Heating in Water Bath and Microwave Irradiation, *Advance Journal of Food Science and Technology*, 12(1), 290–301.

McClements, D. J., and Rao, J. (2011). Food-grade Nanoemulsions: Formulation, fabrication, properties, performance, biological fate, and potential toxicity. *Critical Reviews in Food Science and Nutrition*, 51(4), 285–330.

Mohammed N.K., Muhialdin B.J. and Hussin A.S.M. (2020). Characterization of Nanoemulsion of *Nigella Sativa* Oil and its Application in Ice Cream. *Food Science Nutrition*, 8(6), 2608–2618.

McSweeney P.L.H and J. P. McNamara. (2021). *Encyclopedia of Dairy Sciences*. Academic Press.

Rehman A., Qunyi T., Sharif H.R., Korma S.A., Karim A., Manzoor M.F., Mehmood A., Iqbal M.W., Ali H.R.A. and Mehmood T. (2021). Biopolymer based Nanoemulsion Delivery System: An Effective Approach to Boost the Antioxidant Potential of Essential Oil in Food Products. *Carbohydrate Polymer Technologies and Applications*, 2(100082), 1–16.

Schreiner T.B., Santamaria-Echart A., Ribeiro A., Peres A.M., Dias M.M., Pinho S.P., and Barreiro M.F. (2020). Formulation and Optimization of Nanoemulsions using the Natural Surfactant Saponin from Quillaja Bark. *Molecules*, 25(7), 1538.

Senapati P.C., Sahoo S.K. and Sahu A.N. (2016). Mixed Surfactant-based (SNEDDS) Self-Nanoemulsifying Drug Delivery System Presents Efavirenz for Enhancing Oral Bioavailability. *Biomedicine & Pharmacotherapy*, 80, 42–51.

Wang D., Zhang L., Huang J., Himabindu K., Tewari D., Horbanzuk J.O., Xu S., Chen Z., and Atanasov A. G. (2020). Cardiovascular Protective Effect of Black Pepper (*Piper nigrum* l.) and its Major Bioactive Constituent Piperine. *Trends in Food Science & Technology*, 1–12.

Zhao C., Shen X. and Guo M. (2018). Stability of Lutein Encapsulated Whey Protein Nano-Emulsion During Storage. *PLoS ONE*, 13(2), e0192511.

Developing Modern Livestock Production in Tropical Countries – Adli et al. (eds)
© 2023 The Authors, ISBN 978-1-032-44025-5
Open Access: www.taylorfrancis.com, CC BY-NC-ND 4.0 license

Characteristics of biomass and mineral yeast saccharomyces cerevisiae using soybean meal and fish meal

D. Pantaya, S. Wulandari, M.M.D. Utami*, H. Subagja, A.H. Prayitno & M. Adhyatma
Animal Science Department, Politeknik Negeri Jember, Jember, Indonesia

R. Lestari
Faculty of Biology, Indonesia University, Jakarta, Indonesia

ABSTRACT: The research aimed to analyze the characterization and mineral content of Saccharomyces cerevisiae using soybean meal and fish meal media. The method of research used a completely randomized design using three types of yeast (local yeast, peat soil yeast, and yeast of Food Nutrition Culture Collection [FNCC]). The characterization based on biomass has not been different significantly, but the biomass of all yeast with the soybean meal medium was higher than the fish meal medium. The highest biomass was obtained from local yeast followed by FNCC and peat soil yeast. The mineral content of potassium, sodium, calcium, and magnesium in the FNCC yeast was higher when compared to local and peat soil yeast; on the contrary, the iron content of local yeast was higher than FNCC yeast and peat soil yeast. The result of this study recommends the soybean meal medium for Saccharomyces cerevisiae, and in general, the mineral content of FNCC yeast was higher than local and peat soil yeast.

1   INTRODUCTION

Feed additives are feed ingredients that are needed in the right amount and can improve production performance. Several studies were conducted in the last two decades to evaluate feed additives that use live microbes as microbial supplements specific to ruminant feed (Sundus & Enas 2018). Yeast, as a living microorganism, is widespread in the natural environment. *Yeast Saccharomyces cerevisiae* multiplies as a single cell that divides with buds (Azhar *et al.* 2017). Yeast contains 40% crude protein, vitamins, and minerals that can be used for lamb (Shurson 2018).

Soybean meal is a major source of protein. Soybean meal is an important source of protein for animals due to its excellent amino acid composition and high level of digestibility. The composition of soybean meal is as follows: dry matter 90.0%, crude protein 48.0%, lysine 2.63%, threonine 1.58%, methionine 0,60%, isoleucine 0.61%, tryptophan 0.59, fat 2.5%, available phosphorus 0.24%, and calcium 0.30% (Thormann *et al.* 2004). Fishmeal is a high-quality feed ingredient that is easily digested and palatable by livestock. Fishmeal is an excellent source of protein, lipids, minerals, and vitamins.

The mineral yeast content is very important and affects the quality of yeast used to stimulate the development of microbes in the rumen. There is very limited published information on the mineral content of biomass yeast *Saccharomyces cerevisiae*. This research aimed to analyze the mineral content of yeast Saccharomyces cerevisiae using soybean meal

---

*Corresponding Author: merry.mdu@polije.ac.id

DOI: 10.1201/9781003370048-22
This chapter has been made available under a CC BY NC ND license

and fish meal media. The results of this study will recommend the best medium for yeast growth to produce minerals beneficial for metabolism in the stomach of the livestock

2 MATERIAL AND METHODS

2.1 *Materials*

This study used three types of yeast: local yeast, yeast from peat soil, and yeast from the Food and Nutrition Culture Collection (FNCC) (Table 1). FNCC is one of the divisions of the Center for Food and Nutrition Studies at Gadjah Mada University which focuses on providing microbial cultures or isolates that are used for research and applications in small-scale and industrial food products. The main activities in the FNCC include collecting, characterization, preserving, and distributing microbial cultures. Soybean meal and fish meal are obtained from commercial products.

Table 1. Biomass production of yeast with different media (CFU/g).

Num.	Treatments	Local Yeast	Peat soil Yeast	FNCC Yeast
1	Soybean meal	24.67×10^9	219×10^9	203.67×10^9
2	Fish meal	145×10^9	61.67×10^9	77.67×10^9

2.2 *Methods*

Soybean meal and fish meal were ground with a mesh size of 1 mm using a sample mill (IKA-Werke M20, Germany) to obtain soybean meal and fish meal which are small and uniform in size, the chemical composition of the sample was analyzed using the method of Ferris *et al.* (2003) and Pantaya *et al.* (2022). The sample was then heated for 1 hour at a temperature of 70°C. The tube was weighed before centrifugation, and then centrifuged at 10,000 rpm for 10 min. Next, the precipitate and supernatant were weighed and the weight and volume were recorded. About 1 ml of the solution was homogenized using an ultra turra blender and then stored at -20°C in a polyethylene tube. About 1 ml was poured in a centrifuge tube and vortexed for 2 min and centrifuged 5,000 g, 5 min at -5°C. The method of research used a completely randomized design using three types of yeast (local yeast, peat soil yeast, and yeast of FNCC). If there is a difference in the mean of treatment, the Duncan test is carried out.

3 RESULTS AND DISCUSSION

The results of testing the mineral content of the three yeast groups are shown in Table 2.

Table 2. Mineral contents of yeast.

Num.	Minerals (ppm)	Local Yeast	Peat soil Yeast	FNCC Yeast
1	Potassium (K)	1.2497	1.2010	1.3646
2	Sodium (Na)	0.0181	0.0193	0.0409
3	Calcium (Ca)	0.2932	0.2823	0.3527
4	Magnesium (Mg)	0.1366	0.1124	0.1498
5	Iron (Fe)	0.0795	0.0722	0.0753

4 DISCUSSION

Biomass production using soybean meal media is higher than fish meal. According to Fardiaz and Idiyanti (2002), the use of soybean meal increases the dry weight of yeast due to the availability of peptones in the media, which can increase the amount of yeast production mass. Furthermore, peptone is a nutrient element that is very important for the development of microbes (Taskin *et al.* 2016).

Soybean meal contains more complete ingredients compared to fish meal, especially the amino acid content. Yeast needs amino acid nutrients as a source of protein formation. Another research (Utami *et al.* 2016) reported that yeast contains protein components ranging from 41% so it requires amino acid components to form biomass. The increase in production is also expected to increase the protein content in yeast. From these results, the production of yeast biomass is influenced by the composition of the media, including the content of proteins, sugars, and amino acid content in the media. The highest biomass production was sorted from local yeast, peat soil yeast, and FNCC yeast.

5 CONCLUSION

Biomass production using soybean meal media is higher than fish meal. Biomass production based on the highest yeast type is local yeast followed by FNCC yeast and the lowest biomass from peat soil yeast. The highest mineral content of potassium, sodium, calcium, and magnesium was obtained from FNCC yeast, followed by local yeast and peat soil yeast, while the highest mineral iron content was obtained from local yeast, followed by FNCC yeast and peat soil yeast.

ACKNOWLEDGMENT

We gratefully acknowledge the funding of this research from Politeknik Negeri Jember through the Matching Fund Program 2022.

REFERENCES

Azhar S.H.M., Abdulla R., Jambo S.A., Marbawi H., Gansau J.A., Faik A.A.M. and Rodrigues K.F. (2017). Yeasts in Sustainable Bioethanol Production: A Review. *Biochemistry and Biophysics Reports*, 10, 52–61.

Eruvbetine D. (2003). Canine Nutrition and Health: A Paper Presented at the Seminar Organized by Kensington Pharmaceuticals Nig. *Ltd., Lagos on, 21.*

Fardiaz D. and Idiyanti T. (2002). *Peptone Production From Soybean Press Cake and Yeast Bby Papain Enzyme For The Bacterial Growth Media.*

Ferris D.A., Flores R.A., Shanklin C.W. and Whitworth M.K. (1995). Proximate Analysis of Food Service Wastes. *Applied Engineering in Agriculture*, 11(4), 567–572.

Keddy P.A. (2010). *Wetland Ecology: Principles and Conservation.* Cambridge University Press.

Kogan G. and Kocher A. (2007). Role of Yeast Cell Wall Polysaccharides in Pig Nutrition and Health Protection. *Livestock Science*, 109(1–3), 161–165.

Mohammed S.F., Mahmood F.A. and Abas E.R. (2018). A Review on Effects of Yeast (Saccharomyces Cerevisiae) as Feed Additives in Ruminants Performance. *J. Entomol. Zool. Stud*, 6, 629–635.

Nuyim T. (2003). Peatland Status and Management in Thailand. ASEAN Peatland Management Initiative. 16–17 October. Bogor.

Pantaya D., Pamungkas D., Wulandari S. and Utami M.M.D. (2022, February). Fermentation of Soybean Meal-hydrolysates as the Medium that Treated by Papain Enzyme with Saccharomyces Cerevisiae for Biomass Production. In *IOP Conference Series: Earth and Environmental Science* (Vol. 980, No. 1, p. 012025). IOP Publishing.

Puastuti W. (2009). *Manipulation of Bioprocess in Rumen to Improve Fiber Feed Utilization.*

Rieley J. and Page S. (2016). Tropical Peatland of the World. In *Tropical Peatland Ecosystems* (pp. 3–32). Springer, Tokyo.

Santos A., Marquina D., Leal J.A. and Peinado J.M. (2000). (1→ 6)-β-D-glucan as Cell Wall Receptor for Pichia Membranifaciens Killer Toxin. *Applied and Environmental Microbiology*, 66(5), 1809–1813.

Shurson G.C. (2018). Yeast and Yeast Derivatives in Feed Additives and Ingredients: Sources, Characteristics, Animal Responses, and Quantification Methods. *Animal Feed Science and Technology*, 235, 60–76.

Stivrins N., Ozola I., Galka M., Kuske E., Alliksaar T., Andersen T.J. and Reitalu T. (2017). Drivers of Peat Accumulation Rate in a Raised Bog: Impact of Drainage, Climate, and Local Vegetation Composition. *Mires and Peat*, 1–19.

Taskin M., Unver Y., Firat A., Ortucu S. and Yildiz M. (2016). Sheep Wool Protein Hydrolysate: a New Peptone Source for Microorganisms. *Journal of Chemical Technology and Biotechnology*, 91(6), 1675–1680.

Tian J., Wang H., Vilgalys R., Ho M., Flanagan N. and Richardson C.J. (2021). Response of Fungal Communities to Fire in a Subtropical Peatland. *Plant and Soil*, 466(1), 525–543.

Tiner R.W. (2016). *Wetland Indicators: A Guide to Wetland Formation, Identification, Delineation, Classification, and Mapping.* CRC Press.

Tomé D. (2021). Yeast Extracts: Nutritional and Flavoring Food Ingredients. *ACS Food Science and Technology*, 1(4), 487–494.

Utami M.M.D., Pantaya D., Pamungkas D., Wulandari S. and Febri A. (2016). Optimasi Produksi Pepton dari Bungkil Kedelai Untuk Media Produksi Yeast. *Prosiding.*

Wayan G.I., Ni,K.S. and Putu, S. (2010). The Effects of Minerals on the Chest Circumference, Body Length and Body Height of Male Bali Cattle. *Buletin Veteriner Udayana*, 8(2), 128–134.

Zain M., Sutardi T., Suryahadi. and Ramli N. (2008). Effect of Defaunation and Supplementation Methionine Hydroxy Analogue and Branched Chain Amino Acid in Growing Sheep Diet based on Palm Press Fiber Ammoniated. *Pakistan Journal of Nutrition*, 7(6), 813–816.

Rumen degradation profile of several macroalgae collected from Gunungkidul D.I. Yogyakarta

H. Herdian* & A. Sofyan
Research Center for Animal Husbandry National Research and Innovation Agency (BRIN), Cibinong Indonesia
Animal Feed and Nutrition Modelling (AFENUE) Research Group, Faculty of Animal Science, IPB University, Bogor, Indonesia

A.A. Sakti
Research Center for Animal Husbandry National Research and Innovation Agency (BRIN), Cibinong Indonesia

I.N.G. Darma
Faculty of Animal Science, IPB University, Bogor, Indonesia
Research Assistant of Feed Additive And Supplement Technology Research Group of Research Center for Animal Husbandry National Research and Innovation Agency (BRIN)

Jasmadi, H. Novianty, A.R. Sefrienda, T. Kurniawan & S. Hariyadi
Research Center for Food Technology and Processing, National Research and Innovation Agency (BRIN), Gunungkidul, Indonesia

Nur Adianto
Directorate of Laboratory Management, Research Facilities, and Science and Technology Park National Research and Innovation Agency (BRIN), Gunungkidul, Indonesia

S. Permadi
Research Center for Oceanography, Research Organization for Earth Sciences and Maritime- National Research and Innovation Agency (BRIN), Jakarta, Indonesia

ABSTRACT: Four types of macroalgae, i.e., *Ulva spp.*, *Chaetamorpha spp.*, *Sargassum spp.*, and *Enteromorpha spp.* collected from Gunungkidul D.I. Yogyakarta coastal were evaluated for degradation in the rumen using the in-situ technique. Approximately 5 g of each sample was put in a nylon bag and incubated on the rumen of two male PO cows for 6, 12, 24, 48, and 72 hours. The results of degradation observations were fitting using non-linear regression equations. The response variables calculated were dry matter degradation (DMD), organic matter degradation (OMD), effective degradation of dry matter (EDDM), effective degradation of organic matter (EDOM), and the kinetic degradation profile of each material. The experimental design used a randomized completely block design (RCBD). The cows as a host were not significantly different ($p > 0.05$). The DMD at 72 h incubation value was different between types of algae ($P < 0.05$) with *Ulva spp.* having the highest value of 81.58%, and the lowest was *Sargassum spp.* with 39.46%. Relatively similar results occur in OMD and EDOM values. The highest OMD value was obtained from *Ulva spp.*, and the lowest from *Sargassum spp.* with values 74.28% and 24.62%, respectively, while the highest EDOM value was obtained from *Enteromorpha spp.* = 49.48% and the lowest was obtained from *Sargassum spp.* = 19.24%. The highest EDDM value was obtained from *Ulva spp.* 97.32% and the lowest value was obtained from *Sargassum spp.* = 35.25%. The results

---

*Corresponding Author: hendravit@yahoo.com

DOI: 10.1201/9781003370048-23

showed that the macroalgae being collected had different degradation under rumen fermentation conditions.

Keywords: Macroalgae, insacco, rumen degradation

1 INTRODUCTION

Generally, based on their cellularity, marine algae were separated as micro and macroalgae (Beetul *et al.* 2016) while chemically marine algae consisted of protein, fatty acids, minerals, and vitamins which mainly concern with food purposes and some bioactive compounds which lead to pharmaceutical or other functional materials (El Gamal 2010). The bioactive compounds among them were polyphenols, bromophenols, sulfated polysaccharides, fucoidan, fucosterol, phlorotannins, carotenoid pigments and fucoxanthin (El Gamal 2010). As a result, this plant has antibacterial (Zainuddin *et al.* 2019), antiprotozoal (Torres *et al.* 2014), and antioxidant (Rumengan & Desy 2015) properties while Roque *et al.* (2019) reported decreasing methane production effect for the 5% Asparagopsis taxiformis organic matter supplementation as feed intake. In the study of potential ruminant animal feed, we conduct the research for profiling the rumen degradation of *Ulva spp.*, *Chaetamorpha spp.*, *Sargassum spp.*, and *Enteromorpha spp.*, collected from Gunungkidul D.I. Yogyakarta Indonesia coastal using in situ technique.

2 MATERIALS AND METHODS

Four types of macroalgae, i.e., *Ulva spp.*, *Chaetamorpha spp.*, *Sargassum spp.*, and *Enteromorpha spp.*, were collected from the Gunungkidul D.I. Yogyakarta Indonesia coastal region (8°08′14.9″S 110°34′07.9″E). The collected samples were cut into pieces and then dried in a hot air force oven at 50°C for 3 days. The samples were milled then using a laboratory grinder. The reduced-size samples were filtered using sieve holes with diameters of 1 mm for chemical analysis and 3 mm for in situ analysis.

The in-situ rumen technique was conducted according to Ørskov and Mc. Donald (1979). The samples were incubated in two male fistulated PO cattle. The animals were fed with elephant grass and concentrated at a 60% to 40% ratio, water was delivered ad libitum, and both animals passed the ethical clearing procedure issued by The Ethical Commission of Integrated Research and Testing Laboratory Gadjah Mada University (Certificate#: 00004/04/LPPT/IV/2022). The samples with approximately 5g of weight were then incubated in the rumen for 6, 12, 24, 48, and 72 hours with a duplicate for each. The chemical composition of macroalgae including dry matter (DM), organic matter (OM), crude protein (CP), extract ether (EE), and ash was determined, according to AOAC (1990), while crude fiber (CF) was determined according to Ibrahim (1988).

The design experiment used a randomized completely block design (RCBD). In each withdrawn period, the DMD and OMD disappearance was calculated and fitted by non-linear regression (Ørskov & McDonald 1979) by NewWay (Chen 1997). For every constant reveals the Potential Degradability of Dry Matter (PDDM), Potential Degradability of Organic Matter (PDOM), Effective Degradability of Dry Matter (EDDM), and Effective Degradability of Organic Matter (EDOM) with 0.06 h^{-1} passage rate's constant or rumen particle (Ørskov & McDonald 1979) were measured. Differences in responses were analyzed by the Analysis of Variance (ANOVA) Nested model, while the mean difference was evaluated by the Least Significant Difference (LSD) counted by CoStat.

3 RESULTS AND DISCUSSION

The CP, CF, NFE, and Ash composition of the sample varied (Table 1), except for EE which resumed slight differences. The CP content of the macroalgae appears in the range of 7.95 to 13.90%, and these results were lower than the CP concentration of *Porphyra spp.* with 60.9% (Gülzari *et al.* 2019). Compared with the terrestrial plant, the CP concentration was higher than the tropical Gramineae plant, i.e., *Urochloa hybrid* and *Urochloa brizantha* (Anzueta-Q S. *et al.* 2021). Ash content laid at 28.75% to 51.32%, with *Enteromorpha spp.* having the highest result but the content is still lower than *Laminaria japonica* with 64.30% CP content. This high ash condition occurred probably because of the salt storage treatment (Weihao *et al.* 2022). *Chaetomorpha spp.* has the highest CF content (18.03%). This condition was higher than *E. arborea, M. pyfera, G. robustum,* and *P. torreyi* CP content (4.30–17.6% range), while EE (0.21–0.48% vs 0.4–1.3%) and NFE (52.6 vs 68.2 %) range was lower (Serviere-Zaragoza *et al.* 2002).

Table 1. Chemical Composition (DM %).

Algae	CP	EE	CF	NFE	Ash
Ulva spp.	12.64	0.31	3.73	59.86	35.33
Chaetomorpha spp.	13.90	0.37	18.03	30.62	43.88
Sargassum spp.	7.82	0.48	8.27	65.53	28.75
Enteromorpha spp.	7.95	0.21	3.55	47.28	51.32

CP = Crude Protein, EE = Extract Eter, CF = Crude Fiber, NFE = Nitrogen Free Extract.

The cattle as a host animal contributed a non-significant effect to the incubation of macroalgae in the rumen ($P>0.05$). The type of macroalgae being incubated was significantly different ($P<0.05$) in the matter of DMD or OMD for 72 h rumen incubation. The highest DMD result was obtained from *Ulva spp.* and the lowest was obtained from *Sargassum spp.* with values of 81.58% and 39.46%, respectively. A similar result revealed for OMD with 74.28% for *Ulva spp.* as the highest result and 24.62% for *Sargassum spp.* as the lowest. The pattern for DMD and OMD degradation with 5-point observation was significantly different ($P<0.05$) for each macroalga. As shown in the graph, *Sargassum spp.* has the lowest intercept at 0 h value for OMD and DMD compared with others, with a similar result found at "a" value in Table 2, which shows the lowest "a" value (33.40% and 16.86% for DMD and OMD, respectively). *Chaetomorpha spp.* showed the highest "a" value for DMD (59.68%) and *Ulva spp.* for OMD (34.80%). The DMD potential degradation of *Ulva spp.* has reached the highest one, while *Sargassum spp.* has the highest OMD value (63.13%), and the *Chaetomorpha spp.* has the lowest (10.86% and 20.18%). The highest "c" value for DMD and OMD was achieved by *Enteromorpha spp.* (0.044% and 0.042) while the lowest set by *Sargassum spp.* (0.004% and 0.019%). Potential degradation "a + b" value showed the highest DMD and OMD reached by *Ulva spp.* (92.32% and 89.89%), while the lowest DMD value was reached by *Sargassum spp.* and *Chaetomorpha spp.* (62.20% and 52.88%). The EDDM and EDOM highest values were achieved by *Enteromorpha spp.* (67.37% and 49.48%). *Sargassum spp.* commonly known as brown algae (seaweed) has a potential bioactive activity that could support health and also for food. Some bioactive compounds that could be extracted from sargassum included terpenoids, flavonoids, sterols, sulfated polysaccharides, polyphenols, sargaquinoic acids, sargachromenol, pheophytin (Subhash *et al.* 2014), and L-fucopyranose (Artemisia *et al.* 2019).

Table 2. Dry matter and organic matter degradation for 72-hour rumen incubation.

Algae	72 h[1]	a[2]	b[3]	c[4]	a + b[5]	ED[6]
DMD[7]						
Ulva spp.	81.58[a]	53.86[b]	38.45[a]	0.020[ab]	92.32[a]	62.98[b]
Chaetomorpha spp.	69.15[c]	59.68[a]	10.86[b]	0.031[a]	70.55[ab]	63.31[b]
Sargassum spp.	39.46[d]	33.40[c]	28.80[ab]	0.004[b]	62.20[b]	35.25[c]
Enteromorpha spp.	79.12[b]	58.27[a]	21.87[ab]	0.044[a]	80.14[ab]	67.37[a]
OMD[8]						
Ulva spp.	74.28[a]	34.80[b]	55.09[a]	0.020[ab]	89.89[a]	47.86[b]
Chaetomorpha spp.	47.39[c]	32.69[a]	20.18[b]	0.022[a]	52.88[ab]	37.66[b]
Sargassum spp.	24.62[d]	16.86[c]	63.13[ab]	0.019[b]	79.99[b]	19.24[c]
Enteromorpha spp.	69.88[b]	34.79[a]	37.17[ab]	0.042[a]	71.96[ab]	49.48[a]

Notes
[1] = 72 hours rumen degradation, [2] = rapid soluble component (%), [3] = insoluble but potentially degradable material (%), [4] = constants rate degradation ($\%.h^{-1}$), [5] = potential degradability (%), [6] = effective degradability (%), [7] = dry matter degradation, [8] = organic matter degradation
[a,b,c,d] Different lowercase letters within columns showed differences between mean

4 CONCLUSION

It was concluded that the macroalga being collected have different chemical compositions and different degradation characterization in the rumen.

ACKNOWLEDGMENT

The authors are grateful to the Research Organization for Life Sciences and Environment, the National Research and Innovation (BRIN), for funding the research through Research Program (DIPA Rumah Program 2022).

REFERENCES

Anzueta-Q. S., Isabel C.M.B., Juan S.R.N., Idupulapati R., Ngonidzashe C., Rolando B.R., Jon M. and Jacobo A. (2021). Nutritional Evaluation of Tropical Forage Grass Alone and Grass-Legume Diets to Reduce in vitro Methane Production. *Frontiers In Sustainable Food System*, 5, 663003.
AOAC. (1990). *Association of Official Analytical Chemistry International ed* 16th. England.
Artemisia R., Erna P.S., Ronny M. and Akhmad K.N. (2019). The Properties of Brown Marine Algae *Sargassum turbinarioides* and *Sargassum ilicifolium* Collected From Yogyakarta, Indonesia *Indonesian Journal of Pharmacy*, 30, 1, 43–51.
Beetul K., Gopeechund A., Kaullysing D., Mattan-Moorgawa S., Puchooa D. and Bhagooli R. (2016). *Challenges and Opportunities in the Present era of Marine Algal Applications; Algae-Organisms for Imminent Biotechnology*; Thajuddin N., Dhanasekaran D., Eds.
Chen X.B. (1997). *Neway-Excel Microsoft Office: A Utility for Processing Data of Feed Degradability and In Vitro Gas Production*. England: Rowett Research Institute.
El Gamal A.A. (2010). Biological Importance of Marine Algae. *Saudi Pharmaceutical Journal*, 18(1), 1–25.
Elisa S.Z., Dalia G.L. and German P.D. (2002). *Gross Chemical Composition of Three Common Macroalgae and a Sea Grass on the Pacific Coast of Baja California*, Mexico.
Gülzari Ş.Ö., Lind V., Aasen I.M. & Steinshamn H. (2019). Effect of Supplementing Sheep Diets with Macroalgae Species on in Vivo Nutrient Digestibility, Rumen Fermentation and Blood Amino Acid Profile. *Animal*, 13(12), 2792–2801.

Harrysson H., Krook J.L., Larsson K., Tullberg C., Oerbekke A., Toth G. and Undeland I. (2021). Effect of Storage Conditions on Lipid Oxidation, Nutrient Loss and Colour of Dried Seaweeds, Porphyra Umbilicalis and Ulva Fenestrata, Subjected to Different Pretreatments. *Algal Research*, 56, 102295.

Ibrahim M.N.M. (1988). *Feeding Tables for Ruminants in Sri Lanka*. Animal Feed Advisory Committee Veterinary Research Institute.

Meng W., Mu T., Sun H. and Garcia-Vaquero M. (2022). Evaluation of the Chemical Composition and Nutritional Potential of Brown Macroalgae Commercialised in China. *Algal Research*, 64, 102683.

Ørskov E.R. and McDonald I. (1979). The Estimation of Protein Degradability in the Rumen from Incubation Measurements Weighted According to Rate of Passage. *The Journal of Agricultural Science*, 92 (2), 499–503.

Roque B.M., Brooke C.G., Ladau J., Polley T., Marsh L.J., Najafi N., and Hess M. (2019). Effect of the Macroalgae Asparagopsis Taxiformis on Methane Production and Rumen Microbiome Assemblage. *Animal Microbiome*, 1(1), 1–14.

Serviere-Zaragoza E., Gómez-López D. and Ponce-Díaz G. (2002). Gross Chemical Composition of Three Common Macroalgae and a Sea Grass on the Pacific Coast of Baja California, Mexico. *Hidrobiológica*, 12 (2), 113–118.

Yende S.R., Harle U.N. and Chaugule B.B. (2014). Therapeutic Potential and Health Benefits of Sargassum Species. *Pharmacognosy Reviews*, 8(15), 1.

Zainuddin E.N., Hilal A., Huyyirnah H., Ridha H. and Dolores V.B. (2019) Antibacterial Activity of Caulerpa Racemosa Against Pathogenic Bacteria Promoting Bice-ice Disease in the Red Alga Gracilaria Verrucosa. *Journal of Applied Phycology*, 31, 3201–3212.

Developing Modern Livestock Production in Tropical Countries – Adli et al. (eds)
© 2023 The Authors, ISBN 978-1-032-44025-5
Open Access: www.taylorfrancis.com, CC BY-NC-ND 4.0 license

Association of growth hormone gene polymorphisms with growth traits in texel crossbreed

F.E. Wahyudi, T.E. Susilorini & S. Maylinda
Faculty of Animal Science, Brawijaya University, Malang, East Java, Indonesia

ABSTRACT: The association of growth hormone (GH) gene polymorphisms with growth traits such as body weight (BW), chest girth (CG), body length (BL), and body height (BH) in TC (TC) sheep has an important role in the genetic marker-based selection program (MAS). The study aimed to examine the association of GH genes with the growth traits of TC sheep. The material used is 42 ewes. The research method is a survey. The length GH gene is 661 bp. DNA fragments were amplified, and the genotype was identified using the PCR-RFLP. The results showed that SNP was found at position c.573 G>A. The Hardy–Weinberg equilibrium shows that the population is in balance. The genotype frequencies of AA, AG, and GG were 0.24; 0.55; and 0.21. The frequencies of the A and G alleles were 0.51 and 0.49. There was an association between the genetic diversity of the GH gene and growth traits (p<0.01).

Keywords: TC sheep, Growth Hormone gene, SNP, and Growth Traits

1 INTRODUCTION

The Texel Crossbreed (TC) sheep is a result of a cross between a Texel male sheep from the Netherlands and a local ewe. The advantages of TC sheep are higher productivity and performance than local sheep, high-quality muscle and meat, and low-fat meat. Improving genetic quality is needed to produce superior and high genetic-quality seeds. One of the efforts to improve the genetic quality of livestock is through selection. Selection based on genetic markers has seeds by producing high genetic quality quickly and accurately.

Polymorphism is a genetic variation that occurs at a gene locus, and more than one allele occupies the gene locus in a population. Genetic variation is caused by changes in a nucleotide in the genome caused by mutation, relative or random marriage, migration, and selection. One gene with a high genetic polymorphism is the GH gene. The GH gene is the primary gene that controls the nature of growth, muscle and bone growth, and protein synthesis. Research by Malewa *et al.* (2014) regarding the analysis of GH gene polymorphisms in fat-tailed sheep using PCR-RFLP with the HaeIII enzyme showed polymorphic results due to the AG (AG-CC) to (GG-CC) transition mutation in exon 3. The influence of genetic diversity on the GH gene locus with growth traits such as BW, CG, BL, and BH is expected to be the basis for selection based on genetic markers to produce superior seeds.

2 MATERIAL AND METHODS

The research material used was 40 TC ewe (1-1,5 years) obtained from Agrilestari Farms, Malang, East Java. The method used in this research is observation, and the sample was

DOI: 10.1201/9781003370048-24
This chapter has been made available under a CC BY NC ND license

conducted by purposive sampling. Took blood of ewe from much as 5 mL using a vacutainer, especially in the jugular vein. The variables observed were BW, CG, BL, and BH. The data obtained were then analyzed using analysis of allele and genotype frequencies, heterozygosity and Hardy-Weinberg equilibrium, and associations GH gene genotypes, polymorphisms of GH gene with growth traits of TC analyzed using ANOVA. The frequency of genotypes and alleles can be calculated based on the formula (Nei & Kumar 2000):

$$\text{Genotype frequency}: x_{ii} = \frac{n_{ii}}{N}; \ \text{Allele frequency}: x_i = \frac{2n_{ii} + \sum_{i \neq j} n_{ij}}{2N}$$

3 RESULT AND DISCUSSION

Genetic diversity is indicated by the variation of all alleles and genotypes at a locus. Identification of allele and genotype frequencies aims to determine a population's genetic diversity level. The results of the calculation of the allele frequency and the genotype frequency of the growth hormone (GH) gene can be seen in Table 1.

Table 1. Allele frequency and genotype of TC Sheep.

Genotype Frequency			Allele Frequency	
AA(10)	AG(23)	GG(9)	A	G
0,25	0,58	0,18	0,54	0,46

Based on the results of the study, it was shown that the frequency of the AG genotype was higher than that of the AA and GG genotypes. The frequency of the A allele was higher than that of the G allele. This was due to the selection process, arrangement, and random mating. Gene frequency is influenced by selection, gene mutation, mixing two populations with different gene frequencies, inbreeding, outbreeding, and genetic drift. El-Hanafy et al. (2010) showed that the frequency of the AB genotype was higher than the AA and BB genotypes in Barki goats and Damascus goat crosses with Barki, while the frequency of the A allele was higher than that of the B allele. Polymorphic results can be used for markers of genetic variation within a population and to estimate the level of the kinship of livestock in the population.

The study results showed that the GH gene polymorphism significantly affected body weight, chest girth, body length, and height in Texel crossbred sheep ($p < 0.01$) (Table 2). This is because the GH gene is essential in controlling growth and body metabolism, which can

Table 2. Association polymorphisms of GH gene on growth traits of TC.

Parameter	Genotipe		
	AA (10)	AG (23)	GG (7)
Body Weight (kg)	33,98 ± 2,67[c]	26,27 ± 4,26[b]	17,27 ± 1,72[a]
Chest Girth (cm)	74,60 ± 3,34[b]	68,76 ± 5,61[a]	57,86 ± 5,39[a]
Body Lenght (cm)	59,16 ± 5,69[b]	54,20 ± 4,49[ab]	49,14 ± 2,98[a]
Body Height (cm)	61,75 ± 6,03[b]	57,44 ± 6,32[ab]	51,21 ± 2,68[a]

Notes: [a,b,c] Different superskips on the same line show significant differences ($p < 0.01$).

increase sheep's body weight and linear body measurements. This is comparable to the research of Susilorini *et al.* (2017) that the variation of the GH gene genotype has a very significant effect on body weight at birth, body weight at 100 days of age, and body weight gain. It was added by Depison *et al.* (2017) which state that the restricted GH gene with the MspI enzyme significantly affects body weight, weight gain, chest girth, and body length. Hua *et al.* (2009) stated that the presence of SNPs in the GH gene causes various growth effects. The AA genotype had the best average body weight, chest girth, body length, and body height compared to the AG and GG genotypes because there was a dominant A allele that affected livestock growth so that cattle with the A allele had higher growth than the G allele. Agung *et al.* (2017) stated that alleles and genotypes of the GH gene affect livestock productivity and growth.

4 CONCLUSION

Polymorphisms of the GH gene are associated with growth traits of TC sheep in Agri Lestari Dairy Farm, Pujon District, Malang Regency, East Java. Thus, the GH gene can be used as a genetic marker for selection by the MAS method on the growth traits of TC sheep.

REFERENCES

Agung P.P., S. Anwar, W.P.B. Putra and dan Said S. (2017). Keragaman gen *Growth Hormone* (GH) pada beberapa rumpun sapi lokal Indonesia. *Biodiversitas.* 3(3), 304–308.

Allendoft F.W., Luikar G. and Aitken S.N. (2013). *Conservation and the Genetics of Population.* 2nd ed. UK: Wiley-Blackwell.

Depison, Anwar S., Jamsari, Arnim and Yurnalis. (2017). Association of Growth Hormone Gene Polymorphism with Quantitative Characteristics of Thin-tailed Sheep using PCR-RFLP in Jambi Province. *African Journal of Biotechnology.* 16(20), 1159–1167.

El-Hanafy A.A., El-Saadani M.A., Eissa M., Maharem G.M. and Khalifa Z.A. (2010). Polymorphism of β-lacto Globulin Gene in Barki and Damascus and their Cross Bred Goats in Relation to Milk Yield. *Biotechnology in Animal Husbandry.* 26(1), 1–12.

Hua G.H. Chen S.L. Yu J.N. Cai K.L. Wu C.J., Li Q.L., Geng L.Y. Shen Z. Xu D.Q. and Yang L.G.. (2009). Polymorphism of the Growth Hormone Gene and its Association with Growth Traits in Boer Goat Bucks. *Journal Meat Science,* 81, 391–395.

Malewa A.D., Hakim L. Maylinda S. and Husain M.H. (2014). Growth Hormone Gene Polymorphisms of Indonesia Fat Tailed Sheep using PCR-RFLP and their Relationship with Growth Traits. *Livestock Research for Rural Development,* 26(6), 115–121.

Nei M. and Kumar S. (2000). *Molecular Evolution and Phylogenetics.* New York (USA): Oxford University Press.

Susilorini T.E., Kuswati and Maylinda S. (2017). Polymorphism of Growth Hormone Gene in Selecting Etawah Crossbred (PE) Goats. *Research Journal of Life Science.* 4(2), 153–158.

Developing Modern Livestock Production in Tropical Countries – Adli et al. (eds)

Effect of feeding with different energy levels on intestinal characteristics of crossbreed chicken

S.P. Lestari, M.H. Natsir, O. Sjofjan & Y.F. Nuningtyas
Faculty of Animal Science, Universitas Brawijaya, Malang, East Java, Indonesia

ABSTRACT: This study aimed to determine the effect of feeding with different energy levels on the gut characteristics of villous number, length, and crypt depth of crossbreed chickens. The experiment was conducted in vivo with 162 DOC crossbreed chickens and was maintained for 60 days, 3 treatments with 6 replications. The results showed a significant effect ($P<0.05$) on the villous number average number of villi produced by a treatment E2 (2800 Kcal/kg for the starter and 2950 Kcal/kg for the finisher), which was 58.17 and no significant effect ($P>0.05$) on the villi length of 468.78, and crypt depth was E3 (2900 Kcal/kg for the starter and 3100 Kcal/kg for the finisher), which is equal to 145. Based on the study results, it can be concluded that feeding with different energy levels showed the best results in the average number of villi in intestinal characteristics of crossbreed chicken

Keywords: Crossbreed chicken, ileum villous number, length, and crypt depth

1 INTRODUCTION

The amount of genetically modified foods was increasing in the last 10 years (Siddiqui *et al.* 2022a). A lot of research has been undertaken to seek alternatives to food. One potential that can act as non-genetically modified food were chickens (Siddiqui *et al.* 2022b). Local chickens are raised under an extensive traditional system, where they are free to scavenge forage around. Almost all local chicken breeds are very low in production and reproduction. The growth is relatively slow compared to cross-breed chickens, such as broilers, and has low feed efficiency. Jowo super chicken is a cross between a Bangkok male chicken with a Lohman hen. Free-range chicken is a group of native chickens that have been domesticated and traditionally reared by the general public. Free-range chicken has several advantages, such as having nutritional value, delicious taste, and more disease resistance. Anggraini *et al.* (2019) stated that the superiority possessed by super native chickens is the ability to adapt well to environmental conditions. Feed plays an essential role because it functions for basic life, growth, production, and reproduction. The feed ingredients used must contain sufficient nutrients according to needs and be in a balanced state. If one of these nutrients is lacking, it can cause disturbances in the body of livestock and can reduce productivity. Digestive tract health and nutrition are closely related to each other. Utilization of feed nutrients can only be achieved optimally if the digestive tract is in good health. Intestinal characteristics can be used as an indicator of livestock health where the increase in villi length and crypt depth indicates that an animal has a good health status. The intestine is one of the organs that has an important role in the digestive tract, especially the small intestine, which functions to absorb feed nutrients. Intestinal characteristics are related to the production performance of an animal, whereas good gut characteristics will produce livestock with good production performance as well. Based on this description, this study focuses on the effect of feeding with different energy levels on gut characteristics in crossbreed chickens.

DOI: 10.1201/9781003370048-25

2 MATERIAL AND METHODS

A total of 162 DOC (i.e., day-old chick) non-sexing crossbreed chickens (gender undifferentiated) were used. The chicken was maintained for 60 days and applied to 3 treatments with 6 replications each, with each replication consisting of 9 crossbreed chickens. The cage used in the study used an open house type cage with litter in the form of rice husks replaced every 2 weeks. The cages were made into 30 plots composed of bamboo and wire, equipped with a hygro thermometer, and maintained over 21 days during the brooding period. Each cage plot measures 1 m × 1 m × 2 m and is equipped with one feeder and a chicken drinker. Drink given in the form of clean water was added with vitamins for the first 21 days with a frequency of 2 times a day, in the morning and afternoon. Feed and water are provided ad libitum. The method used in this study was an experiment with a completely randomized design (CRD), three treatments with eight replications (3x6).

Research treatments (Table 1):

E1 = Metabolic Energy 2700 Kcal/kg for the starter and 2800 Kcal/kg for the finisher.
E2 = Metabolic Energy 2800 Kcal/kg for the starter and 2950 Kcal/kg for the finisher.
E3 = Metabolic Energy 2900 Kcal/kg for the starter and 3100 Kcal/kg for the finisher.

Table 1. Feed formulation and nutrition content for the starter phase.

Ingredients	Starter Phase (%)		
	Treatment E1	Treatment E2	Treatment E3
Rice Bran	18.19	9.91	6.22
Soybean meal	18.26	16.19	16.28
Yellow corn	32	37	40
Corn DDGS	5	10	10
Fish flour	10	10	10
Copra meal	5	5	5
Broiler Concentrate	10	10	10
Coconut oil	0.18	0.55	1.48
Salt	0.21	0.21	0.21
Premix	0.98	0.98	0.66
Nutrient content			
PK (%)[1]	22.94	22.79	23.56
BK (%)[1]	88.6	86.8	88.33
KA (%)[1]	11.4	13.2	11.67
LK (%)[1]	5.04	4.01	5.74
SK (%)[1]	6.87	8.82	7.46
Ca (%)[1]	1.71	1.77	1.38
P (%)[1]	0.96%	0.86	0.85
ME (kcal/kg)[1]	2,466	2,246	2,446

3 DATA ANALYSIS

Prior to statistical analysis, data were analyzed using analysis of variance (ANOVA). The results were presented as standard error mean (SEM). Moreover, probability values were

Table 2. Feed formulation and nutrition content for the finisher phase.

Ingredients	Finisher Phase (%)		
	Treatment E1	Treatment E2	Treatment E3
Rice bran	14.69	6.45	0.43
Soybean meal	10.31	10.46	10.57
Yellow corn	38	45	50
Corn DDGS	10	10	10
Fish flour	10	10	10
Copra meal	5	5	5
Concentrate broiler	10	10	10
Coconut oil	0.44	1.56	2.89
Salt	0.1	0.1	0.11
Premix	1.46	1.44	1
Nutrient content			
PK^2 $(\%)^2$	22.62	21.48	21.91
BK^2 $(\%)^2$	90.88	91.21	91.40
KA^2 $(\%)^2$	4.91	5.00	4.59
LK^2 $(\%)^2$	6.03	6.43	7.04
SK^2 $(\%)^2$	6.55	5.11	4.81
ME $(kcal/kg)^3$	2,431	2,651	2,736

Sources: [1]The results of proximate analysis of feed at the Laboratory of Animal Science and Fisheries Laboratory, Blitar; [2]The results of a comparative study of feed at the Laboratory of Nutrition and Animal Feed Science, Faculty of Animal Science, Universitas Brawijaya, Malang; [3]The results of proximate analysis of feed at the Central Laboratory of the University of Muhammadiyah Malang, Malang. Sampling was carried out on the 60th day by cutting 1 chicken from each experimental unit. Before slaughtering, the chicken is weighed first. After the chicken was cut, the small intestine villi were taken by cutting 3 cm from the ileocecal junction to the ileum for disposal, then cutting 4 cm long and removing the digest by flushing using a syringe containing a physiological NaCl solution slowly. The clean intestine sample was then put into a film pot containing 10% formalin solution to make preparations. The number of villi, villi length, and crypt depth were observed in the laboratory.

calculated using the least significant different testing. The following model was used:

$$Yij = \mu + Ti + eij$$

where Yij was the parameters observed, μ was the overall mean, Ti was the effect level of liquid smoke encapsulation, and eij was the amount of error number (Ardiansyah *et al.* 2022; Adli *et al.* 2022).

4 RESULT AND DISCUSSION

4.1 *Effect of feeding with different energy levels on the number of villi of crossed chickens*

Table 3 shows the average number of villi of the small intestine in the ileum in broilers fed with different energy levels. The results of statistical analysis showed a significant difference (P > 0.05) in the number of villi of the small intestine in cross-breed chickens. Feeding resulted in an average number of villi in the ileum as much as 52.17 ± 8.33 in treatment E1, E2 showed an average of 58.17 ± 5.18, and treatment E3 produced an average of

Table 3. Data analysis results in the effect of feeding with different energy levels on the characteristics of crossbred chickens.

Treatments	Villous Number	Villous Length (μm)	Crypt Depth (μm)
E1	52.17 ± 8.33^{ab}	451.73 ± 83.12	121.33 ± 36.81
E2	58.17 ± 5.18^{ab}	462.68 ± 61.67	142.68 ± 46.37
E3	48.33 ± 2.40^{a}	468.78 ± 21.07	145.73 ± 41.48

48.33 ± 2.40. Villi play a role in the process of absorption of feed nutrients. Apriliyani et al (2016) stated that the villi are part of the mucous membrane. Table 3 shows the results of the average length of the villi of the small intestine in cross-bred chickens fed with feed with different energy levels, which showed no significant difference ($P>0.05$) in the length of the villi of the small intestine in cross-breed. The highest mean value was indicated by treatment E3 with an average value of 468.78 ± 21.07, followed by treatment E2 with 462.68 ± 61.67 and E1 with an average value of 451.73 ± 83.12. Small intestinal conditions such as villi height in the small intestine represent areas for wider nutrient absorption. An increase in villous height and villi width is associated with a wider villous surface for the absorption of nutrients into the bloodstream (Jamilah & Mahfudz 2014). Table 3 shows the average small intestine crypt depth results in cross-breed chickens fed with different energy levels. Based on the statistical analysis results, no significant difference ($P> 0.05$) was observed in the depth of crypts of the small intestine of a Bangkok male cross-breeding chicken with a Lohman hen. The highest mean value of cryptography was indicated by treatment E3 with a value of 145.73 ± 41.48, E2 with an average value of 142.68 ± 46.37, and the lowest value was indicated by treatment E1 with a value of 121.33 ± 36.81 (Figure 1). Crypt is considered a villous-forming factory. The deeper the crypt, the faster the tissue turnover that allows the renewal of damaged or inflamed small intestinal villi due to the presence of pathogenic bacteria or some anti-nutrients inhibit (Allahdo *et al.* 2018).

 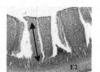

Figure 1. Intestinal histopathology of crossbreeds fed with different energy levels.

5 CONCLUSION

To sum up, feeding with different energy levels showed the best average number of villi in the E2 treatment with metabolic energy of 2800 Kcal/kg for the starter and 2950 Kcal/kg for the finisher. Villi length and crypt depth in treatment E3 with metabolic energy of 2900 Kcal/kg for the starter and 3100 Kcal/kg for the finisher (E3).

REFERENCES

Allahdo P., Ghodraty J., Zarghi H., Saadatfar Z., Kermanshahi H. and Dovom M.R.E. (2018). Effect of Probiotic and Vinegar on Growth Performance, Meat Yields, Immune Responses, and Small Intestine Morphology of Broiler Chickens. *Italian Journal of Animal Science*, 17(3), 675–685.
Adli D.N., Sjofjan O., Irawan A., Utama D.T., Sholikin M.M., Nurdianti R.R. Nurfitriani R.A., Hidayat C., Jayanegara A. and Sadarman S. (2022). Effects of Fibre-rich Ingredient Levels on Goose Growth

Performance, Blood Profile, Foie Gras Quality and its Fatty Acid Profile: A Meta-analysis. *Journal of Animal and Feed Sciences*, 31(4), 301–309.

Anggraini A.D., Widodo W., Rahayu I.D. and Sutanto A. (2019). Effectivity of Adding Javanese Tumeric Powder in Feed to Increase Productivity of Super Native Chicken. 14(2), 222–227.

Apriliyani N.I., Djaelani M.A., dan Tana S. (2016). Profil Histologi Duodenum Berbagai Itik Lokal di Kabupaten Semarang. *Bioma*, 18(2), 144–150.

Ardiansyah W., Sjofjan O., Widodo E., Suyadi S. and Adli D.N. (2022). Effects of Combinations of α-Lactobacillus Sp. and Curcuma Longa Flour on Production, Egg Quality, and Intestinal Profile of Mojosari Ducks. *Adv. Anim. Vet. Sci*, 10(8), 1668–1677.

Bogusławska-Tryk M., Bogucka J., Dankowiakowska A. and Walasik K. (2020). Small Intestine Morphology and Ileal Biogenic Amines Content in Broiler Chickens Fed Diets Supplemented with Lignocellulose. *Livestock Science*, 241.

Jamilah N.S. and Mahfudz L.D. (2014). The Effect of Inclusion of Lime as Acidifier in Step-Down Feeding System on Intestinal Condition of Broiler Chickens. *JITP*, 3(2), 90–95.

Siddiqui S.A., Asif Z., Murid M., Fernando I., Adli D.N., Blinov A.V., Golik A.B., Nugraha W.S., Ibrahim S.A. and Jafari S.M. (2022a). Consumer Social and Psychological Factors Influencing the Use of Genetically Modified Foods—A Review. *Sustainability*, 14(23), 15884.

Siddiqui S.A., Alvi T., Sameen A., Khan S., Blinov A.V., Nagdalian A.A., Mehdizadeh M., Adli D.N. and Onwezen M., (2022b). Consumer Acceptance of Alternative Proteins: A Systematic Review of Current Alternative Protein Sources and Interventions Adapted to Increase Their Acceptability. *Sustainability*, 14 (22), 15370.

Developing Modern Livestock Production in Tropical Countries – Adli et al. (eds)
© 2023 The Authors, ISBN 978-1-032-44025-5
Open Access: www.taylorfrancis.com, CC BY-NC-ND 4.0 license

Semen quality in the freezing process using various diluents in Saanen goats

L. Nisfimawardah, M.N. Ihsan, T. Susilawati & S. Wahjuningsih*
Faculty of Animal Science, Universitas Brawijaya, Jl. Veteran, Malang, Indonesia

A. Firmawati
Faculty of Veterinary Medicine, Universitas Brawijaya, Jl. Puncak Dieng, Malang, Indoensia

C.D. Sulistyowati & Amalia
Singosari Center Artificial Insemination, Malang, Indonesia

ABSTRACT: The purpose of this research was to examine the quality of semen after freezing using tris aminomethane-egg yolk, AndroMed, and OviXcell as the diluents. This research was carried out in the Laboratory Singosari Center Artificial Insemination (SCAI) Malang, East Java, Indonesia. The method used in the study was an experimental laboratory with 3 treatments and 5 replications and the research design used a completely randomized design (CRD). The sample used had criteria for fresh semen from bull Saanen goats with a minimum individual motility of 70%. The treatment in this research was T0 = dilution of semen with tris aminomethane-egg yolk, T1 = dilution of semen with AndroMed, and T2 = dilution of semen with OviXcell. Then, the data obtained were analyzed using Analysis of Variance (ANOVA) with the variables used being individual motility and viability. These results showed no significant difference ($P>0.05$) in individual motility and viability. In conclusion, freezing of goat semen using tris aminomethane-egg yolk, AndroMed and OviXcell diluents had no difference in individual motility and viability.

Keywords: AndroMed, Freezing Semen, OviXcell, Saanen Goats, Tris Aminomethane-egg yolk

1 INTRODUCTION

The livestock industry in Indonesia continues to develop and improve genetic quality. Currently, various efforts to increase reproduction are continuously being carried out and are very advanced. Several reproductive technologies are applied in Indonesia, namely Artificial Insemination (AI) to accelerate livestock productivity. The population of goats in East Java in 2021 is 3.763 million/head. Saanen goats have advantages such as dairy goats producing milk with milk fat reaching 2.5% to 3% (BPS 2021). Artificial Insemination (AI) is a reproductive biotechnology that is carried out by artificial mating using an insemination gun which is inseminated into the rectum to reach the cervix. AI is widely applied to large ruminants, especially cattle, and is still minimally applied to small ruminants. This is influenced by the goals of AI and small ruminant breeders which are not as much as large ruminants (Inounu 2014). Factors that influence the success of AI are semen quality, estrus detection, inseminator technique, and knowledge. The success of AI on semen quality is

---

*Corresponding Author: yuning@ub.ac.id

DOI: 10.1201/9781003370048-26

carried out by conducting a semen quality test. The semen quality test consisted of macroscopic and microscopic tests. A macroscopic test is an evaluation of fresh semen including volume, pH, color, and consistency. The microscopic test is an evaluation that cannot be seen with the naked eye and requires special tools including motility, viability, abnormality, and concentration. Motility is needed to keep spermatozoa alive until they meet oocytes in the female reproductive organs, and undergo capacitation until fertilization occurs into oocytes (Setiyono et al. 2020).

Artificial insemination can be applied to several types of semen including fresh, liquid, and frozen semen using motility, viability, and abnormality parameters. Each semen has weaknesses such as fresh semen does not last long and must be ejaculated immediately, and liquid semen only lasts two to four days at a storage temperature of 4–5°C. Liquid semen cannot be stored for a long time so the quality of liquid semen at the time of storage can be observed based on motility, viability, and membrane integrity (Ratnawati et al. 2017). AI biotechnology is carried out by selecting bulls, semen collection, liquid semen, and frozen semen to evaluate the semen quality. The quality of semen is determined by the type of diluent used consisting of tris aminomethane-egg yolk, AndroMed, and OviXcell. The diluent used must have properties as a nutrient or a source of energy and good preservation of semen viability. Semen dilution was carried out to obtain more semen before insemination and to maintain the quality of the processed semen before freezing (Effendi et al. 2015). In addition, the semen collection technique can determine the quality of fresh semen because it serves as a post-storage place before the process is carried out until the semen is liquid and frozen. The criteria for a good diluent are able to prevent cold shock during cooling so that it reaches the freezing stage if the semen quality is good. Therefore, this study was conducted to determine the quality of Saanen goat's semen with the use of tris aminomethane-egg yolk diluent, AndroMed, and OviXcell.

2 MATERIALS AND METHODS

The research material used was the fresh semen of Saanen goats at Singosari Center Artificial Insemination (SCAI) Malang, East Java, Indonesia. Shelters were carried out once a week using an artificial vagina with 5 shelters during the study. Semen that will be used as research has requirements with minimum individual motility of 70%. Semen was diluted using tris aminomethane-egg yolk, AndroMed (Minitub, Germany), and OviXcell (IMV technologies, France). Fresh semen was tested macroscopically including volume, pH, color, and consistency. Microscopic tests include individual motility and viability in fresh semen, liquid semen, and frozen semen. The study used a laboratory experimental method with 3 treatments with 5 replications and a laboratory experiment using a Completely Randomized Design (CRD). The research design used a completely randomized design (CRD) with 3 treatments and 5 replications. Data analysis used Analysis of Variance (ANOVA) using Microsoft Excel.

3 RESULT AND DISCUSSION

3.1 *Sperm motility*

Motility is the movement or locomotion of spermatozoa which is used as a parameter of semen quality in AI. Success in AI is influenced by the motility of spermatozoa. The progressive motility of fresh semen produced in Saanen goats at the age of 2, 3, and 6 was 67.96%, 69.44%, and 62.70%, respectively (Fitriana et al. 2021). The motility obtained by using various diluents, namely tris aminomethane-egg yolk (T0), AndroMed (T1), and OviXcell (T2) can be seen in Table 1.

Table 1. Sperm motility before freezing and post-thawing motility in various diluents.

Semen Quality	Motility (%)		
	T0	T1	T2
Before Freezing	53 ± 4.5	56 ± 7.4	60 ± 0.0
Post Thawing Motilty	42 ± 4.5	39 ± 2.2	40 ± 0.0

Based on the results, Table 1 shows a decrease in motility values from before-freezing to post-thawing motility. The decrease in motility is caused by the dilution process when liquid semen is processed into frozen semen so that there is a drastic change in temperature from 4–5°C to −196°C. In addition, the decrease in motility was caused by the temperature adaptation process of 37°C to 5°C. The adaptation phase of spermatozoa occurs at the time of equilibration in cold conditions or environments at a temperature of 4–5°C for 2–3 hours. The results of the analysis on individual motility between treatments showed that the effect was not significantly different (T>0.05). The best motility of liquid semen at T2 using OviXcellsemen diluent, in this case, is because OviXcell contains soy lecithin and it has a phospholipid and glycoprotein composition that functions as a cryoprotectant in the cryo-preservation process of semen (Fernandes et al. 2021). At T0 before freezing, 53 ± 4.5% decreased due to spermatozoa using tris aminomethane-egg yolk diluent experiencing cold shock and oxidative stress in tris aminomethane-egg yolk diluent. On the quality of semen during post-thawing motility, the best results were obtained by T0 with a value of 42 ± 4.5% because the tris aminomethane-egg yolk diluent contains egg yolk functions as a cryopro-tectant or prevents cold shock in spermatozoa and contains raffinose as an energy source and prevents lethal effects of freezing.

3.2 Sperm viability

Viability is the survival of spermatozoa to determine the percentage of live and dead sper-matozoa on freezing of Saanen goat semen. Viability can be observed by dripping the dye eosin-nigrosin on the semen and then making a review. The marking of live and dead sper-matozoa was indicated by the percentage of color absorption and not color absorption. If the spermatozoa are alive, it does not absorb color, and if it absorbs color, it is marked with dead spermatozoa. The following is the percentage of viability obtained using various dilu-ents, namely tris aminomethane-egg yolk (T0), AndroMed (T1), and OviXcell (T2) can be seen in Table 2.

Based on Table 2, the results of the spermatozoa viability analysis showed that the results obtained using various diluents were not significantly different (T>0.05). In Table 2, it can be seen that the highest viability percentage was obtained by T2 at 82.10 ± 12.50% before freezing and 73.27 ± 20.69% by T0 at post-thawing motility. The use of OviXcell diluent at

Table 2. Sperm Viability before freezing and post-thawing motility in various diluents.

Semen Quality	Viability (%)		
	T0	T1	T2
Before Freezing	56.80 ± 25.16	81.51 ± 14.62	82.10 ± 12.50
Post-thawing Motilty	73.27 ± 20,69	58.53 ± 4.70	53.90 ± 18.22

T2 affects the survival of spermatozoa when the semen is liquid because lecithin soya contained in OviXcell diluent functions as an extracellular cyoprotectant, as well as egg yolk, substitute to prevent cold shock (Falchi et al. 2018). Meanwhile, during post-thawing the best motility was obtained by tris aminomethane-egg yolk because in the composition of tris aminomethane raffinose was added which functions as an energy source and prevents lethal effects in freezing.

4 CONCLUSION

The results of semen quality at the best motility before freezing at T2 were $60 \pm 0.0\%$ and viability at T2 was $82.10 \pm 12.50\%$. While the results of semen quality at the best motility at the time of post-thawing motility at T0 of $42 \pm 4.5\%$ and viability at T0 of $73.27 \pm 20.69\%$. Based on the results of research frozen semen at the time post-thawing motility, tris aminomethane-egg yolk, and OviXcell diluents are good for the frozen semen process.

ACKNOWLEDGMENT

We thank Faculty Animal Science Universitas Brawijaya for the research granted under the scheme "Hibah Guru Besar" in Community Fund DPA (Dokumen Pelaksanaan Anggaran) Universities with Legal Entity (PTNBH) Universitas Brawijaya with contract No. DPA-FPt-251101/2022-1, for funding this research. Singosari Artificial Insemination Center (SCAI) has provided facilities at the time of research and contribution with the Faculty of Animal Science Universitas Brawijaya.

REFERENCES

BPS. (2021). *Statistik Peternakan dan Kesehatan Hewan 2021*. Direktorat Jenderal Peternakan dan Kesehatan Hewan: Jakarta.

Effendi F.I., Wahjuningsih S., and Ihsan M.N. (2015). Pengaruh Pengencer Tris Aminomethane Kuning Telur Yang Disuplementasi Sari Kulit Manggis (Garcinia Mangostana) Terhadap Kualitas Semen Sapi Limousin Selama Penyimpanan Suhu Dingin 50C. *Jurnal Ilmu-Ilmu Peternakan (Indonesian Journal of Animal Science)*, 25(3), 69–79.

Falchi L., Galleri G., Zedda M.T., Pau S., Bogliolo L., Ariu F., and Ledda S. (2018). Liquid Storage of Ram Semen for 96 h: Effects on Kinematic Parameters, Membranes and DNA Integrity, and ROS Production. *Livestock Science*, 207, 1–6.

Fernandes M., Hernández P.R., Simões J., and Barbas J.P. (2021). Effects of Three Semen Extenders, Breeding Season Month and Freezing–Thawing Cycle on Spermatozoa Preservation of Portuguese Merino Sheep. *Animals*, 11(9), 2619.

Fitriana D., Sumarton and Susilowati S. (2021). Analysis of The Effect of Age on the Quality of Fresh Semen of Saanen Buck. *Jurnal Dinamika Rekasatwa*, 4 (2), 217–223.

Inounu I. (2014). Upaya Meningkatkan Keberhasilan Inseminasi Buatan Pada Ternak Ruminansia Kecil. *Wartazoa*, 24(4), 201–209.

Ratnawati D., Isnaini N., and Susilawati T. (2017). Pemanfaatan Casa Dalam Observasi Motilitas Spermatozoa Semen Cair Sapi Madura Dalam Pengencer Berbeda. *Jurnal Ilmu-Ilmu Peternakan Universitas Brawijaya*, 27(1), 80–95.

Setiyono A., Setiadi M.A., Kaiin E.M., and Karja N.W.K. (2020). Movement Pattern of Bull Sperm Following Incubation in Fertilization Media Supplemented with Heparin and/or Caffeine. *Jurnal Veteriner*, 21(3), 458–469.

Susilawati T. (2011). *Spermatologi*. Indonesia: Universitas Brawijaya Press.

Developing Modern Livestock Production in Tropical Countries – Adli et al. (eds)
© 2023 The Authors, ISBN 978-1-032-44025-5
Open Access: www.taylorfrancis.com, CC BY-NC-ND 4.0 license

Using ensiling coffee skin on growth performance in early periods of sheep

A. Amam*, M.W. Jadmiko & P.A. Harsita
Department of Animal Science, Universitas Jember, East Java, Indonesia

O. Sjofjan & D.N. Adli
Faculty of Animal Science, Universitas Brawijaya, Malang, Indonesia

ABSTRACT: This research was conducted to determine the effect of using ensiling coffee skin on growth performance in early periods of Sheep. A total of 40 heads of crossbreed sheep were used in this study. A randomized block design with five treatments and four replications, each replication consisted two sheep, was employed. The treatment used as follows: T0: 60% commercial feeds and 40% kale straw; T1: 60% commercial feed, 30% kale straw, 10% pollard, and 0.2% ensiling coffee skin; T2: 60% commercial feed, 30% kale straw, 10% pollard, and 0.4% ensiling coffee skin; T3: 60% commercial feed, 30% kale straw, 10% pollard, and 0.6% ensiling coffee skin; and T4: 60% commercial feed, 30% kale straw, 10% pollard, and 0.8% ensiling coffee skin (Table 1). The parameters observed in the early periods stage were growth performance (initial body weight, body weight gain, final body weight, and feed intake). The results were analyzed via one-way ANOVA and if a significant effect was identified, least significant difference (LSD) testing was then applied. The effect of treatment on growth performance and feed conversion did not differ significantly ($p > 0.05$). Since it was early periods, the use of ensiling coffee skin on growth performance in early periods of sheep was continuously investigated.

Keywords: Coffee skin, ensiling, fermented, growth performance, Saccharomyces cerevisiae

1   INTRODUCTION

Sheep can be a source of protein in Indonesia. In 2022, the national production of sheep reached 17 million heads. With this condition, there is a potential for sheep local farmers in Indonesia. However, the sheep local farmers face several problems including feed management. Local farmers still use cut-carry systems in order to fulfill forage intake for sheep. One method that can be implemented is ensiling, since it was low-cost and easy for implementing (Sadarman et al. 2022). Ensiling was the most favorable technique that can help to utilize the problems for local farmer sheep. This is because Indonesia is a tropical area with highly fluctuating temperatures and high humidity cause a high-stress level and discomfort. Under these conditions, there are limitations to providing water for grass areas in Indonesia. The ensiling technique is usually used for forages to make longer during the dry season (San Martin et al. 2021). Each region, including East Java, has a potential agricultural by-product. It is reported that at the end of 2022, the production reached 774.60 thousand tonnes, which is an increase of 1.62 previous from 762.70 thousand tonnes. One of the potential options that can be used is coffee skin. Coffee skin has the potential to use as an

---

*Corresponding Author: amam.faperta@unej.ac.id

DOI: 10.1201/9781003370048-27

Table 1. Feed ingredient and nutrient composition.

	DM (% fresh)	CP (%)	OM (%)	TDN (%)
Commercial feed	87.26	18.23	86.23	74.22
Kale straw	81.23	9.4	80.23	84.23
Pollard	89.22	15.23	86.24	78.25
Coffee skin	78.22	9.94	79.22	79.22
Ensiling coffee skin	81.22	12.24	80.22	84.51

alternative by-product to utilize sheep productivity (Oliveira & Franca 2015). Indonesia has a huge diversity of potential agricultural by-products (Siddiqui et al. 2022a; Sjofjan et al. 2021). It is reported that Indonesia has a huge plantation of coffee, which is can be used in integrated farming systems. Since there is a lack of information regarding the use of coffee skin as silage. This research was conducted to evaluate Ensiling Coffee Skin on growth performance in the early period of Sheep.

2 MATERIALS AND METHODS

2.1 Experimental design

A total of 40 heads of crossbreed sheep were used in this study. A randomized block design with five treatments and four replications was used. Each replication consisted of two sheep was employed after evaluating body weight. The treatment used as follows: T0: 60% commercial feeds and 40% kale straw; T1: 60% commercial feed, 30% kale straw, 10% pollard, and 0.2% ensiling coffee skin; T2: 60% commercial feed, 30% kale straw, 10% pollard, and 0.4% ensiling coffee skin; T3: 60% commercial feed, 30% kale straw, 10% pollard, and 0.6% ensiling coffee skin; and T4: 60% commercial feed, 30% kale straw, 10% pollard, and 0.8% ensiling coffee skin. The sheep were provided with *ad-libitum access* water two times differently for the time given. The preparation of the ensiling coffee was done by following Adli et al. (2020) and Sjofjan and Adli (2021). The coffee skin was sifted to separate the meal from the remaining shells after being carefully evaluated and then placed on the floor that had been coated with trash bags and sacks. Suspensions of *Saccharomyces cerevisiae* and molasses were homogenized in a blender and then added at 40 ml and 20 ml per 1 kg of coffee. The next step was to add *pollard* at 9g per kg of coffee skin. The last step was putting the coffee skin in a sack with holes to allow entry of air and storing it for 6 days at room temperature after which it was wind-dried. The parameters observed in the early periods stage were growth performance (initial body weight, body weight gain, final body weight, mortalities, and intake DM).

2.2 Data analysis

The data analysis was constructed using SAS online edition, using general linear and continued. The differences among treatment means ($p < 0.05$) were determined using the Duncan's multiple range test

$Y_{ij} = B_0 + B_1 X_{ij} + e_{ij}$ (Adli et al. 2022; Ardiansyah et al. 2022).

3 RESULTS AND DISCUSSION

Table 2 presented that using ensiling coffee was significant ($p < 0.05$). The composition of 60% commercial feed, 30% kale straw, 10% pollard, and 0.8% ensiling coffee skin reached

38.75 kg of final body weight when compared with the control (Figures 1 and 2). In contrast, using ensiling coffee were not significantly differed ($p > 0.05$) in the dry matter intake, g/day of sheep. Using ensiling coffee skin did not cause a negative effect on the skip which is presented in the low mortalities (Table 2). If compared with Palinggi et al. (2014), several microorganisms such as *A. niger, S. cerevisiae, Rhizopus sp.*, and *B. subtilis* presented a greater value of crude protein and crude fiber. The use of agro-industrial and by-products with appreciable quantities might provide opportunities to optimize livestock production (Ososanya & Olorunnisomo 2015). Moreover, the feed composition of the intake of sheep was due to the relative humidity and ambient temperature during seasonal (Rathwa et al. 2017; Siddiqui et al. 2022b).

Table 2. Using ensiling coffee skin on growth performance on the early period of sheep.

Parameters	TO	T1	T2	T3	T4	SEM
IW (Kg)	25.00	26.1	25.60	29.20	32.90	2.13
FBW (Kg)	28.70[a]	33.57[b]	34.35[c]	36.57[d]	38.75[e]	3.09
Intake DM, g/day	2.19	2.11	2.22	2.33	2.21	011
Mortalities	0.00	0.00	0.00	0.00	0.00	0.33

DM – Dry matter; IW – Initial body weight; FBW – Final body weight *different superscripts mean significant differences.

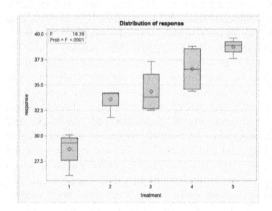

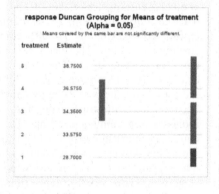

Figure 1. Distribution response of using ensiling coffee on growth performance of sheep.

Figure 2. Response of using ensiling coffee on the growth performance of sheep.

3 CONCLUSION

Since it was early periods, the use of ensiling coffee skin on growth performance in early periods of Sheep was continuously conducted. Using Ensiling Coffee Skin on growth performance in early periods of sheep was positively increasing the final body weight of sheep without any adverse effect. However, since the research was continuously conducted, the dose is dependent.

REFERENCES

Adli D.N., Sjofjan O., Irawan A., Utama D.T., Sholikin M.M., Nurdianti R.R. Nurfitriani R.A., Hidayat C., Jayanegara A., and Sadarman S. (2022). Effects of Fibre-rich Ingredient Levels on Goose Growth Performance, Blood Profile, Foie Gras Quality and its Fatty Acid Profile: A Meta-analysis. *Journal of Animal and Feed Sciences*, 31(4):301–309.

Adli D.N., Sjofjan O., Natsir M.H., Nuningtyas Y.F., Sholikah N. and Marbun A.C. (2020) The Effect of Replacing Maize with Fermented Palm Kernel Meal (FPKM) on Broiler Performance. *Livestock Research for Rural Development*, 32(7):1–4.

Ardiansyah W., Sjofjan O., Widodo E., Suyadi S., and Adli D.N. (2022). Effects of Combinations of α-Lactobacillus sp. and Curcuma Longa Flour on Production, Egg Quality, and Intestinal Profile of Mojosari Ducks. *Advances Animal Veterinary Science*, 10(8):1668–1677.

Hernández-Bautista J., Rodríguez-Magadán H.M., Villegas-Sánchez J.A., Salinas-Rios T., Ortiz-Muñoz I.Y., Aquino-Cleto M., and Lozano-Trejo S. (2018). Health Status and Productivity of Sheep Fed Coffee Pulp During Fattening. *Austral Journal of Veterinary Sciences*, 50(2): 95–99.

Oliveira L.S., and Franca A.S. (2015). An Overview of the Potential Uses for Coffee Husks. *Coffee in Health and Disease Preventi*

Ososanya T.O. and Olorunnisomo O.A. (2015). Silage Characteristics and Preference of Sheep for Wet Brewer's Grain Ensiled with Maize Cob. *Livestock Research for Rural Development*, 27(12) 283–291.

Palinggi N.N., Kamaruddin and Laining A. (2014). Improvement of Coffee Skin Quality Using Fermentation for Livestock Ingredients. *Presiding Forum Inovasi Teknologi Akuakultur*, 633–653.

Rathwa S.D., Vasava A.A., Pathan M.M., Madhira S.P., Patel Y.G. and Pande A.M. (2017). Effect of Season on Physiological, Biochemical, Hormonal, and Oxidative Stress Parameters of Indigenous Sheep. *Veterinary World*, 10(6): 650.

San Martin D., Orive M., Iñarra B., García A., Goiri I., Atxaerandio R., Urkisa Z. and Zufia J. (2021). Spent Coffee Ground as Second-generation Feedstuff for Dairy Cattle. *Biomass Conversion and Biorefinery*, 11 (2), 589–599.

Sadarman I.A., Ridla M., Jayanegara A., Nahrowi R.R., Sofyan A., Herdian H., Darma I.N.Y., Wahyono T., Febrina D., Harahap R.P., Nurfitriani R.A., and Adli D.N. (2022). Influence of Ensiling and Tannins Addition on Rumen Degradation Kinetics of Soy Sauce Residues. *Advances Animal Veterinary Science*, 10 (2), 270–276.

Sjofjan O., Adli D.N., Natsir M.H., Nuningtyas Y.F., Bastomi I., and Amalia F.R. (2021). The Effect of Increasing Levels of Palm Kernel Meal Containing A-B-Mannanase Replacing Maize to Growing-Finishing Hybrid Duck on Growth Performance, Nutrient Digestibility, Carcass Trait, and VFA. *Journal of the Indonesian Tropical Animal Agriculture*, 46(1), 29–39.

Sjofjan O. and Adli D.N. (2021) The Effect of Replacing Fish Meal with Fermented Sago Larvae (FSL) on Broiler Performance. *Livestock Research for Rural Development*, 33(7):1–8.

Siddiqui S.A., Asif Z., Murid M., Fernando I., Adli D.N., Blinov A.V., Golik A.B., Nugraha W.S., Ibrahim S.A. and Jafari S.M., (2022a). Consumer Social and Psychological Factors Influencing the Use of Genetically Modified Foods—A Review. *Sustainability*, 14(23), 15884.

Siddiqui S.A., Alvi T., Sameen A., Khan S., Blinov A.V., Nagdalian A.A., Mehdizadeh M., Adli D.N. and Onwezen M., (2022b). Consumer Acceptance of Alternative Proteins: A Systematic Review of Current Alternative Protein Sources and Interventions Adapted to Increase Their Acceptability. *Sustainability*, 14 (22), 15370.

Developing Modern Livestock Production in Tropical Countries – Adli et al. (eds)
© 2023 The Authors, ISBN 978-1-032-44025-5
Open Access: www.taylorfrancis.com, CC BY-NC-ND 4.0 license

The relationship between body weight and pregnancy rate of fat tail sheep through the introduction of Garut sheep breeds in Probolinggo district

A.R.I. Putri*, A. Budiarto, G. Ciptadi, A.A. Hemiyanti, P. Akhiroh & A.B. Zaman
Faculty of Animal Science, Brawijaya University, Malang, Indonesia

ABSTRACT: The productivity of sheep can be increased, and the genetic quality of their offspring can be improved, and thus increasing farmer profits. One form of maintenance management is to apply the method of Artificial Insemination (AI). With a combination of estrous synchronization methods, AI was performed on 30 productive fat tail sheep using frozen semen obtained from BBIB Lembang, Bandung. The purpose of this study was to determine whether a successful pregnancy rate affected the sheep's body weight. When estrus has been synchronized, most ewes are in estrus within 36–48 hours and ovulate at 60 hours. The results showed that 15 sheep showed the highest yield with body weight above 30 kg, which obtained a percentage of estrus 100% and a pregnancy rate of 80%. In comparison, 15 sheep with a body weight below 30 kilograms received an estrus percentage of 26.66%, and the rate of pregnancy was 12.33%. Based on these results, it was found that body weight in fat-tailed sheep had a very significant effect ($P>0.05$) on the success of AI. The conclusion of this study showed that the body weight of fat-tailed sheep had a significant effect on the success of artificial insemination.

Keywords: artificial insemination, body weight, introduction, pregnancy rate, sheep

1 INTRODUCTION

Forage Fat-tailed (DEG) sheep is a small ruminant that is popular in Indonesia because it is one of the sources of animal protein, so it has the potential to be developed as one of the national meat supply livestock. The high potential for the reproduction of sheep indicates that sheep contribute significantly to the supply of meat for consumption by the people of Indonesia. Besides that, sheep contributed quite a lot to increasing income and improving the economy of the community, especially in rural areas (Udo & Budisatria 2011). One of the efforts to increase the reproduction rate of fat-tailed sheep is to shorten the lambing interval. Increased production of sheep farms in Indonesia has been developed in various ways, one of them being estrus synchronization.

The implementation of natural breeding and or artificial insemination (AI) can be carried out efficiently after prostaglandin F2α treatment, and the results are obtaining offspring of the same age and being able to shorten the calving interval so that the frequency of giving birth is higher also increasing the number of litter sizes. Through AI technology using superior semen quality selected from local sheep breeds, it is possible to spread the genetic quality of sheep, which is better in their appearance, body weight gain, and performance (Ciptadi et al. 2014). Diagnosis of pregnancy in ewes is crucial after mating, either by natural breeding or AI. In

---

*Corresponding Author: ardyah.putri@ub.ac.id

DOI: 10.1201/9781003370048-28
This chapter has been made available under a CC BY NC ND license

general, early pregnancy diagnosis is carried out to determine whether sheep are pregnant or not pregnant immediately after mating, so that lost production time due to infertility can be treated appropriately. Based on previous research, it is known that fertility in livestock is indeed influenced by many factors, including; nutrition, stress, environment, sexual behavior, timing or estrous, etc. Growth in livestock is usually measured by the height and weight of the animal. It is known that even though body height is not significantly affected by a pregnancy, livestock body weight can increase significantly (Petrovic et al. 2012). Based on this, we hypothesize that body weight will affect pregnancy success in livestock.

Reproduction is related to the mechanism of the hormonal system, namely the relationship between the hypothalamic-pituitary hormones, such as gonadotrophin-releasing hormone (GnRH), follicle-stimulating hormone (FSH), and luteinizing hormone (LH). Estrus synchronization involves manipulating the length of the luteal phase of the estrus cycle. The estrus period in sheep occurs simultaneously on the same day or several days later. The length of the luteal phase can be shortened by treatment with prostaglandin F2α or its analogs or it can be lengthened by treatment with exogenous progestogens (Xu 2011). Normally, progesterone is secreted from the corpus luteum in a normal estrus cycle. With the decrease in the progesterone level, the follicles start growing (Dijkstra et al. 1996). The same situation can be mimicked externally. Progesterone can be administered externally for a certain duration, and its withdrawal can cause induction of estrus (Pal & Dar 2020). This method is often used for large numbers of livestock to minimize energy, time, and cost.

Farmers usually use methods to detect pregnancy in the field by observing the behavior of livestock. If the livestock shows no signs of returning to heat after the last marriage, the farmer concludes that the animal is pregnant, and vice versa. Some of the advantages of ultrasonography (USG) include that this tool is non-invasive or does not cause physical trauma to the organs being examined, does not have side effects on animals or examiners, can estimate gestational age, number of developing fetuses and see the development of organs. Fetal organs do not require special space and preparation so that they can be used in the field and is easy, fast, and precise in their use (Streter & Step 2007). The results of this study are to provide information about the effect of body weight on the success of AI in productive DEG so that it can be used to increase the success of AI with reference to livestock body weight.

2 MATERIALS AND METHODS

As many as 30 DEG goats were used from several breeders in Krejengan District, Bantaran District, Kedopok District, and Mayangan District, Probolinggo District. Then, the body weight was weighed and grouped into 2, namely above 30 kg and below 30 kg. Furthermore, estrus synchronization was carried out by giving the hormone PGF2α which was carried out on 30 sheep intramuscularly using the enzaprost-T hormone as much as 1 ml each on day one and observing estrus on days 2 and 3.

All DEG goats showing signs of estrus were artificially inseminated using frozen semen sheep straw obtained from BBIB Lembang City. Ultrasonography examination was performed 60 days after artificial insemination in ewes. The instrument used is ultrasound which consists of a control unit, a monitor screen, and a transducer (probe). For examination of pregnancy, the linear transducers have ultrasound beams that are uniform throughout all tissue levels and do not diverge in deeper tissue. Linear transducers are well-adapted for first-trimester ultrasound imaging and can provide a detailed anatomic evaluation of the fetus.

The observation variable in this study was to see the effect of body weight on the success of the pregnancy rate, which was the object of the research. Body weight is an important aspect of livestock because it can be used to determine feed requirements for livestock. The percentage of lust is the number of sheep that are in estrus after the PGF2α hormone injection treatment with the ratio of sheep that are not in heat or estrus. Lastly, the percentage of pregnancy is the number of sheep that are pregnant after artificial insemination with the ratio of sheep that are not pregnant after artificial insemination. The three data were tabulated and calculated and followed by an unpaired t-test to determine the effect between body weight and the percentage of pregnancy success.

3 RESULTS AND DISCUSSION

The differences in the body weight of sheep in this study can also be influenced by genetic factors, environment, and different feeds in each cage, which causes the livestock to lack nutrition before artificial insemination is carried out. Sheep with a body weight of less than 30 kg had a pregnancy percentage of 12.33%, as many as two heads, while sheep weighing more than 30 kg had a pregnancy percentage of 80%, as many as 12; this indicates that the lack of body weight significantly affects the success of AI (Table 1).

Table 1. Percentage of ewes that experienced post-synchronization estrus and post-AI pregnancy.

No	Body Weight (kg)	N	Estrus (%)	Non-estrus (%)	Pregnancy rate (%)
1	> 30	15	100	0	80
2	< 30	15	26,66	73,34	12,33

Based on the results of this study, sheep with a body weight below 30 kg had a lower percentage of pregnancy than sheep with a weight above 30 kg. This is because a body weight below 30 kg has an unfavorable body condition that causes various reproductive problems such as decreased secretion of steroid and thyroid hormones, percentage of lust, estrus behavior, and increased anestrus and anovulation (Purohit 2022). Steroid hormones are made from fat, so the hormones estrogen and progesterone, which are steroid hormones, are influenced by fat levels in the blood. In thin body conditions, reproductive hormones, especially LH, are lower in concentration in the body, which causes fewer eggs to be produced. Fat in the body of livestock can serve as an energy reserve that can be used when pregnant until giving birth. Liu et al. (2019) stated that the ideal livestock has a body condition value of 3 or the sheep are not too fat and not too thin. In lean body conditions, reproductive hormones, especially LH, are lower in concentration in the body, which causes fewer eggs to be produced.

The success of AI is strongly influenced by the accuracy of lust detection, inseminator skills, and timeliness of AI implementation. With the application of estrus synchronization, the administration of the hormone PGF2α will increase the percentage. The success of sheep reproduction is a supporter of productivity in increasing livestock production and population. The main requirement for the success of AI is detecting signs of estrus. In ewes, signs of estrus are an indication that the ewe is in heat. The signs of estrus in sheep are restlessness, decreased appetite, bleating, silence when a male rides it, the mucus coming out of the vagina, warmth to the touch, and a red and swollen vulva (Sudewo 2008). The males can provoke the beginning of the onset of estrus. The female is willing to be approached and shows interest in the male which is assumed to be the beginning of estrus.

The results of artificial insemination based on the percentage of lust with PGF2α hormone injection treatment intramuscularly in fat-tailed sheep in this study were higher than the results of previous research, which yielded 40% of heat (Parasmawati 2011) and conducted Etawa crossbreed goats (PE) obtained a lust rate of 60% (Hafiziddin et al. 2011). Different body conditions for estrus synchronization prove that the female sheep with a lean body condition have a lower response than the female with a moderate body condition. Failure to achieve proper postpartum estrus in DEG is the result of the lack of guaranteed feed availability which directly affects nutritional intake for postnatal DEG, which supports the emergence of postpartum estrus.

A positive ultrasound result of pregnancy was indicated by the presence of embryonic fluid, embryonic vesicle diameter, uterine diameter, and uterine thickness, as well as the presence of a fetus. The number of pregnant sheep with a weight below 30 kg was 2 (12.33%) while the number of sheep above 30 kg was 12 (80%), which indicated that body weight had an effect on the success of pregnancy. Based on these results, it was found that body weight in fat-tailed sheep had a very significant effect ($P>0.05$) on the success of artificial insemination. Insufficient nutrition of brood stock results in less-than-optimal development of reproductive organs. Hormonal imbalance causes excessive uterine contractions and low concentrations of progesterone required for implantation and maintenance of early pregnancy, resulting in low pregnancy rates.

4 CONCLUSION

Based on the research, it can be said that body weight in productive fat tail sheep (DEG) has a significant effect on the success of estrus and artificial insemination. The use of frozen semen of Garut sheep is considered to have a higher genetic quality so the introduction of Garut sheep will be able to simultaneously improve the performance of local sheep in the Probolinggo area, it is hoped that further research will be carried out in the future to observe the results of the offspring whether they have better potential than their parents. This research still requires a more in-depth study, for example, the maximum weight limit for successful pregnancy in sheep.

REFERENCES

Ciptadi G., Budiarto A., Ihsan M.N., Wisaptiningsih U., Wahjuningsih. 2014. Reproductive Performance and Success of Artificial Insemination in Indonesian Crossbreed Goats in Research versus Small Holder Farm. *American-Eurasian Journal of Sustainable Agriculture* 8:35–38.

Dijkstra G., de Rooij D.G., de Jong F.H. and van den Hurk R. 1996. Effect of Hypothyroidism on Ovarian Follicular Development, Granulosa Cell Proliferation and Peripheral Hormone Levels in the Prepubertal rat. *Eur J Endocrinol.* 134:649–654

Govind and Purohit N. 2022. Vet Gynecology Lecture -2 Hormones in animal reproduction. (PDF) *Vet Gynecology Lecture -2 Hormones in Animal Reproduction are Explained in Details* (researchgate.net).

Hafizuddin W.N., Sari T.N., dan Hamdan S. 2011. Persentase Estrus Dan Kebuntingan Kambing Peranakan Etawa (PE) Setelah Pemberian Beberapa Hormon Prostaglandin Komersial. *Jurnal Kedokteran Hewan* Vol. 5(2), September 2011 ISSN: 1978-225X.

Liu H., Gipson T.A., Puchala R., Goetsch A.L. 2019. Relationships Among Body Condition Score, Linear Measures, Body Mass Indexes, and Growth Performance of Yearling Alpine Doelings Consuming High-forage Diets. *Applied Animal Science* 35: 511–520.

Pal, Prasanna and Dar M.R. 2020. *Animal Reproduction in Veterinary Medicine, chapter: Induction and Synchronization of Estrus*. ISBN 978-1-83881-938-5. InTech Open. DOI: 10.5772/intechopen.90769

Parasmawati F., Suyadi and dan Wahyuningsih S. 2011. Peforman Reproduksi Pada Persilangan Kambing Boer Dan Peranakan Etawa (PE). *Jurnal Ilmu-ilmu Peternakan* 23(1): 11–17.

Petrovic, Milan P., Caro-Petrovic V., Ružić-Muslić D., Maksimovic N., Ilic Z., Milosevic B. and Stojković J. "Some Important Factors Affecting Fertility in Sheep." *Biotechnology in Animal Husbandry* 28 (2012): 517–528.

Streeter R. and Step D.L. 2007. Diagnostic Ultrasonography in Ruminants. The Veterinary Clinics of North America. *Food Animal Practice.* 23. 541–74, vii. 10.1016/j.cvfa.2007.07.008.

Sudewo. 2008. Reproductive Performance and Preweaning Mortality of Peranakan Etawa Goat Under Production System of Goat Farming Group in Gumelar Banyumas. *Animal Production, Mei 2008* Vol 10 (2): 67–70.

Udo H.M.J. and BudisatriaI.G.S. (2011). Fat-tailed Sheep in Indonesia; An Essential Resource for Smallholders. *Tropical animal health and production.* 43. 1411–8. 10.1007/s11250-011-9872-7.

Xu Z.Z., 2011. *Reproduction, Events and Management Control of Estrous Cycles: Synchronization of Estrus. Encyclopedia of Dairy Sciences* (Second Edition). Academic Press; 448–453.

Developing Modern Livestock Production in Tropical Countries – Adli et al. (eds)
© 2023 The Authors, ISBN 978-1-032-44025-5
Open Access: www.taylorfrancis.com, CC BY-NC-ND 4.0 license

Antibacterial activity test of Temulawak (Curcuma xanthorrizha Roxb) encapsulation against the growth of lactic acid bacteria, salmonella, and Escherichia coli

A.D. Santos*, R. Indrati, O. Sjofjan & D.N. Adli
Faculty of Animal Science, Universitas Brawijaya, Malang, Indonesia

ABSTRACT: This study was conducted in vitro with the aim to determine the antibacterial inhibition activity of encapsulated temulawak (Curcuma Xanthorrhiza Roxb) against lactic acid bacteria, Salmonella and Escherichia coli have 6 different treatments to be observed, namely; (T0) negative control (distilled water), (T1) positive control (tetracycline + distilled water), (T2) temulawak encapsulation 25% + distilled water, (T3) temulawak encapsulation 50% + distilled water, (T4) temulawak encapsulation 75% + distilled water, and (T5) temulawak encapsulation 100% + distilled water. The results of the research on the inhibitory power of temulawak encapsulation in the T5 treatment with a concentration of 100% had a diameter of the inhibition zone against E. coli bacterial activity. where there was a very significant difference (P<0.01). This indicates that temulawak encapsulation is effective in inhibiting E. coli bacteria. In contrast, the antibacterial activity of temulawak encapsulation against LAB bacteria and Salmonella has not shown effective results because the highest value is found in the T1 treatment (0.1% antibiotic); for other treatments (T0, T2, T3, T4, and T5), it has a value of 0.0 mm, and there is no significant effect (P<0.05). Therefore, the use of temulawak encapsulation has not given positive results in inhibiting the growth of lactic acid bacteria and Salmonella.

Keywords: temulawak encapsulation, inhibition zone diameter, lactic acid bacteria, salmonella and E. coli

1 INTRODUCTION

Herbal plants are phytobiotics that are inseparable from human needs and are needed in their utilization as traditional medicines for the health and also as herbal plants for food ingredients. In addition, with its properties, the herbal plant temulawak which has antioxidant activity can be used as a feed additive for livestock to overcome the use of feed contaminated with synthetic antibiotics. Temulawak (Curcuma Xanthorrhiza Roxb) belongs to a group of spice plants that have benefits for increasing appetite and as an anticholesterol, anti-inflammatory, antianemia, antioxidant, and antimicrobial. Curcuminoids are the main yellow substance in temulawak known to have many benefits for human and animal health (Khamidah et al. 2017). It can be reported by Masuda et al. (1992) that the active components responsible as antioxidants in temulawak rhizomes are curcumin, demethoxycurcumin, and bisdemethoxycurcumin. Antibacterial is a typical chemical compound produced by living organisms in low concentrations and can inhibit important processes in a microorganism (Rahmawati et al. 2014; Siswandono & Soekardjo 1995). Encapsulation

---

*Corresponding Author: dossantosabilio05@gmail.com

DOI: 10.1201/9781003370048-29

technology is usually done using a spray dryer or vacuum oven at temperatures above 100°C. This can cause a loss of activity of active compounds before or during the encapsulation process. As an alternative, this study uses a microwave oven with a temperature lower than 60°C (Natsir et al. 2017).

2 MATERIALS AND METHODS

The method used in the study was a laboratory experimental method using a completely randomized design (CRD), feed additives in the form of temulawak encapsulation consisting of 6 treatments and 4 replicates, so there were 24 experimental units as follows: T0: Negative control (distilled water), T1: Positive control (tetracyclin 0.1 mg), T2: 25% temulawak encapsulation + distilled water, T3: 50% temulawak encapsulation + distilled water, T4: 75% temulawak encapsulation + distilled water and T5: Encapsulated temulawak 100% + distilled water. Tools used in in vitro testing for antibacterial activity are autoclave, analytical balance, petri dish, test tube, measuring cup, glass jar, erlenmeyer, incubator, 1 ml micropipette, waterbath, electric stove, tweezers, stirring rod, bunsen, spirtus, caliper, blue tips, scissors, and test tube rack. The materials used were distilled water, 70% alcohol, antibiotics (tetracycline), temulawak encapsulation, LAB suspension with Mann Rogosa Sharpe Agar (MRS-A) test media, E. Coli bacteria with Nutrient Agar (NA) test media and Salmonella bacteria using Muller Hilton Agar (MHA) test media, label paper, disc paper, tissue, petromax plastic, aluminum foil, cotton, masks, gloves, mattress straps, and corn paper. The data obtained from the study were tabulated using excel and analyzed with ANOVA (Analysis of Variance), the design used is a completely randomized design (CRD), if there are differences between treatments can be continued with further tests, namely Duncan's Multiple Range Test (DMRT) (Adli et al. 2021; Harsojuwono et al. 2011).

3 RESULTS AND DISCUSSION

The effect of using temulawak encapsulation on antibacterial activity, namely, lactic acid bacteria, Salmonella, and E. Coli, has been studied. Temulawak, a herbal plant, has antioxidant compounds against bacteria. The bioactive compound of temulawak (*Curcuma Xanthorrhiza Roxb*), namely xanthorrhizol, known as an antibacterial and can be used in the prevention of diseases in livestock. This bioactive ingredient can inhibit the growth of pathogenic bacteria (Alipin et al. 2017). Furthermore, Bayoa et al. (2014) added that temulawak is one of the herbal plants that can be used as a feed additive in broiler rations containing essential oils, curcumin, and xanthorizol, which can suppress fungi, increase appetite and animal performance. Curcumin is a derivative of phenolic compounds. The mechanism of phenolic compounds functions as an antimicrobial substance by damaging proteins in bacterial cells, causing leakage of nutrients from the cells, which causes bacterial cells to die or inhibit their growth (Sunanti 2007). Bacterial parameters used in this study were LAB (gram-positive bacteria), salmonella, and E. coli (gram-negative bacteria). It aims to determine the comparison of the magnitude of the inhibition of gram-positive and gram-negative bacteria. The inhibition zone of diameter of lactic acid bacteria, Salmonella and E. coli can be seen in Table 1.

Encapsulation of temulawak in treatment T5 with 100% concentration has an inhibition zone diameter against Escherichia coli bacterial activity with a value of 11.01 ± 0.38 mm, compared to other treatments (T0, T2, T3, and T4), although the value is still low against treatment T1 (0.1% antibiotic) which is 33.81 ± 2.59 mm, where there is a very significant difference compared to treatment T1 positive control (P<0.01). These results indicate that temulawak encapsulation is effective in inhibiting the growth of E. coli bacteria. so that the higher the concentration of antimicrobials contained in temulawak encapsulation, the

Table 1. Inhibition zone diameter of Lactic Acid Bacteria, Salmonella, and E. coli.

Treatment	Inhibition zone diameter (mm)		
	Lactic acid bacteria	Salmonella	Escherichia coli
T0 (aquades)	$0 \pm 0,00^a$	$0 \pm 0,00^a$	$0 \pm 0,00^a$
T1(antibiotic)	$52.33 \pm 2,59^b$	$27.56 \pm 0,88^b$	$33.81 \pm 2,59^f$
T2	$0 \pm 0,00^a$	$0 \pm 0,00^a$	$5.36 \pm 0,76^b$
T3	$0 \pm 0,00^a$	$0 \pm 0,00^a$	$8.03 \pm 0,32^c$
T4	$0 \pm 0,00^a$	$0 \pm 0,00^a$	$8.78 \pm 1,49^{cd}$
T5	$0 \pm 0,00^a$	$0 \pm 0,00^a$	$11.01 \pm 0,38^e$

Notes: Different notations (a, b, c, cd, d, e, and f) in the same column indicate a significant effect (P<0.01).

greater the diameter of the inhibition zone produced. Curcumin contained in temulawak rhizomes is effective as the E. coli antibacterial with a concentration of 100% in the Minimum Inhibition Concentration (MIC) test (Ananggia & Murnah 2007). Furthermore, the temulawak rhizome is categorized as very strong in inhibiting the growth of Escherichia coli bacteria (31.56 mm) because it exceeds the standard inhibition category ≥ 20 mm (Adila et al. 2013). Another thing temulawak encapsulation in treatment T1 (0.1% anti-biotic) can form the diameter of the inhibition zone with the highest average value on lactic acid bacteria and salmonella, respectively, 52.33 ± 2.59 mm and 27.56 ± 0.88 mm, and treatment T2, T3, T4, T5 and negative control (T0) there is no diameter of the inhibition zone formed. The antibacterial activity of temulawak encapsulation against LAB bacteria and salmonella cannot show effective results because the average value for other treatments (T0, T2, T3, T4, and T5) has the lowest value of 0.0 ± 0.0 mm which has no inhibition compared to the control T1 treatment (antibiotics). These results contradict other research conducted by Retnaningsih (2015) on the inhibitory power of temulawak rhizomes which showed an inhibition zone of 15.5 mm of temulawak juice to inhibit *Salmonella typhi* after an incubation time of 24 hours. Davis and Stout (1971) stated that a clear zone diameter of 10–20 mm has strong inhibition, a clear zone diameter of 5–10 mm has moderate inhibition and a clear zone diameter <5 mm has weak inhibition, against LAB, Salmonella and E. coli. The results showed that temulawak encapsulation in various treatments had no significant effect (P<0.05), which means that there was no difference in the diameter of the inhibition zone from the six treatments compared to the control T1 treatment (antibiotics). Because from the results of the study, the diameter of the inhibition zone in the treatment of T2, T3, T4, T5, and negative control (distilled water) is the same, namely 0 mm, so it cannot inhibit the growth of lactic acid bacteria and salmonella.

4 CONCLUSION

Temulawak encapsulation is effective in inhibiting E. coli bacteria in treatment T5 which has strong inhibition, although the value is still low against the control treatment T1 (0.1% antibiotic), so it is said that the higher the concentration of antimicrobials contained in temulawak encapsulation, the greater the diameter of the resulting inhibition zone. While the encapsulation of temulawak on LAB bacteria and salmonella did not form the diameter of the inhibition zone because the T2, T3, T4 and T5 treatments had a value of 0 (zero) compared to the T1 treatment, so it could not inhibit LAB and Salmonella bacteria.

REFERENCES

Adli D.N., Sjofjan O., Irawan A., Utama D.T., Sholikin M.M., Nurdianti R.R. Nurfitriani R.A., Hidayat C., Jayanegara A., and Sadarman S. (2022). Effects of Fibre-rich Ingredient Levels on Goose Growth Performance, Blood Profile, Foie Gras Quality and its Fatty Acid Profile: A Meta-analysis. *Journal of Animal and Feed Sciences*, 31(4):301–309.

Ardiansyah W., Sjofjan O., Widodo E., Suyadi S., Adli D.N. (2022). Effects of Combinations of α-Lactobacillus sp. and Curcuma Longa Flour on Production, Egg Quality, and Intestinal Profile of Mojosari Ducks. *Adv. Anim. Vet. Sci*, 10(8):1668–1677.

Adila R., Nurmiati and Agustien A. (2013). Antimicrobial Test of Curcuma spp. Against the Growth of Candida albicans, Staphylococcus aureus and Escherichia coli. *Journal of Biology, Andalas University*, 2 (1):1–7.

Alipin K., Safitri R., and Kartasudjana R. (2017). Probiotic and Temulawak Supplementation in Broilers on Salmonella sp Population and Blood Cholesterol. *Veterinary Journal*, 17(4):582–586. https://doi.org/10.19087/jveteriner.2016.17.4.582.

Ananggia S.A., and Murnah. (2007). *Chromatogram Profile and Antibacterial Activity of ethanol extract of Temulawak rhizome against Escherichia coli Growth in vitro*. Medical Faculty, Diponegoro University.

Bayoa D.L.M., Sarayar C.L.K., Najoan M., and Utiah W. (2014). The Addition Effectiveness of Curcuma Xanthorrhiza Roxb and Curcuma Zedoaria Rox Flours in Commercial Ration on Performances og Broilers. *Zootek Journal*, 34(May):85–94.

Davis W.W., and Stout T.R. (1971). Disc Plate Method of Microbiological Antibiotic Assay. I. Factors Influencing Variability and Error. *Applied Microbiology*, 22(4):659–665. https://doi.org/10.1128/aem.22.4.659-665.1971.

Harsojuwono B.A., Arnata I.W., and Puspawati G.A.K.D. (2011). *Experiment Design: Theory, SPSS and Excel Applications*. Lintaskata Publishing, March, 126.

Khamidah A., Antarlina S.S., and Sudaryono T. (2017). Variety of Temulawak Processed Products to Support Food Diversity. *Journal of Agricultural Research and Development*, 36(1):1. https://doi.org/10.21082/jp3.v36n1.2017.p1-12.

Masuda T., Isobe J., Jitoe A., and Nakatani N. (1992). Antioxidative Curcuminoids From Rhizomes of Curcuma Xanthorrhiza. *Phytochemistry*, 31(10):3645–3647. https://doi.org/10.1016/0031-9422(92)83748-N

Natsir M.H., Hartutik, Sjofjan O., Widodo E., and Widyastuti E.S. (2017). Use of Acidifiers and Herb-acidifier Combinations with Encapsulated and Non-encapsulated Intestinal Microflora, Intestinal Histological and Serum Characteristics in Broilers. *AIP Conference Proceedings*, 1844 (May). https://doi.org/10.1063/1.4983423.

Rahmawati N., Sudjarwo E., and Widodo E. (2014). Test of Antibacterial Activity of Herbal Extracts Against Escherichia coli Bacteria. *Indonesian Journal of Animal Science*, 24(3):24–31. https://jiip.ub.ac.id/index.php/jiip/article/view/184.

Retnaningsih A. (2015). Inhibition Test of Turmeric Rhizome (Curcuma domestica Val) and Temulawak Rhizome (Curcuma xanthorriza roxb) Against Salmonella thypi Bacteria. *Journal of Holistic Health*, 9 (3):158–160.

Siswandono and Soekardjo B. (1995). Medical Chemistry. Airlangga University Press. Surabaya. *Application of Antimicrobial Substrate From Lactic Acid Bacteria as Biopreservative in Beef Meatballs with Cold Storage*. Thesis. Department of Animal Product Technology. Faculty of Animal Husbandry. Institute of Agriculture Bogor.

Developing Modern Livestock Production in Tropical Countries – Adli et al. (eds)
© 2023 The Authors, ISBN 978-1-032-44025-5
Open Access: www.taylorfrancis.com, CC BY-NC-ND 4.0 license

Reproductive index of female Kacang goat managed by smallholder in Talawi district, Indonesia

Lendrawati & E. Ratni
Department of Animal Production and Technology of Andalas University, Padang, Indonesia

ABSTRACT: This study was conducted to evaluate the reproduction index of the mature female Kacang goat managed by smallholders in Talawi district, West Sumatera Province, Indonesia. A total of 281 Kacang does data were purposively selected and collected from around 1,028 Kacang goat population through surveys and interviews with 128 farmers. All of the data were analyzed descriptively. The result showed that the Kacang goat delivered single kids as much as 45.45%, twins as 53.03%, and 1.51% as triplets per birth, with the average litter size, was 1.51. The pre-weaning mortality is 21.86%. The kidding interval and days open were 7.61 and 2.61 months, respectively. Moreover, the results also showed that the Kacang had a reproduction index of 1.87. The research concluded that Kacang goats are well adapted and suitable to be reared by Talawi District smallholders regarding performance and reproduction index.

1 INTRODUCTION

Goat population in Indonesia increased of 539,000 heads or 2,88% between 2020 (18,690,000 heads) and 2021 (19,229,000 heads). West Sumatra Province's goat population was 254,502 head, with the most goat breed being Kacang goat. As a local genetic resource, Kacang goat is important to conserve and develop to serve as a local genetic resource for good goat farming development in the future. Goats are small livestock that provides benefits to fulfill meat demand. A border community reared Kacang goats for their beneficial properties, such as easy to breed, quick to reach sexual maturity, relatively easy maintenance, low space requirement, low capital for breeding, and ease of development. However, measurement of the reproductive performance of Kacang goats reared by smallholders should be done to understand and ensure goat farming sustainability and to maintain the Kacang goat conservation. Thus, this study aims to evaluate the reproduction index of female Kacang goats managed by smallholders in Talawi district, Sawahlunto Regency, West Sumatera Province, Indonesia.

2 MATERIALS AND METHODS

The study was conducted in smallholder farming in Talawi District, Sawahlunto Regency. There were 128 goat farmers in this area, with the total population being around 1,028 Kacang goats. Purposive sampling was done to select the study's sample, including 128 goat farmers with 281 mature female Kacang goat were selected. The Kacang goat population structure is presented in Table 1.

DOI: 10.1201/9781003370048-30

Table 1. Structure population of Kacang goat in Talawi District.

No.	Structure population	Number	Percentage
1	Pre-weaning	183	33.57
2	Weaning	81	14.86
3	Mature	281	51.56
	Total	545	

The Kacang goats were reared under a semi-intensive farming system. The feeding was done thoroughly free grazing from 09.00 AM to 17.00 PM without any concentrate feed addition. Over the night, the goat stays back in the housing.

The observed variables in this study were litter size, pre-weaning mortality, kidding interval, days open, and reproduction index of mature female goat. All of the data were collected through surveys and interviews, with questionnaires as the primary data and farmers' recording sheets as the secondary data.

The litter size, kidding interval, days open, pre-weaning mortality, and reproduction index were analyzed descriptively and measured as follows:

$$\text{Pre-weaning mortality (\%)} : \frac{\text{the total pre-weaning kids} \times 100}{\text{the total of delivered kids}}$$

$$\text{Reproduction index} : \frac{\text{litter size } (1 - \text{pre-weaning mortality})}{\text{Kidding interval (year)}}$$

3 RESULT AND DISCUSSIONS

3.1 Litter size

The result of litter size measurement in this study is presented in Table 2. It can be seen that the kidding type in one birth of Kacang goat in this study can be divided into three groups, which were single, twins, and triplets. The Twins kidding is shown to be mostly occurring (53.03%), and then followed by single (45.45%) and triplet (1.51%) kids. Moreover, the average litter size of Kacang goat in this study was 1.51 ± 0.53. The result was higher than Suyadi et al. (2019), which showed that the average litter size of Kacang goat reared under a closed population in Sidoarjo was 1.31 ± 0.51. However, Nasich *et al.* (2019) showed higher results, with the average litter size of Kacang goat reared in the highlands area around 1.6.

The total of successful ovulation and embryonal mortality affected litter size. The small litter size of the livestock could also be affected by the given feed and genetic factors. The nutrition consumed will affect on body growth and reproductive hormone. added that the litter size of goats would be highly affected by the number of parities, body conformation, ages of dams, genetic factors, seasons, and nutrition intakes. In this study, the Kacang goat

Table 2. Kidding type and average litter size of Kacang goat.

Kidding type	The percentage of kids (%)	Number delivered kids (heads)
Single	45.45	128
Twin	53.03	149
Triple	1.51	4
Average litter size	1.51 ± 0.53	

dams in the study area were freely grazing field grass around the fishpond without any feed addition. It could be predicted that the mature goat received inadequate feed in both quality and quantity. An approach to improve the litter size of Kacang goat dams in this study might be made by giving more qualified feeds and better breeding management.

3.2 Pre-weaning mortality

The pre-weaning mortality indicates the mothering ability of the goat and the kids' ability to adapt to the environment. The pre-weaning mortality is affected by several factors, such as bad pre-weaning management, low colostrum intake, housing condition, and farm hygiene condition (Widaningsih & Nurdiani 2000). Pre-weaning mortality, days open, kidding interval, and reproduction index of mature Kacang goats are presented in Table 3.

Table 3. Pre-weaning mortality, days open, kidding interval, and reproduction index.

Variable	Value
Pre-weaning mortality (%)	21.86
Days open (months)	7.61 ± 0.99
Kidding interval (months)	2.61 ± 0.99
Reproduction index	1.87

In this study, the pre-weaning mortality was 21.86%. These findings lower than Elieser *et al.* (2012) showed that pre-weaning mortality of Kacang goats was 23.6% and higher than Suryadi *et al.* 2019 stated pre-weaning mortality was 20.7%. The pre-weaning mortality of Kacang goats in this study would affect the farming sustainability, thus urging proper improvements in management. According to Hasibuan and Mahmilia (2010), pre-weaning mortality at 10% would be enough to harm farming efficiency.

4 CONCLUSIONS

The research concludes that Kacang goats were well adapted and suitable to be managed by smallholders in Talawi District regarding its reproductive performances. However, efforts to improve the reproduction index are suggested to improve farming efficiency, thus ensuring the conservation of Kacang goats as local resources in Indonesia.

ACKNOWLEDGEMENT

This research has been supported by PNBP of Andalas University 2022 with contract number: T/104/UN.16.17/PT.01.03/Pangan-RPT/2022.

REFERENCES

Budiarsana I.G.M. and Sutama I.K. (2001). Fertilitas Kambing Peranakan Etawah Pada Perkawinan Alami dan Inseminasi Buatan. Hlm. 85–92. In *Prosiding Seminar Nasional Peternakan dan Veteriner. Pusat Penelitian dan Pengembangan Peternakan*, Bogor.

Directorate General of Livestock and Animal Health, Ministry of Agriculture 2021 Livestock and Animal Health Statistic 2021. Jakarta: *Directorate General of Livestock and Animal Health Ministry of Agriculture*: Jakarta.

Elieser S., Sumadi S., Budisatria G.S. and Subandriyo S. (2012). Productivity Comparison between Boer and Kacang Goat dam. *Journal of the Indonesian Tropical Animal Agriculture*, 37(1), 15–21.

Hasibuan M.S. and Mahmilia F. (2010). *Mortalitas Prasapih Kambing Kacang dan Boerka di Stasiun Percobaan Loka Penelitian Kambing Potong Sei Putih. In Seminar Nasional Teknologi Peternakan dan Veteriner*. Stasiun Percobaan Loka Penelitian Kambing Potong Sei Putih, Galang, Sumatera Utara.

Kaunang D., Suyadi S. and Wahjuningsih S. (2013). Analisis Litter Size, Bobot Lahir dan Bobot Sapih Hasil Perkawinan Kawin Alami dan Inseminasi Buatan Kambing Boer dan Peranakan Etawah (PE). *Jurnal Ilmu-Ilmu Peternakan (Indonesian Journal of Animal Science)*, 23(3), 41–46.

Mahmilia F. (2007). Reproduction Performance of Boer, Kacang and its Crosses does that Crossed with Boer. *Seminar Nasional Teknologi Peternakan dan Veteriner*, 485–490.

Nasich M., Sarah O.L., Ciptadi G., Busono W. and Budiarto A. (2019, March). The Productivity of Kacang Goat Pre-weaning Period in Low-land and High-land in West Timor, Timor Island Indonesia. In *IOP Conference Series: Earth and Environmental Science* (Vol. 247, No. 1, p. 012017). IOP Publishing.

Widaningsih. and Nurdiani Y. (2000). The Strategy for Decreasing Pre-weaning Mortality of Kids in Goats and Sheep. Bogor: *Balai Penelitian Ternak*.

Developing Modern Livestock Production in Tropical Countries – Adli et al. (eds)
© *2023 The Authors, ISBN 978-1-032-44025-5*
Open Access: www.taylorfrancis.com, CC BY-NC-ND 4.0 license

The effect of breed and growth hormone receptor genotype on the heat tolerance coefficient in dairy cow at Grati

Sucik Maylinda*
Staff member in Faculty of Animal Science Brawijaya University, Malang, Indonesia

Ali Mahmud
Staff member in Faculty of Animal Science at University of Muhammadiyah Malang, Malang, Indonesia

ABSTRACT: This study aims to compare the Heat Tolerance Coefficient (HTC) of local and imported dairy cattle from New Zealand reared in Grati Pasuruan, and to determine the effect of the Growth Hormone Receptor (GHR) genotype on cattle's HTC. The research was conducted in Grati-Pasuruan, East Java. The research material was 31 cows (local and imported) from lactation I to II. Variables measured were respiratory frequency, rectal temperature, and HTC calculation using the equation: (Tf/Ti + Rf/Ri). Polymorphism analysis in GHR gene using PCR-RFLP (Polymerase Chain Reaction)-(Restricted Fragment Length Polymorphism) technique; PCR was performed with 386 bp amplification in the flanking region using primer F: 5′ TGCGTGCAC AGCAGCTCAACC and R: 5′ AGCAACCCCACTGCTGGGCAT and fragment digestion using restriction enzyme Alu1. Polymorphism analysis used the formula PIC (Polymorphic information content): $1 - \Sigma p2$ ij. One-way ANOVA was used to analyze the genotype effect on HTC. Polymorphism is 44.88 %. All alleles were in the Hardy-Weinberg equilibrium. Statistically, local breeds have better adaptability than imported cattle (P<0.01). All genotypes caused almost the same HTC (CC = 3.64, CD = 3.78, DD = 3.58). The conclusion is that local cattle had better adaptability than imported cattle, and the CC, CD, and DD genotypes caused the same adaptability.

Keywords: Breed, GHR-genotype, Local cattle, Imported cattle, HTC

1   INTRODUCTION

Dairy cows in Indonesia are generally from the Friesian Holstein breed, which was imported from the Netherlands in the 17th century. The history of Holstein cattle is according to Sudono et al. (2003), Holland Fries cattle (FH) from the Province of the North of the Netherlands and the Province of West Friesland. called Friesian. This breed of cattle is quite productive with good adaptability in tropical environments. Many studies show that this breed is still producing quite well in tropical areas, especially in dairy cattle breeding areas in Indonesia which have a cool climate, such as in Pujon, Batu, Boyolali, and Lembang. Moreover, areas where the environmental temperature is quite hot, such as Pasuruan, Grati, Surabaya, and Jakarta, there is a slight decrease in production. Because this cow is so well known in Indonesia, its production capability in the tropics should be evaluated not only for its milk production, but also for its adaptability. The ability to adapt to heat is generally done by evaluating the HTC (Heat Tolerance Coefficient).

---

*Corresponding Author: sucik@ub.ac.id

DOI: 10.1201/9781003370048-31

The objectives of the research were to analyze the phenotypic and genetic diversity (genetic polymorphism) at the Growth Hormone Receptor locus which is thought to have a relationship with good capability in adaptation to a hot environment according to the HTC value. The problems of the research were in line with the increase in demand for milk, and it is thought that the fulfillment of this demand is getting harder because demand is increasing but the speed of supply is not fast enough. This condition requires the selection to produce productive dairy cows. There are two types of selection, namely (a) conventional selection and (2) marker-based selection (Marker Assisted Selection). Mapping of genes in the cow's genome makes new horizons in the field of livestock breeding.

2 MATERIAL AND METHODS

The research was done at Grati sub-district, Pasuruan-East Java. Thirty-one cows (imported and local dairy cows) were used. Imported cows were purebred from New Zealand, and Local cows are the Friesian Holstein Crossed or FH Grade. Variables measured were Respiratory Frequency, Rectal Temperature, and the HTC and the calculation using the Benezra equation: $T_f/T_i + R_f/R_i$, where T_f is the average body temperature at noon (°C); T_i is the average body temperature in the morning (°C); Rf is the average respiration rate at noon (breaths per minute), and R_i is the average respiration rate in the morning (breaths per minute) (Yosit et al. 2016).

The research was conducted in two steps: (1) This stage is to collect data in the field in the form of respiratory frequency and body/rectal temperature in the morning and afternoon (at 12.00); (2) to collect blood samples in each cow as much as 5 Ul by using a venoject in the jugular vein. The research was done at Genomic Laboratory to conduct PCR (Polymerase Chain Reaction) and RFLP.

PCR was done using the primer as below (Aggrey et al. 1998):

- primer F : 5' TGCGTGCAC AGCAGCTCAACC
- primer R : 5' AGCAACCCCACTGCTGGGCAT

The protocol for PCR was:

Steps	Temperature (oC)	Duration	Cycle (X)
Predenaturasi	94	5 minutes	1
Denaturasi	92	1 minute	
Annealing	66	80 seconds	26
Elongation	72	2 minutes	
Extension	4	Until next process	

3 DATA ANALYSIS

Data were obtained and the HTC and were calculated using the Benezra equation: $T_f/T_i + R_f/R_i$. HTC data are tabulated with the main factor being the breed of cattle and the second factor being the genotype of the cattle. Data were analyzed using ANOVA with a Nested design model. The mathematical model in the data analyzing is: $Y_{ijk} = \mu + a_i + g_{(j)i} + e_{ijk}$ where Y_{ijk} is the measurements in i-breed, j-genotype, and k-cows, μ is the population mean, a_i is the effect of i-breed and j-genotype, and e_{ijk} is sampling error in i-breed and j-genotype (Steel & Torrie 1981).

4 RESULT AND DISCUSSION

Based on the result listed in Table 1, the polymorphism of the population was calculated using the PIC calculation = 1 –Σp2 ij. = 44.88 %). The figure of the Agarose Electrophoresis can be seen in Figure 1.

Table 1.   PCR-RFLP Result and its relationship with HTC of cow (using Alu1 enzyme) in Imported cattle and Local cattle in HTC.

Cattle breed	N	CC genotype	CD genotype	DD genotype	Overall
Imported	14	4.07	4.02	4.1	4.054[b]
Local	17	2.99	3.71	3.39	3.34[a]
Allele	Allele C = p = 0.34				
Frequency	Sllele D = q = 0.66				
Overall	31	3.643	3.78	3.58**)	

Note: The different superscripts in the same column mean that HTC is statistically different (P < 0.01) between Imported and Local cattle. **the HTC of all genotypes is almost the same.

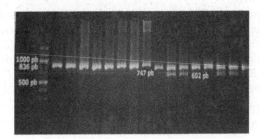

Figure 1.   The result of agarose electrophoresis of the PCR-RFLP product.

The polymorphism is calculated based on the result of PCR-RFLP that can be seen in Figure 1.

- Statistically, local breeds have better adaptability than imported cattle (P<0.01). Local FH has better adaptability (HTC = 3.34) and the Imported FH (purebred FH) has worse adaptability (HTC = 4,054). (See Table 1.)
- All genotypes caused almost the same HTC (CC = 3.64, CD =3.78, DD = 3.58). The conclusion is that local cattle had better adaptability than imported cattle and all genotypes give almost the same HTC.

The results in this study are possible because the genes that cause adaptive traits are not in the GHR locus but rather in the coding for adaptive traits. Some alternatives for studying marker genes, for example, the study in microsatellite sequence, because as reported by Saeed, Wajid, Abas, and Ayub (2021), three microsatellite markers were detected within the bovine HSP70 gene. As known that the HSP70 is the gene for adaptability in cattle.

5 CONCLUSION

More research is needed to evaluate the effect of genotypes in other regions for example in DNA-microsatellite with more cows to obtain more accurate results.

REFERENCES

Aggrey S.E., Yao J., Zadworny D., Hayes J.F., and Kuhnlein U. (1998). Synergism Between Genetic Markers in the Growth Hormone and Growth Hormone Receptor Genes in Influencing Milk Related Traits in Holsteins. *Journal Dairy Science*, 80(1), 229–232.

Saeed A., Wajid A., Abbas K., Ayub G., Din A.M., Ain Q., and Hussain T. *Novel Polymorphisms in Complete Coding Region of Heat Shock Protein 70.1 Gene in Subtropically Adapted Red Sindhi Cattle Breed.*

Steel R.G.D., and Torrie J.H. (1986). *Principles and Procedures of Statistics: A Biometrical Approach.* New York, NY, USA: McGraw-Hill.

Sutarno S., and Setyawan A.D. (2016). The Diversity of Local Cattle in Indonesia and the Efforts to Develop Superior Indigenous Cattle Breeds. *Biodiversitas Journal of Biological Diversity*, 17(1).

Yosi F., Prajoga S.B.K., and Natawiria E.M. (2019). Heat Tolerance Identification on Adult Madura Breeds Cow According to Rhoad and Benezra Coefficient. *Ecodevelopment*, 2(2).

131

Developing Modern Livestock Production in Tropical Countries – Adli et al. (eds)
© 2023 The Authors, ISBN 978-1-032-44025-5
Open Access: www.taylorfrancis.com, CC BY-NC-ND 4.0 license

Quality semen of Boer goat using coconut water diluent during cold storage

D.C. Pinto, N. Isnaini & T. Susilawati*
Faculty of Animal Science, Brawijaya University, Malang, Indonesia

ABSTRACT: Artificial insemination using liquid semen is an appropriate method for improving genetic quality in areas This study aims to find a combination of coconut water and egg yolk that can be used as a semen diluent during cold storage in Boer goats. Boer goats used were 3–4 years old and semen collected for 1 week 2 times using an artificial vagina. The method used is an experimental laboratory, and the design used is Randomised Design Group using 4 treatments and 10 replicates of each treatment as a group. Semen was diluted with coconut water and egg yolk diluent with the ratio of dilution composition in each treatment as follows: First treatment as control (P0) = CEP-3 + 10% egg yolk + 0.4% egg white, Second treatment (P1) = 90% coconut water + 10% egg yolk, Third treatment (P2) = 85% coconut water + 15% egg yolk and fourth treatment (P3) = 80% coconut water + 20% egg yolk. The variables observed in the study were the quality of spermatozoa, that is the percentage of individual motility, viability, and abnormality of spermatozoa. The data were analyzed using Analysis of Variance and there were differences between treatments then continued with Duncan Multiple Range Test. The results showed that the quality of semen in fresh semen was a volume namely: 0.99 ± 0.11 ml, with a yellowish white color, motility of spermatozoa = 73 ± 3.5%, the viability of spermatozoa: 77.19 ± 4.54%, abnormality of spermatozoa = 8.96 ± 1.05 and spermatozoa concentration 4,120 ± 441.46 million/ml. It was concluded that the addition of 20% egg yolk can maintain the motility of spermatozoa until the third day with individual motility >40.41%.

Keywords: Liquid semen, boer goat, coconut water, egg yolk, semen quality and artificial insemination

1 INTRODUCTION

Boer goats are a type of goat that has long been recognized and maintained by society. Efforts can be made to improve the productivity and genetic quality of Boer goats using artificial insemination (AI) technology (Heriyanta et al. 2013). Artificial insemination can be done using liquid semen and frozen semen. Artificial insemination using frozen semen has long been widely recognized by farmers, but in practice, there are still obstacles experienced by farmers and technical personnel in remote areas, especially since the availability of liquid nitrogen (liquid N2) is very limited. In addition, the process of making frozen semen is very complicated (Sholikah & Susilawati 2020). Efforts to overcome these obstacles require various methods to replace chemicals with local diluents, namely using coconut water and egg yolk as alternative diluents, for the manufacture of liquid semen. Coconut water has the potential to be utilized as a semen diluent because coconut water is very easy to obtain and widely available in rural areas at a relatively low price compared to imported synthetic

---

*Corresponding Author: tsusilawati@ub.ac.id

DOI: 10.1201/9781003370048-32

chemical diluents. Young coconut water contains sugar such as glucose, fructose, and sucrose which are needed by spermatozoa (Yong et al. 2009). The use of coconut water is not able to maintain semen quality during cold storage, so it needs to be combined with egg yolk because the egg yolk contains lipoproteins, which play a role as an extracellular cryoprotectant in spermatozoa (Dwitarizki et al. 2015). In connection with this description, research was conducted on the use of young green coconut water (*Cocos viridis*) diluent and local chicken egg yolk as an alternative diluent for Boer goat liquid semen diluent.

2 MATERIALS AND METHODS

This research was implemented at the Laboratory of Reproduction and Animal Breeding and Field Laboratory, Faculty of Animal Science, Brawijaya University, from the 1st of August to the 24th of September 2022. The materials used were fresh semen of 2 heads of Boer goats aged 3–4 years. Coconut and streptomycin water used was green coconut (*Coconut viridis*), NaHCO3, penicillin, CEP-3, and eosin negrosin. The method used is an experimental laboratory, with Randomised Design Group using 4 treatments and 10 replicates of each treatment as a group. Semen was diluted with coconut water and egg yolk diluent with the ratio of dilution composition in each treatment as follows: First treatment as control (P0) = CEP-3 + 10% egg yolk + 0.4% egg white, Second treatment (P1) = 90% coconut water + 10% egg yolk, Third treatment (P2) = 85% coconut water + 15% egg yolk and fourth treatment (P3) = 80% coconut water + 20% egg yolk. The variables observed in the study were the quality of spermatozoa, that is the percentage of individual motility, viability, and abnormality of spermatozoa. Data on liquid semen quality were analyzed using Analysis of Variance, with a very significant $P<0.01$ and a significantly different $P<0.05$. If there were differences between treatments then continued with the Duncan Multiple Range Test t (Sudarwati et al. 2019).

3 RESULTS AND DISCUSSION

In one of the efforts to maintain the quality of fresh semen of Boer goats, it is necessary to test the quality of macroscopic and microscopic before dilution and preservation listed in Table 1.

Table 1. The average fresh semen of Boer goat.

Semen quality test	Observation result
Macroscopic	
Volume (ml)	0.99 ± 0.10
Color	Yellowish milky white
Odor	Typical of goat semen
Consistency	Spoon-thick
pH	$6,59 \pm 0,18$
Microscopic	
Mass motility	2+
Individual motility (%)	$73 \pm 3,50$
Viability (%)	$77,19 \pm 4,54$
Abnormality (%)	$8,96 \pm 1,05$
Concentration (x 107) of spermatozoa million/ml	$4.120 \pm 441,46$
Total spermatozoa million/ml	$4090 \pm 724,93$
Total motile spermatozoa million/ml	$298.706 \pm 56.534,73$

Based on the result of the fresh semen quality test in Table 1, it is shown that the average volume of fresh semen of Boer goat namely: 0.99 ± 0.10 ml, this result is not different from the results of research by Sholikah and Susilowati (2020) namely: 0.93 ± 0.16. Susiliwati (2013) mentioned that the volume of goat semen once ejaculated has an average of 1 ml with a range of 0.5–1.2 ml. The color of fresh semen is milky white and has a medium and thick consistency. Susiliwati (2013) stated that the consistency of semen is positively correlated with the concentration of spermatozoa with a relative assessment, namely: dilute, medium, and thick (concentrated) and has a pH of 6.59 ± 0.18 according to the opinion of Susilawati (2011), the pH of fresh semen is between 6.2 and 6.8. The results of examining the quality of fresh semen microscopically showed mass motility 2+, this result is in accordance with the research of Sholikah and Susilawati (2020), namely 2+. The average individual motility is $73 \pm 3.50\%$, viability, $77.19 \pm 4.54\%$, and abnormality, namely $8,96 \pm 1,05\%$. The average semen concentration obtained in the results of this study is $4,120 \pm 441.46$ million/ml. The results obtained in this study were lower than the research of Audia et al. (2017) namely: $5293,3 \pm 188,92$. The average total spermatozoa was 4090 ± 724.93 million/ml, and the total motile spermatozoa were $298,706 \pm 56,534.73$ million/ml. Based on macroscopic and microscopic semen quality tests, it is shown that Boer goat semen has met the criteria for further processing into liquid semen for artificial insemination. According to Susiliwati (2013), the quality of fresh semen is good for diluting is semen that has a percentage of spermatozoa motility of 70–90% and abnormality <20%.

Observation of the motility of spermatozoa after a 5°C temperature drop, starting at hour 0 and repeated every 24 hours, until a decrease in the percentage of individual motility until 40%. The percentage of individual motility with different treatments is listed in Table 2.

Table 2.   The average of individual motility spermatozoa of Boer goat liquid semen after treatment.

Treatment	Length of observation day (%)		
	D1	D2	D3
P0	$68,40 \pm 3,04^{b}$	$60,50 \pm 6,44^{c}$	$54,00 \pm 5,66^{b}$
P1	$58,60 \pm 9,64^{a}$	$48,70 \pm 9,81^{a}$	$34,08 \pm 7,99^{a}$
P2	$60,90 \pm 8,02^{a}$	$51,63 \pm 7,32^{ab}$	$36,83 \pm 2,84^{a}$
P3	$63,20 \pm 6,63^{ab}$	$52,75 \pm 6,90^{b}$	$40,41 \pm 5,81^{a}$

Note: Different notations in the same column indicate very significant differences ($P < 0.01$)

Based on the result of the Analysis of Variance shown in Table 2, it is shown that the use of coconut water as a spermatozoa diluent gives a very significantly different ($P<0.01$) in the motility of Boer goat liquid semen on the first, second, and third day. The average value of individual motility on the third day showed the highest percentage value of motility found in P0 namely: $54.00 \pm 5.66\%$, and P3 which is: $40.41 \pm 5.81\%$, while the lowest percentage value was found in the P1 and P2 treatments, namely: $34.08 \pm 7.99\%$ and $36.83 \pm 2\%$. The P3 treatment gave the best results compared to the P1 and P2, except for the control treatment (P0). These results indicate that the storage of liquid semen until 3 days for P1 and P2 is categorized as not suitable for use for AI because the motility is below <40%, but in the P3 treatment can still be used until the third day because the motility is above >40.41%. The results of this study indicate that individual motility is not much different from research (Sholikah & Susilawati 2020) using green coconut water and egg yolk which can maintain individual motility of 42% during cold storage until the third day. The addition of 20% egg yolk percentage in P3 treatment proved to be better and able to maintain the motility of liquid semen spermatozoa at 3–5°C temperature storage until 3 days.

The viability of spermatozoa is one indicator that has a very important role in determining the number of live and dead spermatozoa. The viability of Boer goat liquid semen spermatozoa during cold storage decreased dramatically in all treatments listed in Table 3.

Table 3. The average viability spermatozoa of Boer goat liquid semen after treatment.

Treatment	Length of observation day (%)		
	D1	D2	D3
P0	$74,69 \pm 7,59^c$	$71,01 \pm 9,11^b$	$62,04 \pm 6,45^b$
P1	$67,51 \pm 11,18^a$	$61,32 \pm 11,25^a$	$46,14 \pm 9,70^a$
P2	$68,43 \pm 8,81^{ab}$	$60,54 \pm 9,57^a$	$47,05 \pm 5,86^a$
P3	$70,80 \pm 7,66^b$	$64,16 \pm 9,14^a$	$51,75 \pm 6,75^a$

Note: different notations in the same column indicate very significant differences ($P < 0.01$)

The result of the Analysis of Variance in Table 3 showed that the use of coconut water as a spermatozoa diluent has a very significant effect ($P < 0.01$) on the viability of Boer goat liquid semen spermatozoa on the first, second, and third day. The average percentage of viability on the third day showed the highest value in the control treatment (P0), namely: $62.04 \pm 6.45\%$, followed by P3 treatment, namely: $51.75 \pm 6.75\%$, P2 treatment, namely: $47.05 \pm 5.86\%$ and P1 which is $46,14 \pm 9,70\%$. These results indicate that the viability of spermatozoa on the first until the third day of storage in the P3 treatment gave better results compared to the P1 and P2, except for the control treatment (P0). This is probably because the source of nutrients in the form of simple carbohydrates and flavonoid elements contained in coconut water is still available for spermatozoa. According to Salim et al. (2018), the content of flavonoid as an antioxidant from the enzyme group contained in coconut water plays a role in maintaining membrane stability from oxidative damage due to the influence of lipid peroxidation. While in the egg yolk, there is a lecithin compound that can protect spermatozoa from cold shock, it is in line to the opinion of Coester et al. (2019) that lecithin contained in egg yolk plays an important role in coating the spermatozoa cell membrane by maintaining the phospholipid bilayer of spermatozoa cells.

4 CONCLUSION

Based on the result of this study, it can be concluded that the addition of 20% egg yolk to green coconut water diluent can maintain the quality of liquid semen of Boer goat at 3–5°C until the third day with motility above >40.41%.

REFERENCES

Audia R.P., Salim M.A.., Nurul I. and Susilawati T. (2017). Effect of Different Maturity of Green Coconut Water as a Diluent Added with 10% Egg Yolk on the Quality of Liquid Semen of Boer Goats. *Journal of Tropical Livestock*, 18(1), 58–68.

Coester J.S., Sulaiman A. and Rizal M. (2019). Viability of Limousin Cattle Spermatozoa Preserved with Tris Diluent and Various Concentrations of Soybean Juice. *Journal of Tropical Livestock Science and Technology*, 6(2),175–180.

Dwitarizki N.D., Ismaya and Asmarawati W. (2015). Effect of Sperm Dilution with Coconut Water and Duck Egg Yolk and Storage Duration on Motility and Viability of Garut Sheep Spermatozoa at 5°C Storage. *Livestock Bulletin*, 39(3), 149–156.

Heriyanta E., Ihsan M.N. and Isnaini N. (2013). Effect of Age of Peranakan Etawah (Pe) Goats on Fresh Semen Quality. *Journal of Tropical Livestock*, 14(2), 1–5.

Sholikah N. and Susilowati S. (2020). Effect of Egg Yolk Composition in Green Coconut Water Diluent on Boer Goat Liquid Semen Quality. *Journal of Tropical Livestock Science and Technology*, 7(2), 152–157.

Sudarwati H., Natsir M.H. and Nurgiartiningsih V.M.A. (2019). Statistics and Experiment Design Application in the Field of Animal Husbandry.

Susilawati T. (2011). *Spermatology*. Universitas Brawijaya Press.

Susilawati T. (2013). *Pedoman Inseminasi Buatan Pada Ternak*. Universitas Brawijaya Press.

Yong J.W., Ge L., Ng Y.F., & Tan S.N. (2009). The Chemical Composition and Biological Properties of Coconut (Cocos nucifera L.) Water. *Molecules*, 14(12), 5144–5164.

Developing Modern Livestock Production in Tropical Countries – Adli et al. (eds)

Fermentative gas production of different feeds collected during wet and dry seasons when incubated with rumen fluid from Timor deer (*Cervus timorensis*)

M.S. Arifuddin*, Damry, M. Mangun & Mirajuddin
Study Program of Animal Science, Faculty of Animal Husbandry and Fisheries, Tadulako University, Palu, Indonesia

R. Utomo & H. Hartadi
Faculty of Animal Science, Gadjah Mada University, Yogyakarta, Indonesia

ABSTRACT: An experiment was done to investigate microbial fermentation of various feeds commonly given to Timor deer (*Cervus timorensis*) using the in vitro gas production technique. Seven forage feed samples (Sesbania grandiflora, Leucaena leucocephala, Glyricidia sepium, Zea mays, Ipomea aquatica, Pennisetum purpureum, and native grass) were collected during dry and wet seasons and three concentrate feed samples (rice bran, copra meal, and tofu waste) were dried and ground. The feed sample (200 g) was transferred into an incubation syringe which was then added to the incubation medium (mixture of rumen fluid and buffer solution). The rumen fluid was collected from two Timor deer using a trocar technique. Incubation was run for 72 h, and gas production was read at 2, 4, 6, 12, 24, 48, and 72 h of incubation. Data were fitted to an exponential equation generally used in similar in vitro gas production studies. Results of the study indicated that there was an effect of season on fermentation parameters (values of a, b, or c) for the same feed, but this effect was not consistent from one feed to another. From data of total and cumulative gas productions, it was indicated that Zea mays in the either dry or wet season showed the highest, while Leucaena leucocephala exhibited the lowest, gas production compared to other feeds tested.

Keywords: Cervus timorensis, gas production, wet season, dry season, fermentation

1 INTRODUCTION

Microbial digestion in the rumen of feed substances consumed by ruminants involves the degradation of the feed into simpler components and subsequent fermentation of the resulting products. Degradation results in the formation of monomers, such as glucose produced from carbohydrate degradation and amino acids formed from peptides or proteins. These degradation end products then undergo microbial fermentation which results in the production of volatile fatty acids (VFA), adenosine triphosphate (ATP), and gas. The ATP generated during fermentation is the main energy source used by the rumen microbes. Gas mainly methane (CH_4) and carbon dioxides (CO_2) produced normally leaves the rumen via eructation. From the nutritional point of view, the formation of gas during microbial fermentation is a loss of potential energy which may otherwise be available to animals.

---

*Corresponding Author: sadik_arifuddin@yahoo.com

DOI: 10.1201/9781003370048-33

Gas produced during the fermentation of a feed in the rumen is closely related to the degradation of the feed and it has thus been used as an indicator of microbial feed degradation in the rumen. Gas production technique has been developed in such as a way to obtain more reliable and accurate predictions of feed degradation in the rumen. For example, a pressure transducer was introduced by Theodorou et al. (1994) into the gas production technique to determine the dynamics of fermentation. Besides serving as a technique for estimating feed degradation, gas production has also been used to indicate microbial activities and the environment in the rumen. This is particularly true for wild ruminants where conventional feed degradation studies are more difficult to conduct than for domesticated ones because of, for example, the limited availability of animals as rumen fluid donors.

Timor deer (*Cervus timorensis*) is a wild ruminant that has gained more attention due to its economic potential. However, limited study has been done to address the fermentation pattern of feed in the rumen of Timor deer. This present study was designed to investigate microbial degradation in the rumen of Timor deer of different feeds commonly feed to this animal, using the in vitro gas production technique.

2 MATERIAL AND METHODS

Seven forage feed samples (*Sesbania grandiflora, Leucaena leucocephala, Glyricidia sepium, Zea mays, Ipomea aquatica, Pennisetum purpureum*, and native grass) were collected during dry and wet seasons in Palu as well as three concentrate feed samples (rice bran, copra meal, and tofu waste). All the feed samples were dried (60°C, 48 h). The dried samples were then grounded (1 mm sieve) and brought to the Department of Animal Feed and Nutrition, Gadjah Mada University for in vitro gas production studies.

Rumen fluid was obtained from two adult Timor deer (*Cervus timorensis*). Prior to rumen fluid collection, the donor animals were separated from their counterparts and kept on a feed consisting of Zea mays leaves and rice bran. The forage feed as well as fresh drinking water were provided ad libitum, while the rice bran supplement was given once daily in the morning. The rumen fluid was collected using a trocar technique and the collected rumen fluid was transferred into a container and placed in a thermos.

The incubation medium was prepared by mixing (1:2) rumen fluid and a buffer solution. The solution was placed on a hot plate set at 38°C and was thoroughly mixed with an aid of a magnetic stirrer. The solution was flushed with CO_2 and added with more reducing solution until the total volume of reducing solution used was 49.5 ml. Mixing was continued until the solution was colorless and rumen fluid (457.5 ml) was then finally included in the solution. All the process was done under anaerobic condition (Menke & Steingass 1988).

A total of 30 ml of incubation solution was placed in the incubation syringe containing 200 g of the ground feed sample. Carbon dioxide was once more flushed into the syringe before its plunger and lid were carefully placed in position. The initial plunger position on the syringe scale was then read as zero time (V_0) and the incubation syringe was placed at a temperature of 39°C. A blank incubation syringe (syringe containing incubation medium only) was also included in the run. The incubation was run for 72 h, and the amount of fermentation gas produced was read at 2, 4, 6, 12, 24, 48, and 72 h of incubation.

Data of fermentative gas production were fitted with the following exponential equation (Orskov & McDonald 1979):

$$P = a + b(1 - e^{-ct})$$

Where

P = volume (ml) of gas produced at t time
a = volume (ml) of gas produced from rapidly degradable feed components

b = volume (ml) of gas produced from less rapidly degradable feed components
c = rate of gas production
t = incubation time

3 RESULTS AND DISCUSSION

3.1 *Fermentation parameters*

Data of gas production parameters for feed samples commonly fed to Timor deer when incubated with rumen fluid are presented in Table 1.

Fraction a indicates the amount of gas produced from a rapidly fermented fraction of a feed sample. This is the fraction that rumen microbes first ferment for them to obtain energy for immediate requirements. The results of this study indicated that there was a difference in the value between the wet and dry seasons for the same forage feed sample. Generally, the a value for a feed sample collected during the wet season was higher than the one obtained during the dry season, while the a value for the dry season often exhibited a negative value. The higher value for wet than for dry feed samples could be interpreted that there was a more degradable fraction of feed in wet than in dry season. Since the more degradable feed component consists mainly of rapidly available carbohydrates located inside the plant cells, the plant appears to switch its metabolic pathways to store more degradable carbohydrate inside the cell rather than structural components of the cell wall. Negative a values were observed for some feeds from samples collected during the dry season. This is not correct but it may have indicated the very small amounts of the fraction that was rapidly degradable and fermentable in these samples Orskov dan Ryle (1990). A practical implication we may draw

Table 1. Gas fermentation parameters of different feed samples collected during wet and dry + seasons when incubated with rumen fluid from Timor deer (*Cervus timorensis*).

No.	Feed Samples	a (ml/200 mg DM)	b (ml/200mg)	c (ml/h)	a + b (ml/ 200mg DM)
			Parameters		
1	Sesbania grandiflora (dry)	−1.769	72.169	0.063	70.399
2	Sesbania grandiflora (wet)	1.379	63.900	0.059	65.279
3	Leucaena leucocephala (dry)	4.642	49.041	0.035	53.683
4	Leucaena leucocephala (wet)	5.287	52.487	0.047	57.775
5	Glyricidia sepium (dry)	1.975	65.126	0.063	67.101
6	Glyricidia sepium (wet)	2.348	62.201	0.061	64.549
7	Zea mays (leaves, dry)	4.924	105.826	0.044	110.749
8	Zea mays (leaves, wet)	5.877	83.343	0.039	89.219
9	Water spinach, Ipomea aquatica (dry)	−4.995	74.487	0.057	69.491
10	Water spinach, Ipomea aquatica (wet)	5.877	83.343	0.039	89.219
11	King grass, Pennisetum purpureum (dry)	−1.579	73.233	0.038	71.653
12	King grass, Pennisetum purpureum (wet)	6.353	74.852	0.041	81.205
13	Native grasses (dry)	1.614	66.482	0.039	68.096
14	Native grasses (wet)	2.348	62.201	0.061	64.549
15	Rice bran	4.769	54.969	0.060	59.738
16	Copra meal	2.401	68.816	0.063	71.217
17	Tofu waste	−1.923	83.018	0.054	81.094

from this data is that there may be a need to provide more digestible and fermentable substrate for rumen microbes during dry season feeding.

Fraction b in this study indicates the proportion of feed organic matter that is degradable and fermentable at slower rates compared to the fraction a. This is the fraction that rumen microbes ferment after the rapidly fermentable organic matter has been depleted and become the major source of gas generated during the course of fermentation. In this study, there was no distinctive difference in the value of fraction b between forage feed samples collected during the wet and dry season, with a mean of 70.62 ($\pm$ 14.234) ml/200 g DM. For concentrate feeds, the mean ($\pm$ STDEV) value of b fraction was 68.93 ($\pm$ 14.025) ml/200 g DM. Fraction c indicates the mean rate of fermentative gas production from degraded feed organic matter, and in this study is expressed in ml per h. This fraction can be taken to reflect rates of feed breakdown in the rumen due to microbial degradation. (Please refer/discuss your data with the previous newest published report with the same ingredients, which can be compared with rumen fluid from cattle or other ruminants.)

3.2   Total and dynamics of gas production

Total gas production at the endpoint of 72 h fermentation and cumulative gas production profile during the course of fermentation are presented in Figures 1 and 2, respectively. The cumulative gas production profile is particularly helpful in making an overall comparison of

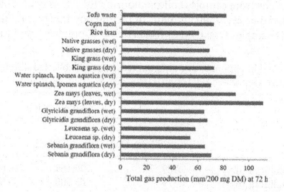

Figure 1.   Total fermentative gas production at 72 h of incubation with rumen fluid from Timor deer (*Cervus timorensis*) of different feed samples collected during wet and dry seasons.

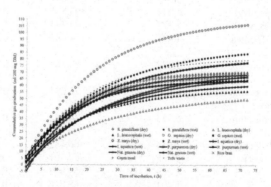

Figure 2.   Cumulative gas production profiles of different feed samples collected during wet and dry seasons when incubated with rumen fluid from Timor deer (*Cervus timorensis*) for 72 h.

the dynamics of gas production generated by different feeds during a given course of fermentation.

It can clearly be seen from both figures that Zea mays leave collected during the dry season produced the highest volume of fermentative gas and this was followed by the same feed collected during the wet season, while Leucaena leucocephala in the dry season generated the least volume of fermentative gas. The highest gas volume produced from Zea may leaves was probably due to adaptation developed by the rumen microbial consortium to degrade and ferment this feed. Animals used as rumen fluid donors were maintained on a diet based on Zea mays leaves, and it is expected that the microbial population in the rumen has adapted to this feed profile. Differences in the fermentative gas production between dry and wet seasons for Zea mays leaves may have been due to the feed factor in that there was more fermentable fraction present in this feed during the dry than the wet season.

The lowest gas production was observed for Leucaena leucocephala, either collected in the wet or dry season. This was probably due to the presence of secondary components in this tree legume, i.e., tannin and mimosine, which prevent optimum fermentation of the feed by the rumen microbes. Gas productions for other feeds, including three concentrate feed samples tested, were in between those for Zea mays leaves and Leucaena leucocephala.

4 CONCLUSION

It can be concluded that fermentation and degradation of feed in the rumen of Timor deer (Cervus timorensis) are different during wet and dry seasons, but the effect of season on feed fermentability varies from one feed to another. Among the common feeds given to Timor deer (Cervus timorensis) tested in the present study, the highest gas production was obtained for Zea mays leaves while the lowest one was exhibited by Leucaena leucocephala.

REFERENCES

Chen B.X. (1995). *Neway Exel: An Axel Application Programme for Processing Feed Degradability Data: User Manual.* UK: Rowet Research Institute Buckburn

Menke K.H. (1988). Estimation of the Energetic Feed Value Obtained From Chemical Analysis and in vitro Gas Production Using Rumen Fluid. *Animal research and development,* 28, 7–55.

Orskov E.R. (1992). *Protein Nutrition in Ruminant,* 2nd edition. UK: Academic Press Limited.

Orskov E.R. and Ryle M. (1990). *Energy Nutrition in Ruminants.* UK: Elsevier Applied Science

Orskov E.R. and McDonald I. (1979). The Estimation of Protein Degradability in the Rumen From Incubation Measurements Weighted According to Rate of Passage. *Journal of Agricultural Science,* 92, 499–503.

Puttoo M., Dryden G.M., and McCosker J.E. (1998). Performance of Weaned Rusa (Cervus timorensis) Deer Given Concentrates of Varying Protein Content with Sorghum Hay. *Australian Journal of Experimental Agriculture,* 38(1), 33–39.

Puttoo M., and Dryden G.M. (1998). Response of Rusa Deer Yearlings to Forage and Forage/concentrate Diets. *Animal Production in Australia,* 22, 336–336.

Theodorou M.K., Williams B.A., Dhanoa M.S., McAllan A.B., and France J. (1994). A Simple Gas Production Method Using a Pressure Transducer to Determine the Fermentation Kinetics of Ruminant Feeds. *Animal Feed Science and Technology,* 48(3–4), 185–197.

Developing Modern Livestock Production in Tropical Countries – Adli et al. (eds)
© 2023 The Authors, ISBN 978-1-032-44025-5
Open Access: www.taylorfrancis.com, CC BY-NC-ND 4.0 license

Factors affecting the production of pig farming in Minahasa Regency, North Sulawesi Province

M.A.V. Manese, N.M. Santa & P.O.V. Waleleng
Faculty of Animal Science, Universitas Sam Ratulangi, Manado City, North Sulawesi, Indonesia

ABSTRACT: This study aims to analyze the factors that affect the production of pig farming in Minahasa Regency. This research was conducted in Minahasa Regency with locations determined by purposive sampling method in West Kakas and Kakas Subdistricts, with the consideration that these locations have a high population of pigs and have more than one model of pig farming. The sample was determined by the total quota sampling method, so that there were 80 pig farmers respondents. The data were analyzed using multiple linear regression equation model with natural logarithms, to analyze the factors that affect the production of pigs. The results showed that there were 2 models of pig farming, the breeding model and the fattening model. The fattening model resulted in a higher number of pig production than the breeding model. Factors that affect the production of pig farming in Minahasa Regency, North Sulawesi Province are feed, body gain of piglets, labor, level of education. The amount of production in fattening model of pig farming is higher than breeding model.

Keywords: body weight gain, labor, pig, production

1 INTRODUCTION

The agricultural sector plays a very important role for the Indonesian economy, because of its contribution to the country's economic development. Agricultural businesses are generally cultivated by rural communities because they are able to provide food as well as absorb labor and contribute to household income. Pig farming is one of the businesses in the agricultural sector which is also able to provide food in the form of pork while absorbing family labor. People are interested in pig farming because in addition to meeting the needs of meat for the community, it also increases family income. If managed properly, pig farming can provide benefits for farmers, because pigs can be sold at weaning age (5–6 weeks) and 8–9 months with a body weight of 90–110 kg. In addition, the reproductive cycle and growth rate of pigs are relatively fast and require attention in aspects of maintenance management and feeding. Minahasa Regency has a fairly high population of pigs, especially in Sonder District, West Kakas District and Kakas District. (Thus, pig farming is one of the businesses carried out by the majority of rural communities in Minahasa. Pigs are also kept by the community for generations, although in general it is only done as a side business. Kakas Barat Subdistrict and Kakas Subdistrict are two subdistricts which are located close together, have the same regional characteristics because both are expansion areas of Kakas Subdistrict. Availability of feed is a major problem in pig farming because 70–80% of the costs incurred are feed costs (Kojo *et al.* 2014; Hardyastuti 2011; Santa *et al.* 2018; Sarajar *et al.* 2019; Sinulingga *et al.* 2020; Suranjaya, *et al.* 2017). The use of factory feed by farmers in West Kakas and Kakas Sub-districts causes farmers' dependence on the availability of feed and affects input costs. The behavior of farmers who use factory feed has an effect on

DOI: 10.1201/9781003370048-34

the fattening period of pigs. This study aims to analyze the factors of feed, body weight of piglets, labor, experience in raising livestock, and age of the breeder on the amount of production of fattening pigs in Kakas and Kakas Barat Districts, Minahasa Regency.

2 MATERIALS AND METHODS

The research location was carried out in West Kakas District and Kakas District during March – June 2022. The data used in this study are primary data and secondary data. Primary data is the result of observations and interviews with pig farmers as respondents. Secondary data in the form of data from the Central Bureau of Statistics and journals related to research. Determination of sub-districts using the purposive sampling method (Silalahi, 2015) in Kakas District and West Kakas District, with the consideration that the area has the largest population of pigs and is a fattening models of pig farm and breeding models. The sample of pig farmers was determined using total quota sampling so that there were 80 pig farmers.

2.1 Data analysis

To analyze the factors that affect the production of pigs, using the multiple linear regression equation according to Sujarwo (2019) which was modified with several related studies and adapted to pig farming, so that it is explained in the logarithmic model as follows.

$$\ln Y = b_0 + b_1 \ln X_1 + b_2 \ln X_2 + b_3 \ln X_3 + b_4 \ln X_4 + b_5 \ln X_5 + b_6 \ln X_6 + dD1 + e \quad (1)$$

where Y = production (kg/year); b0 = constant; b1, ... b7, d = regression coefficient; X1 = feed (kg/year); X2 = body gain of piglets (head/year); X3 = labor (HOK/year); X4 = farmer's age (years); X5 = level of education; X6 = farming experience (years); D = dummy variable; and e = error.

Statistical testing of the regression equation, using the F test and t test. To determine the effect of the independent variables (feed, body gain of piglets, labor, farmer's age, level education, and farming experience) on the dependent variable (amount of pig production), the F test was used (Winarno, 2015). The next test using the t test was used to determine the effect of each independent variable (feed, piglets, labor, farmer age and farming experience) partially on the dependent variable (amount of pig production) (Winarno, 2015).

3 RESULTS AND DISCUSSION

3.1 Pig farming characteristics

The characteristics of pig farming in Kakas District and West Kakas District are explained based on the use of feed, labor, cages and production of pigs. These characteristics explain the traditional way of pig farming on fattening models and breeding models. Pigs are raised intensively by farmers in cages. The function of the cage is to keep it easy to monitor and care for pigs. Based on research, the walls of the pigsty are made of concrete with a zinc roof and a cement floor. According to the farmer, the cage is made so that the pigs are safe and comfortable during pig farming. The area of the fattening pig pen is 200 cm × 300 cm and can accommodate 5 pigs. According to Kojo et al. (2014), the maintenance management carried out by farmers is an intensive handling pattern and in general the cages are made of concrete, both cage walls and floors. The results showed that only 23.33% of farmers used bamboo-walled cages, due to the limited capital of farmers to build concrete-walled cages. The results of the regression analysis of the factors that affect the production of pigs in

Kakas District and West Kakas District are described above. Based on the regression, model has an R-square value = 0.9878 which means that the variation of feed (X1), body gain of piglets (X2), labor (X3), farmer's age (X4), level of education (X5), farming experience (X6), dummy variable (D), can explain variation in pig production (Y) by 98.78%, while the remaining 1.22% variation is explained by variables not examined. The calculated F-value is 603.865 which is greater than the F-table, meaning that the variables feed (X1), body gain of piglets (X2), labor (X3), farmer's age (X4), level of education (X5), farming experience (X6), dummy variable (D) has a significant effect on pig production (Y). The factors that affect the amount of production of pigs are described as follows. The feed variable had a very significant effect on the swine production variable (P<0.001) with a regression coefficient of 1.1060. The regression coefficient of the feed variable is positive and in accordance with the expectation sign, meaning that for every 10 percent increase in the amount of feed consumed by livestock, the production of pigs will increase by 11.06%. This situation is in accordance with the research of Widayati *et al.* (2018) and Sani *et al.* (2020) that feed factors have a positive effect on pig production. Based on the research, it is known that the adequacy of feed, both in quality and quantity will determine the success of the production and reproduction of pigs. possible for farmers to increase the amount of feed to increase the amount of fattening pig production. The amount of feed given to livestock is already excessive, partly due to the wasted feed while farmers feed the pigs. The wasted feed is still counted as the total feed consumed by the pigs, resulting in a higher feed conversion value.

4 CONCLUSION

Factors that affect the production of pig farming in Minahasa Regency, North Sulawesi Province are feed, body gain of piglets, labor, level of education. The amount of production in fattening pig farming is higher than breeding pig farming.

REFERENCES

Dewantari M., Parimartha I.K. & Sukanata I.W. (2017). Profile Usaha Peternakan Babi Skala Kecil di Desa Puhu Kecamatan Payangan Kabupaten Gianyar. *Majalah Ilmiah Peternakan*, 20(2), 79–83.

Hardyastuti (2011). Kajian Biaya Produksi Pada Usaha Peternakan Babi. *Jurnal Sosek Peternakan Unibraw Malang*, 12 (1).

Kojo R.E., Panelewen V.V., Manese M.A. & Santa N. (2014). Efisiensi Penggunaan Input Pakan dan Keuntungan Pada Usaha Ternak Babi di Kecamatan Tareran Kabupaten Minahasa Selatan. *Zootec*, 34 (1), 62–74.

Sani A.S., Makandolu S.M. and Sogen J.G. (2020). Efficiency of Using Production Factors on Pig Household Scale Business in Ende Timur District, Ende Regency. *Jurnal Nukleus Peternakan*, 7(1), 41–50.

Santa N.M. & Wantasen E. (2018). Profit Analysis of Pig Farming in Rural Comunities in Minahasa Regency of North Sulawesi. *JITAA*, 43(3), 289–295.

Sarajar M.J., Elly F.H., Wantasen E. & Umboh S.J. (2019). Analisis Usaha Ternak Babi di Kecamatan Sonder Kabupaten Minahasa. *Zootec*, 39(2), 276–283.

Silalahi U. (2015). *Metode Penelitian Sosial Kuantitatif*. Indonesia: Refika Aditama Press.

Sinulingga Y.P., Santa N.M., Kalangi L.S. & Manese M.A. (2020). Analisis Pendapatan Usaha Ternak Babi di Kecamatan Tombulu Kabupaten Minahasa. *Zootec*, 40(2), 471–481.

Sujarwo. (2019). *Ekonomi Produksi, Teori dan Aplikasi*. Indonesia: UB Press.

Sukanata I., Suciani P. & Suranjaya I. (2014). Analisa Pendapatan dan EfisiensiEkonomis Penggunaan Pakan pada USAhatani Penggemukan Sapi Bali (Studi Kasus di Desa Lebih, Kabupaten Gianyar). *Majalah Ilmiah Peternakan*, 17(1), 164239.

Widayati T.W., Sumpe I., Irianti B.W., Iyai D.A. & Randa S.Y. (2018). Faktor-faktor Yang Mempengaruhi Produksi Usaha Ternak Babi di Teluk Doreri Kabupaten Manokwari. *Agrika*, 12(1), 73–82.

Winarno W.W. (2015). *Analisis Ekonometrika dan Statistika Dengan Eviews*. Indonesia: Upp Stim Ykpn.

Developing Modern Livestock Production in Tropical Countries – Adli et al. (eds)
© 2023 The Authors, ISBN 978-1-032-44025-5
Open Access: www.taylorfrancis.com, CC BY-NC-ND 4.0 license

Evaluation of forage production, feed supply, and quality measure standard at Bali cattle breeding center in Pulukan, Bali Province

R. Malindo, H.A.D. Wicaksono & Maskur
Directorate of General of Livestock and Animal Health Services, Ministry of Agriculture Republic of Indonesia, Jakarta, Indonesia

A. Jayanegara
Department of Nutrition and Feed Technology, Faculty of Animal Science, Bogor Agricultural University, Bogor, Indonesia

O. Sjofjan & S. Chuzaemi
Faculty of Animal Science, Universitas of Brawijaya, Malang, Indonesia

ABSTRACT: This study aimed to evaluate the current feed production, both forage and concentrate, and the nutritional status of Bali cattle the breeding center in Pulukan, Bali Province. This study was conducted using a survey. Data were collected through questionnaires and data analysis was conducted descriptively. Variables measured were the supply of dry matter (DM), crude protein (CP), and total digestible nutrients (TDN). The results showed that the Bali cattle population during 2019–2021 increased by 5.09%/yr. Based on forage production, the average supply of DM, CP, and TDN was 22.8%, 25.8%, and 24.3% of the demand, respectively. The average concentrate supply of DM, CP, and TDN was 29.1%, 45.2%, and 46.4% of the demand, respectively. Thus, the average feed (both forage and concentrate) supply was 52.2%, 70.6%, and 70.7% of the cattle requirements for DM, CP, and TDN, respectively. In conclusion, the current forage production and feed supply still did not me the cattle requirements for DM, CP, and TDN.

Keywords: forage production, feed supply, nutritional status, Bali cattle

1 INTRODUCTION

Bali cattle is one of the essential beef cattle breeds contributing to the developing livestock production in Indonesia. Bali cattle are indigenous beef cattle with a high potential for producing quality beef under local conditions. According to BPS (2020), there are currently 17 million heads of local beef cattle in Indonesia, divided among a variety of breeds, with Bali cattle having the largest population (34.9%). Feed is a significant factor in the success of cattle production because it provides nutrients needed to meet its nutrient requirements during production (Obese *et al.* 2013). Based on data from BPS (2017), feed is the most significant expense in beef cattle production, accounting for over 57 percent of total production costs. Challenges exist in any pasture-based system (Wilkinson *et al.* 2020) and crop-based systems, such as grass deficits which require flexible approaches and adaptive management. Forage deficits arise for various reasons, such as season, weather, and soil characteristics (Hurtado-Uria *et al.* 2013). Farmers may use higher concentrate supplementation to reduce the demand for forage during deficit periods. The nutritional status of the cattle needs to be closely monitored. Feed quantity, quality, and nutrient adequacy affect the productivity of beef cattle (Barbero *et al.* 2020). Thus, this study is needed to evaluate the

DOI: 10.1201/9781003370048-35

145

current feed production and the nutritional status of Bali cattle at the breeding center in Pulukan, Bali Province.

2 MATERIALS AND METHODS

This study was conducted at the Bali cattle breeding center of BPTU-HPT Denpasar in Pulukan, Jembrana Regency, Bali Province. The study was conducted using a survey from April to July 2022. The data were collected through direct interviews using questionnaire sheets, and the data type was quantitative. The data included cattle population structure, cattle body weight, cropland production, pasture production, concentrate feeding, and feed quality. The feed quality data included contents of dry matter (DM), organic matter (OM), neutral detergent fiber (NDF), non-fiber carbohydrate (NFC), ether extract (EE), crude protein (CP), and total digestible nutrients (TDN). The NDF grass and legume were calculated by using the equation of INRA (2018) as: NDF (g/kg) = 260 + 1,14 × CF (gr) and NDF (g/kg) = 320 + 0,575 × CF (gr), respectively. The NFC is calculated as: NFC = OM − (NDF + EE + CP). The TDN in forage and concentrate were calculated by using the equation of Jayanegara *et al.* (2019) as: TDN = 0.479 NDF + 0.704 NFC + 1.594 EE + 0.714 CP and TDN = 0.323 NDF + 0.883 NFC + 1.829 EE + 0.885 CP, respectively. Bali cattle nutrient requirements were calculated using the daily nutrient requirements of cattle in developing countries of Kearl (1982), presented in Table 1. Variables measured were the supply of DM, CP, and TDN. Data analysis was conducted descriptively.

3 RESULTS AND DISCUSSION

3.1 *Results*

Table 1 shows the population of Bali cattle in Pulukan has increased by 5.09% year^{-1}. The population increased from 1,084 heads in 2019 to 1,197 heads in 2021. The population structure was dominated by adult cattle which reached 61.1–74.0% of the total population, compared to young cattle 13.8–21.6% and calves 12.2–17.4%. Figure 1 shows the average body weight for calves, young, and adults were 92.8 ± 24.2 kg; 173.6 ± 47.5 kg; and 255.7 ± 82.7 kg, respectively. According to the cattle population, the average nutrient requirements of DM, CP, and TDN were 2,125.4 tons year^{-1}, 202.1 tons year^{-1}, and 983.8 tons year^{-1}, respectively.

Table 1. Population structure and the average body weight of Bali cattle based on age and sex.

Cattle Population	2019		2020		2021	
	Heads	Mean BW (kg)	Heads	Mean BW (kg)	Heads	Mean BW (kg)
Calf	132	93.8 ± 22.3 (n = 130)	171	96.4 ± 26.8 (n = 262)	208	85.9 ± 19.3 (n = 161)
– Male	61	94.5 ± 24.6 (n = 60)	91	100.0 ± 29.2 (n = 141)	101	86.0 ± 19.4 (n = 83)
– Female	71	93.2 ± 20.4 (n = 70)	80	92.2 ± 23.2 (n = 121)	107	85.8 ± 19.4 (n = 78)
Young	150	177.8 ± 49.1 (n = 240)	247	161.5 ± 44.8 (n = 179)	258	178.9 ± 46.1 (n = 210)
– Male	82	200.0 ± 54.7 (n = 123)	121	177.8 ± 46.7 (n = 93)	142	183.7 ± 50.0 (n = 121)
– Female	68	154.5 ± 27.5 (n = 117)	126	143.9 ± 35.2 (n = 86)	116	172.4 ± 39.6 (n = 89)
Adult	802	261.8 ± 76.3 (n = 188)	730	237.6 ± 89.8 (n = 152)	731	264.8 ± 80.9 (n = 178)
– Male	251	297.6 ± 76.8 (n = 104)	145	262.8 ± 107.8 (n = 87)	152	318.9 ± 82.4 (n = 83)
– Female	551	217.6 ± 47.0 (n = 84)	585	203.7 ± 37.3 (n = 65)	579	217.4 ± 39.3 (n = 95)
Total	1,084		1,148		1,197	

BW, body weight; calf, <1 year; young, 1–2 years; adult, >2 years (BPS, 2017).

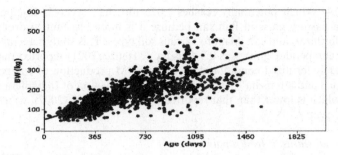

Figure 1.   Distribution of body weight based on age.

3.2 *Discussion*

3.2.1 *Bali cattle population*
This study indicated that the calves and young cattle population increased during 2019–2021, while adult cattle decreased from 802 heads in 2019 to 731 heads in 2021. The population of female cattle is higher than the population of male cattle. The ranges ratio of males to females is 31:69–36:64. The ratio of adult males to adult females is 1:3. The ratio of adult cattle is higher than the ratio recommended by Kementan (2006), which is 1:10. Timlin *et al.* (2021) reported that the average ratio of bulls to cows was 1:20–1:30, and a decrease in the ratio 1:60–1:72 did not cause a decrease in pregnancy rates. A decrease in the ratio of males and females can increase the economic value of livestock business because it is associated with lower costs for maintaining bulls.

3.2.2 *Current forage production*
The forage feeding system in Pulukan has been dependent on king grass (*Pennisetum purpuphoides*) which produced 86.7% of the forage crop production (Table 2). Another forage crop is a legume, i.e., Indigofera (*Indigofera zollingeriana*), and in the form of pasture, i.e., competidor grass (*Paspalum notatum cv. competidor*); their proportions were 4.6% and 8.7%, respectively. The fresh production of king grass in this study was lower than that reported by

Table 2.   Forage cropland and pasture production in Pulukan.

Forage	2019	2020	2021	Mean
Cropland:				
Grass, King grass				
– Land area (ha)	24.0	24.0	24.0	24.0
– Fresh forage production (ton)	2,145.4	2,681.3	2,896.8	2,574.5 ± 315.9
– Productivity (ton ha^{-1})	89.4	111.7	120.7	107.3 ± 13.2
– Contribution to forage supply (%)	85.1	87.6	87.4	86.7
Legume, Indigofera				
– Land area (ha)	2.5	2.5	2.5	2.5
– Fresh forage production (ton)	142.4	120.1	141.3	134.6 ± 10.2
– Productivity (ton ha^{-1})	56.8	48.0	56.4	53.7 ± 4.1
– Contribution to forage supply (%)	9.2	8.4	8.3	8.6
Pasture:	5.6	3.9	4.3	4.6
Competidor grass				
– Land area (ha)	70.0	70.0	70.0	70.0
– Fresh forage production (ton)	232.3	258.5	274.5	255.1 ± 21.3
– Productivity (ton ha^{-1})	3.3	3.7	3.9	3.6 ± 0.3
– Contribution to forage supply (%)	9.2	8.4	8.3	8.7

Suyitman (2014), which potentially reaches 1,076 tons ha^{-1} year^{-1}. Competidor grass is cultivated as a pasture grass in Pulukan because it is more resistant to drought, does not require much fertilizer, and can adapt to various soil types. This study's average annual DM production of competidor grass was 0.9 tons ha^{-1}. Heuzé (2021) reported that under rain-grown moderately fertilized conditions, the annual DM production of competidor grass is mostly between 3 and 8 tons ha^{-1}. The average DM production of Indigofera was 17.3 tons ha^{-1} year^{-1}, which is lower than that reported by Tarigan *et al.* (2007), which could reach 33.3 tons ha^{-1} year^{-1}.

3.2.3 *Nutritional status of feed supply*

Forage supply derived from grass and legumes provided DM, CP, and TDN on average 22.8%, 25.8%, and 24.2%, respectively. Thus, the feed was supplemented by concentrate to minimize the nutrient requirements gap. The average supply of DM, CP, and TDN from concentrate was 29.1%, 45.1%, and 46.4%, respectively. Supplementing concentrate in feed increased the provision of DM, CP, and TDN to 52.1%, 70.6%, and 70.6%, respectively. The nutrient supply of both forage and concentrate had not been able to meet the nutrient requirements of Bali cattle. Then, efforts must be made to increase the forage supply as the primary feed for ruminants.

4 CONCLUSION

The current forage production and feed supply still did not meet the cattle requirements for DM, CP, and TDN. Further improvement of cropland and pasture is required for forage production. Long-term strategies are necessary to promote sustainable forage production in the Pulukan breeding center.

REFERENCES

Barbero R.P., Malheiros E.B., Aguilar N.M., Romanzini E.P., Ferrari A.C., Nave R.L.G., Mullinks J.T., and Reis R.A. (2020). Supplementation Level Increasing Dry Matter Intake of Beef Cattle Grazing Low Herbage Height. *Journal Applied Animal Research*, 48(1), 28–33.

BPS. (2020). *Result of Intercostal Agricultural Survey 2018*. Jakarta: BPS-Statistics Indonesia.

BPS. (2017). *Result of Cost Structure of Livestock 2017*. Jakarta: BPS-Statistics Indonesia.

Heuzé V., Tran G., and Lebas F. (2021). Bahia Grass (Paspalum Notatum). *Feedipedia, a Programme by Inrae, Cirad, Afz and Fao.*

Hurtado-Uria C., Hennessy D., Shalloo L., O'Connor D., and Delaby L. (2013). Relationships between Meteorological Data and Grass Growth Over Time in the South of Ireland. *Irish Geography*, 46(3), 175–201.

[INRA] Institut National De La Recherche Agronomique. (2018). Alimentation Des Ruminants. Edition Quae. Versailles, France, p.728.

Jayanegara A., Ridla M., Nahrowi and Laconi E.B. (2019). Estimation and Validation of total Digestible Nutrient Values of Forage and Concentrate Feedstuffs. *IOP Conference Series: Materials Science and Engineering, 546*(4).

Kearl L.C. (1982). *Nutrient Requirements of Ruminants in Developing Countries*. International Feedstuffs Institute, Utah State University, Logan.

Kementan. (2006). *Peraturan Menteri Pertanian Nomor 54 Tahun 2006, tentang Pedoman Pembibitan Sapi Potong yang Baik (Good Breeding Practices)*. Jakarta: Kementerian Pertanian.

NRC. (2000). *Nutrient Requirements of Beef Cattle*, 7th Revised Edition. Washington D.C: National Academy Press.

Obese F., Acheampong, D. and Darfour-Oduro, K. 2013. Growth and Reproductive Traits of Friesian x Sanga Crossbred Cattle in the Accra Plains of Ghana. *African Journal of Food, Agriculture, Nutrition and Development*, 13(57), 7357–7371.

Suyitman. (2014). Produktivitas Rumput Raja (Pennisetum Purpupoides) Pada Pemotongan Pertama Menggunakan Beberapa Sistem Pertanian. *Jurnal Peternakan Indonesia*, 16(2), 119–127.

Tarigan A., Abdullah L., Ginting S.P. and Permana, D.I.G. (2010). Produksi dan Komposisi Nutrisi Serta Kecernaan in-vitro Indigofera sp. Pada Interval dan Tinggi Pemotongan Berbeda. *J. Ilmu Ternak and Veteriner*, 15(3), 188–195.

Timlin C.L., Dias N.W., Hungerford L., Redifer T., Currin J.F. and Mercadante V.R.G. (2021). A Retrospective Analysis of Bull:Cow Ratio Effects on Pregnancy Rates of Beef Cows Previously Enrolled in Fixed-time Artificial Insemination Protocols. *Translational Animal Science*, 5(3), 1–9.

Wilkinson J.M., Lee M.R.F., Rivero M.J. and Chamberlain A.T. (2020). Some Challenges and Opportunities for Grazing Dairy Cows on Temperate Pastures. *Grass Forage Science*, 7591, 1–17.

Developing Modern Livestock Production in Tropical Countries – Adli et al. (eds)
© 2023 The Authors, ISBN 978-1-032-44025-5
Open Access: www.taylorfrancis.com, CC BY-NC-ND 4.0 license

Breeding value estimation using an animal model for selecting Saburai goats based on weaning and yearling weight

A. Dakhlan, P.E. Santosa & D. Kurniawati
Department of Animal Husbandry, Faculty of Agriculture, Universitas Lampung, Bandar Lampung, Lampung, Indonesia

ABSTRACT: This research was conducted with aiming to estimate genetic parameters (heritability, genetic correlation) and breeding value using an animal model to select Saburai goats based on weaning and yearling weight. Data on weaning and yearling weight of fifty Saburai goats generated from nine bucks and eleven dams were used in this study. Heritability, genetic, and phenotypic correlation were estimated using animal models with the help of the WOMBAT program. The results showed that heritability estimates for weaning and yearling weight were moderate to high category (0.34 ± 0.18 and 0.44 ± 0.15, respectively). Genetic and phenotypic correlation between weaning and yearling weight was categorized as a high positive value (0.45 ± 0.16 and 0.56, respectively). The moderate to high heritability and positive genetic correlation between weaning and yearling weight implied that selection for either weaning weight or yearling weight would succeed.

Keywords: Breeding value, genetic parameters, Saburai goat, Weaning weight, yearling weight

1 INTRODUCTION

Saburai goat is one of the local goats in Lampung Province, resulting from grading up to Boer goat with the terminal composition of 75% Boer goat and 25% Ettawa grade (EG) goat (Dakhlan *et al.* 2021, 2022). This new meat type goat was established by the Ministry of Agriculture as a local goat of Lampung Province in 2015 (Sulastri *et al.* 2018). Improvements in the genetic quality and productivity of Saburai goats continue to be carried out. The selection program is one of the efforts to improve the genetic quality and productivity of Saburai goats. The selection program needs genetic parameters such as heritability estimates and genetic correlation between traits and also estimated breeding value (EBV) of the traits that we are interested in. The genetic parameters are used to predict direct and correlated responses to selection for improving the traits in the future (Javed *et al.* 2004). Research on genetic parameters for weaning and yearling weight, especially in Saburai goats was still limited. Beyleto *et al.* (2010) reported that heritability estimates for weaning and yearling weight of Boerawa (Boer goat × Ettawa Grade goat) estimated using paternal half-sib correlation were 0.30 ± 0.17 and 0.80 ± 0.04, respectively, with a genetic correlation between the two traits was 0.21 ± 0.03. Sulastri *et al.* (2018) reported that heritability estimates for weaning and yearling weight in Saburai goats using the variance analysis method recommended by Becker (1992) were 0.24 ± 0.08 and 0.29 ± 0.17, respectively. Different authors (Adhianto *et al.* 2022) also reported that the genetic and phenotypic correlation between weaning and yearling weight of female Saburai goats using paternal half-sib correlation was 0.30 and 0.27, respectively. These different results of genetic parameters might be due to different time and different method analysis. Breeding value estimation using an

DOI: 10.1201/9781003370048-36

animal model for weaning and yearling weight in Saburai goats have not been performed. Therefore, the present study was conducted to estimate genetic parameters and breeding value of weaning and yearling weight using animal model and used these parameters to select Saburai goat based on the weaning and yearling weight.

2   MATERIALS AND METHOD

Weaning (3 months of age) and yearling weight data of fifty male and female Saburai kids generated from nine bucks and eleven dams were used in this study. Co(variance) components were estimated using an animal model with the help of the WOMBAT program (Meyer 2007). Univariate analysis based on best linear unbiased prediction (BLUP) was used to get the EBV of individual goats and heritability estimates, while for estimating the genetic and phenotypic correlation between weaning and yearling weight we applied bivariate analysis. The animal model for univariate analysis is formulated as follows:

$$y = Xb + Z_1a + Z_2m + e$$

where y is the vector of observations for weaning weight and yearling weight, b is fixed effects (sex, birth type, and birth year), and a is random direct additive genetic effects of the goats. While m is random maternal genetic effects and e is the random residual error. Furthermore, X, Z_1, and Z_2 are incidence matrices related to fixed, additive genetic, and maternal genetic effects, respectively. It was assumed that zero was set for the covariance of the direct and maternal genetic effects.

3   RESULTS AND DISCUSSION

3.1   *Weaning weight and yearling weight of Saburai goat*

The results of this research showed that the weaning and yearling weights of Saburai goats were 16.63 ± 3.00 kg and 36.88 ± 9.01 kg, respectively. The weaning weight and yearling weight of the Saburai goat in this study were similar to those reported by Adhianto *et al.* (2016) who concluded that the weaning and yearling weight of male Saburai goats in two different locations were 16.22 ± 3.77 kg and 36.56 ± 4.85 kg, respectively, in Gisting district, and 16.85 ± 2.58 kg and 38.30 ± 5.35 kg, respectively, in Sumberejo district. Adhianto *et al.* (2022) reported that the weaning weight and yearling weight of female Saburai goats were 16.4 ± 2.0 kg and 36.9 ± 2.5 kg, respectively. The weaning weight of this result is also similar to the weaning weight of the Saburai goat reported by Adhianto *et al.* (2016) which was 16.85 ± 2.58 kg, and reported by Pratama *et al.* (2020) was 17.20 ± 1.69 kg and 17.36 ± 2.24 kg, respectively, for the weaning weight at the first and second parity. A bit different in results of this study and previous study might be due to different times, sex, location, genetics, and environment.

3.2   *Heritability estimates of weaning weight and yearling weight*

The result of this study showed that heritability estimates for the weaning and yearling weight of Saburai goats were 0.34 ± 0.18 and 0.44 ± 0.15, respectively. The results of the present study were higher than those reported by Sulastri *et al.* (2018) which were 0.24 ± 0.08 and 0.29 ± 0.17, respectively, and reported by Beyleto *et al.* (2010) which were 0.30 ± 0.17 and 0.80 ± 0.04, respectively in Boerawa (Boer goat × Ettawa Grade goat). However, the result of the present study was lower than those reported by Hasan *et al.* (2014) that the heritability estimates of weaning and yearling weight of Ettawa Grade goat were 0.35 ± 0.07 and 0.68 ± 0.16, respectively, and reported by Bhattarai *et al.* (2017) that heritability estimates for weaning weight of Khari goats were 0.42 ± 0.13.

3.3 Genetic and phenotypic correlation between weaning weight and yearling weight

The genetic and phenotypic correlation between the weaning weight and yearling weight of Saburai goats of this research were 0.45 ± 0.16 and 0.56, respectively. The result of the genetic and phenotypic correlation of the present study was higher than those reported by Adhianto *et al.* (2022) which were 0.30 and 0.27, respectively, in Saburai goat, and reported by Beyleto *et al.* (2010) in Boerawa goat which was 0.21 ± 0.03. However, the results of this study were lower than those reported by Hasan *et al.* (2014) which were 0.708 and 0.653, respectively in Ettawa Grade goat. This difference in the genetic and phenotypic correlation was maybe because of different methods applied.

3.4 Breeding value of weaning and yearling weight

The estimated breeding value (EBV) of weaning and yearling weight is shown in Figure 1. It can be seen that the variation of EBV both for weaning and yearling weight was quite high. There were 22 individuals with EBV based on weaning weight higher than the average EBV (0.1164, red line in Figure 1) and there were 11 kids with top 25% EBV (blue line in Figure 1), so did for yearling weight there were 22 individuals with EBV higher than the average EBV (0.3493) and there were 11 kids with top 25% EBV.

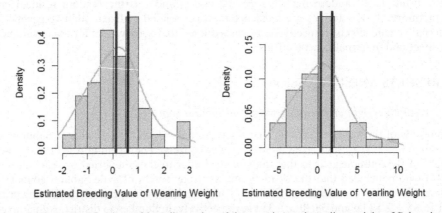

Figure 1.   Histogram of estimated breeding value of the weaning and yearling weight of Saburai goat.

The result of this research showed that the selection program would be successful because the variation of EBV for both weaning and yearling weight was quite high and the heritability estimate for both traits was also moderate to high category (0.34 ± 0.18 and 0.44 ± 0.15, respectively). In addition, selection program would be successful as well either for weaning weight or yearling weight because the genetic correlation between the two traits was positive (0.45 ± 0.16) meaning that improvement of weaning weight will be followed by the improvement of yearling weight.

Response to the selection of weaning and yearling weight were increased with increasing selection intensity ranging from 0.20 kg to 1.79 kg and 0.77 kg to 6.96 kg for weaning and yearling weight, respectively, at 90% to 10% selection proportion. Furthermore, the expected correlated response to selection for yearling weight by directly selecting first for weaning weight ranged from 0.31 kg to 2.75 kg at a selection proportion of 90% to 10%. This study indicated that direct selection of yearling weight (0.77 to 6.96 kg selection response per generation) was better than indirect selection by selecting weaning weight first (0.31 kg to 2.75 kg selection response per generation).

4 CONCLUSION

The selection program of Saburai goats based on weaning weight and yearling weight would be quite successful because of moderate to high heritability estimates and a quite high variation of the goat breeding value. Improvement of weaning weight would be followed by the improvement of the yearling weight of the Saburai goat because of the positive genetic and phenotypic correlation between the two traits. Indirect selection to improve yearling weight by improving weaning weight first would result in lower responses to selection compared to direct selection to yearling weight of Saburai goat.

ACKNOWLEDGEMENT

The authors are very grateful to the Directorate General of Higher Education of the Ministry of Education, Culture, Research, and Technology of the Republic of Indonesia who has funded this research, namely the national competitive basic research scheme with contract number 2152/UN26.21/PN/2022.

REFERENCES

Adhianto K., Hamdani M.D.I., Sulastri S., and Listiana I. (2016). Performan Produksi Kambing Saburai Jantan Pada Dua Wilayah Sumber Bibit di Kabupaten Tanggamus. *Sains Peternakan: Jurnal Penelitian Ilmu Peternakan*, 14(2), 22–29.

Adhianto K., Lenanto S.I., Dakhlan A., and Hamdani M. (2022). Genetic and Phenotypic Correlation of Weaning and Yearling Weight of Female Saburai Goats in Sumberejo District, Tanggamus Regency, Lampung Province, Indonesia. *Advances in Animal and Veterinary Sciences*, 10(2), 42-1-426.

Becker A. (1992). *Manual of Quantitative Genetics*, 5th ed. Pullman, USA: Academic Enterprises.

Beyleto V.Y., and Hartatik T. (2010). Estimasi Parameter Genetik Sifat Pertumbuhan Kambing Boerawa di Kabupaten Tanggamus Propinsi Lampung (Genetic Parameters Estimation on Growth Traits of Boerawa Goat at Tanggamus Regency Lampung Province). *Buletin Peternakan*, 34(3), 138–144.

Bhattarai N., Kolachhapati M.R., Devkota N.R., Thakur U.C., and Neopane S.P. (2017). Estimation of Genetic Parameters of Growth Traits of Khari Goat Kids (Capra hircus L.) in Nawalparasi, Nepal. *International Journal Livestock Research*, 7(1), 80–89.

Dakhlan A., Hamdani M.D.I., Putri D. R., Sulastri S., and Qisthon A. (2021). Prediction of Body Weight Based on Body Measurements in Female Saburai Goat. *Biodiversitas Journal of Biological Diversity*, 22(3).

Dakhlan A., Qisthon A., and Hamdani M. (2022). Genetic Evaluation and Selection Response of Birth Weight and Weaning Weight in Male Saburai Goats. *Jurnal Agripet*, 22(1), 17–25.

Hasan F., and Gunawan A. (2014). Genetic and Phenotypic Parameters of Body Weight in Ettawa Grade Goats. *Media Peternakan*, 37(1), 8–8.

Javed K., Abdullah M., Akhtar M., and Afzal M. (2004). Phenotypic and Genetic Correlations Between First Lactation Milk Yield and Some Performance Traits in Sahiwal Cattle. *Pakistan Veterinary Journal*, 24(1), 9–12.

Meyer K. (2007). WOMBAT—A Tool for Mixed Model Analyses in Quantitative Genetics by Restricted Maximum Likelihood (REML). *Journal of Zhejiang University Science B*, 8(11), 815–821.

Pratama A.G., Dakhlan A., Sulastri S., and Hamdani M.D.I. (2020). Seleksi Induk Kambing Saburai Berdasarkan Nilai Most Probable Producing Ability Bobot Lahir dan Bobot Sapih. *Jurnal Ilmiah Peternakan Terpadu*, 8(1), 33–40.

Sulastri S., Siswanto S., and Adhianto K. (2018). Genetic Parameter for Growth Performance of Saburai Goat in Tanggamus District, Lampung Province, Indonesia. *Advances in Animal and Veterinary Sciences*, 6(11), 486–491.

Developing Modern Livestock Production in Tropical Countries – Adli et al. (eds)
© 2023 The Authors, ISBN 978-1-032-44025-5
Open Access: www.taylorfrancis.com, CC BY-NC-ND 4.0 license

SNP profile of c.400G>A, c.4905C>G, and c.4957C>G of the MSTN genes in Bali cattle using PCR-RFLP technique

A. Fahira, R. Maulidah, I. Kariemah, S.N. Sadrina, R.R. Noor, C. Sumantri, Muladno & Jakaria*
IPB University, Bogor, Dramaga, Indonesia

ABSTRACT: The myostatin (MSTN) gene is one of the genes that influence the growth of beef cattle that can improve the quality and quantity of meat. This study aimed to analyze the polymorphism of the MSTN gene in Bali cattle using PCR-RFLP. The total DNA sample used was 120 samples consisting of 50 Bali cattle from BPTU-HPT Denpasar, 50 Bali cattle from BPT-HMT Serading, and 20 Limousine cattle from BPTU-HPT Padang Mangatas. The polymorphism of SNPs c.400G>A, c.4905C>G, and c.4957C>G of the MSTN gene was analyzed using PCR-RFLP. Therefore, Hind-III, BsrI, and Alu-I enzymes were used as restriction enzymes. Genotype and allele frequencies, heterozygosity, and Hardy–Weinberg equilibrium were analyzed using Popgene32. The results show that SNPs c.400G>A and c.4905C>G of the MSTN gene have 2 alleles. Based on the results, it can be concluded that the SNPs c.400G>A of the MSTN gene were polymorphic, while SNPs c.4905C>G and c.4957C>G were monomorphic.

Keywords: Bali cattle, myostatin gene, PCR-RFLP, polymorphism

1 INTRODUCTION

Indonesia has a variety of animal genetic resources that can be used to increase its productivity and population. Beef cattle, for example, are bred for meat production. According to Statistics Indonesia (2021), the population of beef cattle in Indonesia has reached 18,053,710 heads, an increase of about 3.51% over the previous year's population of 17,440,393 heads. However, this increase has not been sufficient to meet the national meat consumption. The annual beef and buffalo production in Indonesia has reached 458,755 tons (BPS 2021), while beef and buffalo consumption reached 717,150 tons per year. Several studies of MSTN gene polymorphisms in beef cattle have been carried out, including the first generation of Belgian blue cattle in Indonesia (Agung et al. 2016), Belgian blue crossbreed cattle (Jakaria et al. 2021), and Bali cattle (Khasanah et al. 2016). According to Aliyya's et al. (2020) study on the MSTN gene polymorphism, 18 SNPs were found in the MSTN gene in Bali cattle using a sequencing technique, and SNPs c.400G>A, c.4905C>G, and c.4957C>G were three of them that affected cattle growth and carcass. Therefore, it is necessary to analyze the polymorphisms of the three SNPs (c.400G>A, c.4905C>G, and c.4957C>G) of the MSTN gene in Bali cattle because there has not been any study yet.

---

*Corresponding Author: jakaria@apps.ipb.ac.id

DOI: 10.1201/9781003370048-37

2 MATERIALS AND METHODS

This study was carried out at IPB University's Faculty of Animal Science's laboratory of animal molecular genetics. This study used 120 DNA samples consisting of 50 Bali cattle from BPTU-HPT Denpasar, 50 Bali cattle from BPT-HMT Serading, and 20 Limousine cattle from BPTU-HPT Padang Mangatas.

The primers used for the SNP c.400G>A were forward primers (5'- CAA GTT GTC TCT CAG ACT GG-3') and reverse primers (5'- GAG GAG GAA TGT ATG TTG GG-3') referring to the study of Aliyyah et al. (2020), which will amplify exon 1 of the MSTN gene and produced a 608 bp PCR product. The National Center for Biotechnology Information (NCBI) provided the primer sequence used for the SNPs c.4905C>G and c.4957C>G in this study under the accession number AY794986.1. Primer3 Program was used to create the primer design, and Primer Stat was used to evaluate the primer design with forward and reverse primers (5'-CTC TTC TTT CCT TTC CAT ACA GAC-3' and 5'-AGG GGA AGA CCT TCC ATG TT-3') which will amplify exon 3 of the MSTN gene and produced a 451 bp PCR product.

DNA amplification was carried out using an Applied Biosystems PCR Thermal Cycler. According to the PCR conditions that matched the MSTN gene fragment, the DNA amplification condition consisted of three stages: denaturation, annealing, and extension. 1 μL of the extracted DNA sample was transferred to a 0.2 mL tube. DNA amplification reagent consisting of 7.5 μL of PROMEGA Green Master Mix, 6.1 μL of Nuclease Free Water, 0.2 μL of forward primer, and 0.2 μL of reverse primer was placed in a 1.5 μL tube and homogenized the reagent. PCR reagents were distributed to the DNA samples, then homogenized using a rotary mixer and placed into the PCR machine. DNA amplification was carried out under conditions of 95°C predenaturation for 1 minute, 95°C denaturation for 15 seconds, 55°C (c.400G>A) and 58°C (c.4905C>G & c.4957C>G) annealing for 15 seconds, and 72°C extension for 10 seconds. The DNA amplification process was repeated for up to 35 cycles. The PCR products were then electrophoresed on a 1.5% agarose gel to confirm the PCR results.

SNP c.400G>A, c.4905C>G, and c.4957C>G of the MSTN gene were genotyped using PCR-RFLP. Hind-III, BsrI, and Alu-I enzymes were used as restriction enzymes. A total of 5 μL of PCR product was transferred to a 0.2 ml tube. The tube was inserted, then the mixing was made. The mixture consists of 0.9 µl of DW, 0.4 µl of SaqI enzyme, and 0.7 µl of SacI enzyme buffer. The mixture was incubated in an incubator at 65°C for 4 hours. 7 µl of incubated DNA was visualized using a 2% agarose gel. Genotype and allele frequency observed and expected heterozygosity, and Hardy–Weinberg equilibrium were calculated using Popgene32 program (Yeh et al. 2000).

3 RESULTS AND DISCUSSION

The myostatin gene was amplified at an annealing temperature of 55°C for exon 1 and 58°C for exon 3. The amplification obtained a PCR product length of 608 bp and 451 bp as shown in Figure 1.

The Popgene32 program was used to calculate the MSTN gene analysis polymorphism in Bali and Limousine cattle. Genotype and allele frequencies, heterozygosity, and χ^2 value of the SNP c.400G>A of the MSTN gene are shown in Table 1.

The GG genotype was the highest genotype frequency in Bali cattle at BPTU HPT Denpasar and BPT-HPT Serading, while the GA genotype had a low frequency, with the highest allele being the G allele. The allele of the MSTN gene in Bali cattle was polymorphic, while in Limousine cattle was monomorphic because it has only one allele. A population is said to be polymorphic if it has more than one allele at a single locus (Ismail & Essawi 2012). The mutation in the SNP c.400G>A of the myostatin gene was a transition mutation at the

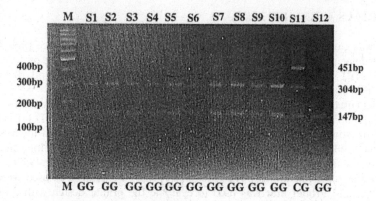

M   S1 S2 S3 S4 S5   S6   S7 S8 S9 S10 S11 S12

400bp   451bp
300bp   304bp
200bp
                                                                     147bp
100bp

M GG GG GG GG GG GG GG GG GG GG CG GG

Figure 1.   The exon 3 of MSTN|Hind-III gene genotype product visualization (line S1-S12 = analyzed samples and M = marker 100 bp).

Table 1.   Genotype and allele frequencies, heterozygosity, and χ^2 value of the SNP c.400G>A of the MSTN gene.

Cattle Breeds	N	Genotype frequency			Allele frequency		He	Ho	χ^2 value
		GG	GA	AA	G	A			
Bali BPTU-HPT Denpasar	50	0.94	0.06	0.00	0.97	0.03	0.05	0.06	0.03[ns]
Bali BPT-HMT Serading	50	0.92	0.08	0.00	0.96	0.04	0.07	0.08	0.04[ns]
Limousin BPTU Padang Mangatas	20	1.00	0.00	0.00	1.00	0.00	0.00	0.00	na

N = number of cattle, ns = not significant (P-value > 0.05), na = not analyzed

400 bases from the guanine base (G) to the adenine base (A) (Aliyya et al. 2020). Table 1 shows that the heterozygosity value in the two Bali cattle populations (BPTU-HPT Denpasar and BPT-HMT Serading) is less than 0.5, whereas the heterozygosity value in limousine cattle is zero. A heterozygosity value of less than 50% (0.5) indicates that the variation of a gene in the population is low (Dorji et al. 2012). Heterozygosity value is influenced by several factors, including mutation rate, effective population size, random or selected mating patterns, migration, and selection (Rell et al. 2013).

Genotype and allele frequencies, heterozygosity, and χ^2 value of the SNPs c.4905C>G and c.4957C>G of the MSTN gene are shown in Table 2.

Based on the results of the MSTN gene genotype identification in Bali cattle, two genotypes (GG and CG) and two alleles (C and G) were obtained. The GG genotype had the highest genotype frequency on SNP c.4905C>G in Bali cattle, with the highest allele is the G allele. The SNP c.4957C>G in Bali cattle and limousine cattle were monomorphic because they only had one allele. The SNP c.4905C>G in Bali cattle is also monomorphic because a gene is said to be polymorphic if one of its alleles is less than 99% or more than 1% (Nei & Kumar 2000).

The observed heterozygosity (Ho) and expectation heterozygosity (He) value of the SNP c.4905C>G in Bali cattle from BPTU-HPT Denpasar had the same value (0.02), while the heterozygosity value in Bali cattle from BPTU-HPT Serading showed that the MSTN gene in Bali cattle was monomorphic where the heterozygosity value showed 0.00. The low value of heterozygosity in a population will affect the sustainability of the population due to the presence of homozygous alleles (Allendorf et al. 2013). According to Dorji et al. (2012), a

Table 2. Genotype and allele frequencies, heterozygosity, and χ^2 value of the SNP c.4905C>G and c.4957C>G of the MSTN gene.

Cattle Breeds	N	SNP	Genotype frequency			Allele frequency		He	Ho	χ^2 value
			CC	CG	GG	C	G			
Bali BPTU-HPT Denpasar	50	c.4905C>G	0.00	0.02	0.98	0.01	0.99	0.02	0.02	0.005[ns]
		c.4957C>G	1.00	0.00	0.00	1.00	0.00	0.00	0.00	na
Bali BPT-HMT Serading	50	c.4905C>G	0.00	0.00	1.00	0.00	1.00	0.00	0.00	na
		c.4957C>G	1.00	0.00	0.00	1.00	0.00	0.00	0.00	na
Limousin BPTU Padang Mangatas	20	c.4905C>G	0.00	0.00	1.00	0.00	1.00	0.00	0.00	na
		c.4957C>G	1.00	0.00	0.00	1.00	0.00	0.00	0.00	na

N = number of cattle, ns = not significant (P-value > 0.05), na = not analyzed

heterozygosity value of less than 50% (0.5) indicates that the variation of a gene in the population is low.

4 CONCLUSION

The SNP c.400G>A of the MSTN gene in Bali cattle was polymorphic, with 2 alleles G and A, and was in Hardy--Weinberg equilibrium. The SNPs c.4905C>G and c.4957C>G of the MSTN gene Bali cattle were monomorphic.

REFERENCES

Agung P.P., Said S., & Sudiro A. (2016). Myostatin Gene Analysis in the First Generation of the Belgian Blue Cattle in Indonesia. *Journal of Indonesian Tropical Animal Agriculture*, 41(1), 13–20.

Allendorf F.W., Luikart G. & Aitken S.N. (2013). *Conservation ang the Genetics of Populations*. 2nd Ed. United Kingdom: Willey and Blackwell.

Aliyya W.L.N., & Noor R.R. (2020, April). Exploring SNPs (Single Nucleotide Polymorphisms) of Myostatin Gene in Coding Region in Bali Cattle. In *IOP Conference Series: Earth and Environmental Science* (Vol. 492, No. 1, p. 012064). IOP Publishing.

Dorji N., Duangjinda M., & Phasuk Y. (2012). Genetic Characterization of Bhutanese Native Chickens Based on an Analysis of Red Junglefowl (Gallus gallus gallus and Gallus gallus spadecieus), Domestic Southeast Asian and Commercial Chicken Lines (Gallus gallus domesticus). *Genetics and Molecular Biology*, 35, 603–609.

Ismail S., & Essawi M. (2012). Genetic Polymorphism Studies in Humans. *Middle East Journal of Medical Genetics*, 1(2), 57–63.

Jakaria J., Aliyya W.L.N., Ismail R., Siswanti S.Y., Ulum M.F., & Priyanto R. (2021). Discovery of SNPs and Indel 11-bp of the Myostatin Gene and its Association with the Double-muscled Phenotype in Belgian Blue Crossbred Cattle. *Gene*, 784, 145598.

Khasanah H., Gunawan A., Priyanto R., Ulum M. F., & Jakaria J. (2016). Polymorphism of Myostatin (MSTN) Promoter Gene and its Association with Growth and Muscling Traits in Bali Cattle. *Media Peternakan*, 39(2), 95–103.

Nei M., & Kumar S. (2000). *Molecular Evolution and Phylogenetics*. Oxford University Press, USA.

Rell F., Widyastuti S.K. & Wandia I.N. 2013. Polimorfisme Lokus Mikrosatelit D10S1432 Pada Populasi Monyet Ekor Panjang di Sangeh. *Jurnal Ilmu dan Kesehatan Hewan*, 1(1), 16–21.

Statistics Indonesia. (2021). *Statistik Indonesia 2021*. Jakarta: Statictics Indonesia.

Yeh F., Yang R.C., Boyle T.B.J., Ye Z., Xiyan J., Yang R. & Boyle T.J. (2000). *PopGene32, Microsoft Windows-based Freeware for Population Genetic Analysis*. Version 1.32.

Developing Modern Livestock Production in Tropical Countries – Adli et al. (eds)
© 2023 The Authors, ISBN 978-1-032-44025-5
Open Access: www.taylorfrancis.com, CC BY-NC-ND 4.0 license

Influence of different prolonged aging times on the goat milk kefir quality

A.K. Umam, L.E. Radiati* & A.M. Wati

Lecturer of Animal Product Technology Department, Faculty of Animal Science, Brawijaya University, Malang, Indonesia

M.R. Rifano

Student of Animal Product Technology Department, Faculty of Animal Science, Brawijaya University, Malang, Indonesia

D.A.A. Putri

Student of Animal Product Technology Department, Faculty of Animal Science, Brawijaya University, Kediri, Indonesia

ABSTRACT: Kefir is a fermented beverage containing lactic acid bacteria as a natural starter combined with yeast. The lactic acid and alcoholic fermentation processes continuously throughout the kefir production process. The culture fermentation is finished after 12 to 24 hours, cooled to 10 to 15 degrees, and kept for several days as part of the aging process. Factors influencing Goat Milk Kefir quality prolonged aging times of 7, 14, and 21 days were studied to develop a Goat Milk Kefir production method. The experimental design was a completely randomized design (CRD) with four treatments and three replications. Duncan Multiple Range Test (DMRT) was used for further statistical analysis. The results show that the best taste and texture were found with Prolonged Aging Time at 14 days. Under aging process conditions for 21 days, goat Milk kefir gave the best flavor and pH value. Fermentation without Prolonged Aging Time resulted in significant results in water-holding capacity.

Keywords: Aging Process, Goat milk kefir, Quality

1 INTRODUCTION

Since the beginning of the twenty-first century, the benefits of probiotics microbiota on the human gut have considerably raised public interest in scientific research. Probiotics are live bacteria that provide the host health benefits when taken at the appropriate level (Hill *et al.* 2014). Fermentation procedures using Lactic Acid Bacteria (LAB) as probiotic bacteria could increase nutritional quality by enhancing the products' texture and preventing the multiplication of food pathogens (Umam *et al.* 2019). Kefir is a fermented milk beverage with kefir grains or kefir cultures containing yeasts and molds. Certain species of yeasts and molds can convert complex molecules into simpler ones, allowing the human body to absorb fermented foods efficiently and also aiming to enhance the quality of food (Radiati *et al.* 2020). According to a study (Baniasadi *et al.* 2022), Kefir contains probiotics and has a more potent antioxidant activity than yogurt. The antioxidant activity of fermented milk products containing Lactobacillus bulgaricus and Streptococcus thermophilus as probiotics ranged

---

*Corresponding Author: lilik.eka@ub.ac.id

DOI: 10.1201/9781003370048-38

from 61.73% to 85.27% after 21 days of storage (Khoirul Umam *et al.* 2018). The lactic acid and alcoholic fermentation processes continuously throughout the kefir production process. The culture fermentation is finished after 12 to 24 hours, cooled to 10 to 15 degrees, and kept for several hours as part of the aging process. In addition, the aging process increases the lactose fermented by the lactase enzyme, hence increasing the quantity of lactic acid produced (Triwibowo *et al.* 2020). The prolonged aging times probably affect the quality of Goat milk kefir products. This research purpose is to study the length of aging times of goat milk kefir based on pH value, water-holding capacity, and sensory quality during 21 days of aging times.

2 MATERIALS AND METHODS

The materials used in manufacturing kefir include goat milk, skim milk powder, L. bulgaricus 12297, and S. thermophilus 14086 combined with kefir grain. Additional equipment used for analysis were Aventru pH Meter AS218 and Centrifugation tools.

The kefir goat milk was made by (1) mixing 3 g of kefir grains into 100 ml of fresh goat's milk (2) incubating the combination of culture at 37°C for 12 to 24 hours (3) opening and stirring the kefir, (4) cooling to 10 to 15 degrees, and (5) aging for 0, 7, 14, and 21 days. After sterilizing the equipment, the kefir was collected and placed in sample bottles at 4°C. Kefir samples were gathered and calculated after 0, 7, 14, and 21 days. Kefir's pH was determined using an Aventru pH Meter AS218. Before using the pH meter on the sample, it was calibrated with pH four and pH seven buffer standards and adequately cleaned with distilled water. A 50 mL sample was placed in a beaker glass and then inserted into an auto-mode pH meter, with pH values recorded in triplicate. The water-holding capacity of the kefir samples was tested using the centrifugation method (Li *et al.* 2014). The profiling method was used for sensory analysis (Bielska *et al.* 2021). A completely randomized design (CRD) with four treatments and three replications was used in this study. The Duncan Multiple Range Test (DMRT) was performed for further statistical analysis.

3 RESULTS AND DISCUSSION

The observations (Table 1) revealed that the prolonged aging time treatment had a significant ($P<0.05$) effect on the pH value. Kefir with a 21-day aging time had the highest pH (5.41), while kefir with no aging time had the lowest (4.81). The role of Lactic Acid Bacteria and Yeast elevated the pH of kefir during the prolonged aging time. The increased acidity of kefir will encourage the growth of lactic acid bacteria. The activity of lactic acid bacteria

Table 1. The pH, WHC, and sensory quality in goat milk kefir with different prolonged aging time.

Aging Time (days)	pH	WHC (%)	Sensory Quality		
			Texture	Flavor	Taste
0	4.81 ± 0.6^a	88.16 ± 0.1^d	2.87 ± 0.3^{ab}	2.40 ± 0.7^a	2.53 ± 0.6^{abc}
7	5.01 ± 0.3^b	84.13 ± 0.5^b	3.07 ± 0.2^{abc}	3.06 ± 0.7^{ab}	2.40 ± 0.6^{ab}
14	5.10 ± 0.4^c	85.09 ± 0.2^c	3.86 ± 0.3^d	3.66 ± 0.6^{bc}	3.46 ± 0.5^d
21	5.41 ± 0.6^d	80.97 ± 0.6^a	2.66 ± 0.6^a	4.13 ± 0.5^{cd}	2.33 ± 0.6^a

[a-d] Different superscript letters in the same column mean significantly different ($P<0.05$) that sorted from lowest to highest

began to stabilize at 36 hours and dropped between 48 and 72 hours after fermentation. However, maturing the kefir for an extended time reduces the acidity level because the alcohol created by yeast activity lowers the pH value of the kefir. Furthermore, Umam *et al.* (2018) demonstrated that a phenolic compound or any other microorganism during the post-acidification period could inhibit the growth of starter bacteria, resulting in a decrease in the total amount of lactic acid bacteria in yogurt products and an increase in pH value. The same authors (Khoirul Umam *et al.* 2022) proved that when the pH falls below 4, LAB activity decreases. Yeast uses this condition to grow and oxidize glucose, causing the alcohol level of kefir to increase rapidly.

WHC changes will be identified during incubation, and WHC influences the level of consumer preference. Kefir made from goat milk has higher WHC levels than cow milk. Gomes *et al.* (2013) claimed that buffalo and cow milk contain more casein micelles than goat milk because the protein network has smaller pores and a higher density, resulting in a higher WHC value. The results suggest that the prolonged age time treatment has a significant effect on kefir WHC (P0.05). The treatment without the aging process had the highest WHC, 88.16%, while the lowest WHC was 21 days of aging time, with an average of 80.97%. WHC decreases as the fermentation period increases, and WHC follows an unstable pH value during fermentation. The pH value affects the WHC value, when the pH of kefir drops, the demineralization of casein micelles occurs. Casein micelles begin to swell below pH 5.5, and almost all of the colloidal calcium phosphate decomposes, precipitates, and causes a decrease in the volume of casein micelles, forming a gel with a three-dimensional network). At the same time, the separated milk serum is made up of whey protein, lactose, and salt, and it is trapped as a liquid phase (Körzendörfer *et al.* 2019). These findings support the results of Jaros and Rohm (2003) who discovered that increasing acidification to a pH below 4.0 might cause damage to the physical qualities and texture of milk, such as gel shrinkage and syneresis. When the pH returns to normal, the milk serum can be reabsorbed by the gel at the same rate as the acidity. Fat is one of the substances that aid in this reabsorption. The surface of fat globules can absorb proteins to create tissues, which influences the WHC content of fermented products.

The evaluation of rheological properties is essential for identifying the numerous interactions in kefir samples. Maintaining the right texture of fermented milk in commercial manufacturing of alternative fermented dairy products can be tricky. As demonstrated in Table 1, statistically significant differences ($P<0.05$) were discovered in this study's investigation of Texture, Flavor, and Taste in goat milk kefir.

The kefir texture on the 21-day aging time was unacceptable to panelists because it was firm, whereas other treatments were softer. The texture score of the kefir sample after 0 days, 7 days, 14 days, and 21 days of aging (2.87, 3.07, 3.86, and 2.66 scores, respectively). Kefir will have a thicker texture as its aging time is longer. However, it will synergize or separate whey from the curd. The texture of Kefir will thicken as it ages because the lactic acid produced by lactose will thicken the casein in milk (Stadie *et al.* 2013). However, the longer the aging period, the greater the syneresis induced by reduced air binding of the protein network, which results in the separation of curd and whey in Kefir due to tissue protein rearrangements. The longer the aging time, the less milky the flavor gets, and the more acidic and slightly alcoholic the flavor has become. The 21-day aging time had the highest value, with a score of 4.13. some Panelists dislike goat milk because it has a goaty or milky flavor. The longer the aging time, the more the LAB and yeast in kefir affect the content of goat milk. Several chemicals formed during fermentation, including lactic acid, acetic acid, pyruvic acid, hippuric acid, propionic acid, butyric acid, diacetyl, and acetaldehyde, influence the scent and flavor of kefir (Rosa *et al.* 2017). Kefir's taste is influenced by chemicals created during fermentation, such as lactic acid, CO_2, and ethanol derived from Lactobacteria's fermentation process. Kefir also contains formic, propionic, succinic acids, aldehydes, acetone isoamyl alcohol, and different folates. Kefir has a low pH and a sour taste due to the acid generated during fermentation. The longer the fermentation time, the lower the pH and the stronger the sour taste of the kefir. With a 14-day age period, the kefir receives high marks for its sour taste. As a result, the assumption that the prolonged aging time of 21 days is too long and that the prolonged aging time of 7 days is more favorable for customers of different genders. Kefir can be characterized by qualities of the best taste (sour), with a score of 3.46 after a 14-day aging period. Long-fermented goat milk kefir has a bitter taste, a lactic acid level of 0.9–1.1%, an alcohol content of 0.5–1%, and a minor amount of CO_2. The pH dropped after 14 days due to a decrease in the activity of lactic acid bacteria. This drop was caused by a reduction in lactose as an energy source. Furthermore, yeast growth inhibits the growth of lactic acid bacteria, and yeast creates alcohol, which reduces the acidity of kefir (Wati *et al.* 2022).

4   CONCLUSION

With a prolonged aging time of 14 days, kefir can be characterized by taste (sour) and Texture (soft) attributes. It is assumed that the sour taste indicated by the significance of pH value and soft Texture has the most significant impact on consumers' assessment of their acceptability. Moreover, under aging process conditions for 21 days, goat Milk kefir gave the best flavor. Fermentation without prolonged aging time resulted in significant results in water-holding capacity.

REFERENCES

Baniasadi M., Azizkhani M., Saris P.E.J., & Tooryan F. (2022). Comparative Antioxidant Potential of Kefir and Yogurt of Bovine and Non-bovine Origins. *Journal of Food Science and Technology*, 59(4), 1307–1316.
Bielska P., Cais-Sokolińska D., Teichert J., Biegalski J., Kaczyński Ł.K. & Chudy S. (2021). Effect of Honeydew Honey Addition on the Water Activity and Water Holding Capacity of Kefir in the Context of its Sensory Acceptability. *Scientific Reports*, 11(1), 1–9.
Gomes J.J.L., Duarte A.M., Batista A.S.M., de Figueiredo R.M.F., de Sousa E.P., de Souza E.L. & do Egypto R.D.C.R. (2013). Physicochemical and Sensory Properties of Fermented Dairy Beverages Made with Goat's Milk, Cow's Milk and a Mixture of the Two Milks. *LWT-Food Science and Technology*, 54(1), 18–24.
Hill C., Guarner F., Reid G., Gibson G.R., Merenstein D.J., Pot B., Morelli L., Canani R.B., Flint H.J., Salminen S., Calder P.C., & Sanders M.E. (2014). Expert Consensus Document. The International Scientific Association for Probiotics and Prebiotics Consensus Statement on the Scope and Appropriate Use of the Term Probiotic. *Nature reviews. Gastroenterology & Hepatology*, 11(8), 506–514.
Jaros D., & Rohm H. (2003). Controlling the Texture of Fermented Dairy Products: The Case of Yoghurt. *Dairy Processing: Improving Quality*, 1, 155–184.
Körzendörfer A., Schäfer J., Hinrichs J., & Nöbel S. (2019). Power Ultrasound as a Tool to Improve the Processability of Protein-enriched Fermented Milk Gels for Greek Yogurt Manufacture. *Journal of Dairy Science*, 102(9), 7826–7837.
Li C., Li W., Chen X., Feng M., Rui X., Jiang M., & Dong M. (2014). Microbiological, Physicochemical and Rheological Properties of Fermented Soymilk Produced with Exopolysaccharide (EPS) Producing Lactic Acid Bacteria Strains. *LWT-Food Science and Technology*, 57(2), 477–485.
Radiati L.E., Umam A.K., Susilo A., & Thoifi A.A. (2020, April). Effect of Lactobacillus Plantarum Concentration Level on Physicochemical Properties of Fermented Goat Meat Dendeng. In *IOP Conference Series: Earth and Environmental Science* (Vol. 478, No. 1, p. 012038). IOP Publishing.
Rosa D.D., Dias M.M., Grześkowiak Ł.M., Reis S.A., Conceição L.L., & Maria do Carmo G.P. (2017). Milk Kefir: Nutritional, Microbiological and Health Benefits. *Nutrition Research Reviews*, 30(1), 82–96.
Stadie J., Gulitz A., Ehrmann M.A., & Vogel R.F. (2013). Metabolic Activity and Symbiotic Interactions of Lactic Acid Bacteria and Yeasts Isolated From Water Kefir. *Food Microbiology*, 35(2), 92–98.
Triwibowo B., Wicaksono R., Antika Y., Ermi S., Jarmiati A., Setiadi A.A., & Syahriar R. (2020). The Effect of Kefir Grain Concentration and Fermentation Duration on Characteristics of Cow Milk-based Kefir. In *Journal of Physics: Conference Series* (Vol. 1444, No. 1, p. 012001). IOP Publishing.

Umam A.K., Lin M.J., Radiati L.E., & Peng S.Y. (2018). The Utilization of Canna Starch (Canna edulis Ker) As a Alternative Hydrocolloid on the Manufacturing Process of Yogurt Drink. *Jurnal Ilmu dan Teknologi Hasil Ternak (JITEK)*, 13(1), 1–13.

Umam A.K., Lin M.J., Radiati L.E., & Peng S.Y. (2019). The Capability of Canna edulis Ker Starch as Carboxymethyl Cellulose Replacement on Yogurt Drink During Cold Storage. *Animal Production*, 20(2), 109–118.

Umam A.K., Radiati L.E., Susila A., & Hapsari R.N. (2019). Chemical and Microbiological Quality of Fermented Goat Meat Dendeng with Different Levels of L. plantarum. In *IOP Conference Series: Earth and Environmental Science* (Vol. 387, No. 1, p. 012012). IOP Publishing.

Umam A.K., Radiati L.E., Suwondo K.H.P., & Kholidah S.N. (2022, February). Study of Antioxidant Activity, Peptides, and Chemical Quality of Goat Milk Kefir on the Different Post-Acidification Periods During Cold Storage. In *9th International Seminar on Tropical Animal Production (ISTAP 2021)* (pp. 178–181). Atlantis Press.

Wati A.M., Lin M.J., & Radiati L.E. (2022). Effect of Different Incubation Time on Goat's Milk Dadih on Thorny Bamboo (Bambusa stenostachya Hackel). *Jurnal Ilmu dan Teknologi Hasil Ternak (JITEK)*, 17 (2), 74–82.

Developing Modern Livestock Production in Tropical Countries – Adli et al. (eds)
© 2023 The Authors, ISBN 978-1-032-44025-5
Open Access: www.taylorfrancis.com, CC BY-NC-ND 4.0 license

Broiler productive performance in partnership system during the Covid-19 pandemic

N. Febrianto*, P. Akhiroh & B. Hartono
Faculty of Animal Science, Universitas Brawijaya, Malang, East Java, Indonesia

ABSTRACT: The Covid-19 pandemic has had an economic impact. This study aims to analyze the production costs, revenues, profits, and performance of broiler production. The research location was determined purposively in Kediri Regency. The research was carried out using a survey method. A total of 45 broiler breeders are members of 9 partner companies and each company was represented by 5 broiler breeders used in this research. Data analysis used input-output and business productivity performance. The results showed that the lowest average cost of livestock production was 15,509 IDR/kg and the highest was 18,414 IDR/kg with an average farmer's income of 3,119 IDR/kg/BB. The lowest BEP value was 15,509 IDR/kg and the highest was 18,414 IDR/kg. The results showed average mortality (4.04%), FCR (1.60), and IP (372.8). In conclusion, broiler farming is still profitable, and production performance is by production standards although management needs to be improved.

Keywords: broiler, Covid-19, partnership, performance

1 INTRODUCTION

The Covid-19 pandemic has caused many companies to reduce the number of workers to prevent the spread of the disease. As a result, people limit the expenditure of their needs, so that the purchasing power or consumption level of the community decreases. Putri *et al.* (2020) stated that the stay-at-home policy made many economic activities temporarily halt. This policy causes many new problems to arise like termination of employment (PHK), and also has an impact on lower-middle businesses, including broiler farms. In the livestock sector, the economic impact caused by Covid-19 begins with the Indonesian rupiah (IDR) exchange rate which tends to decline against foreign currencies and affects the price of imported raw materials for the livestock industry, especially poultry, dairy cattle, and beef cattle. Sihaloho (2020) stated that the exchange rate of 1 USD against IDR on March 2, 2020, was 14,265.00, as of today April 9, 2020, the exchange rate of 1 USD against IDR is 15,880.004. So the IDR weakened by 1.615 points or weakened by 11.32% in 39 days. The worst weakening of the IDR until April 10, 2020, occurred on March 23, 2020, with the exchange rate of 1 USD against IDR of 16,575.00 or weakened by 16.19%. The Covid-19 outbreak felt by farmers was a reduction in the selling price of livestock products, especially carcass and chicken meat due to low purchasing power. Based on research conducted by Wakhidati *et al.* (2020) as many as 95% of respondents stated that it was difficult to get profits during the Covid-19 pandemic even though they were part of a partnership. Other impacts felt by farmers were a decrease in income, a decrease in the selling price of broilers, a decrease in the population of livestock kept, a decrease in consumers, and an increase in

---

*Corresponding author email: nanangfeb@ub.ac.id

DOI: 10.1201/9781003370048-39

This chapter has been made available under a CC BY NC ND license

production costs. Therefore, the research was conducted to analyze production costs, revenues, profits, and production performance of broiler chickens.

2 MATERIAL AND METHODS

The research was conducted on a partnership broiler farming business in the Kediri district. The location selection was done by the purposive sampling method. The determination of the research location was based on the consideration that the Kediri district is one of the areas with a large population of broiler livestock in East Java with a population of 11,445,031 heads (BPS East Java 2020). Another consideration is that the people in this area have broiler livestock which acts as their main and side jobs. The research was carried out using a survey method. A total of 45 broiler breeders are members of 9 partner companies, PT. Anugerah Kartika Agro (A), PT. Intan Permata (B), PT. Charoen Pokphand Indonesia (C), PT. Andalan Ternak Makmur (D), PT. Andalan Yasa Mitra (E), PT. Jaguar Sejahtera (F), PT. Sentra Unggas Perkam (G), PT. Sinar Sarana Sentosa (H), and PT. Star feed (I). The sample was selected purposively with certain considerations (Sugiyono 2017) so that each company was represented by 5 broiler chicken farmers. The data were analyzed by calculating the input-output and business productivity performance. The calculation of input-output includes production costs, revenues, and profits. Productivity performance includes Break Event Point (BEP), Feed Conversion Ratio (FCR), Performance Index (IP), and Mortality.

3 RESULT AND DISCUSSION

3.1 *Operating income analysis*

Operational costs are non-fixed costs paid by farmers personally that are not provided by the company, such as electricity costs, transportation, communication, employee salaries, gas brooder, husks, and others. The number of broiler populations that are kept can affect the production costs paid by farmers. The difference in the price of DOC and feed in each partnership causes the production costs to be different for each farm because the feed cost is the biggest cost that must be paid by farmers in each period, which is around 60–80% and the cost of purchasing DOC is around 10–20%. In Table 1 it is known that the lowest average cost of livestock production is the Partnership of PT. F 15.509 IDR/kg/period, because

Table 1. Production cost, revenue, and profit (IDR/kg/BW).

Company	Fix cost	Variable cost	Total cost	Revenue	Profit
PT.A	202	16.716	16.918	19.103	2.184
PT.B	169	17.108	17.277	18.534	1.258
PT.C	162	17.001	17.163	18.525	1.361
PT.D	164	15.808	15.971	18.121	2.150
PT.E	78	18.336	18.414	18.955	541
PT.F	140	15.369	15.509	18.628	3.119
PT.G	188	17.097	17.285	18.167	881
PT.H	110	15.701	15.812	18.723	2.911
PT.I	168	17.764	17.931	18.949	1.018

Source: primary data processed 2022Note: A = PT. Anugrah Kartika Agro; B = PT. Intan Permata; C = PT Charoen Pokphand Indonesia; D = PT. Andalan Ternak Makmur; E = PT. Andalan Yasa Mitra; F = PT. Jaguar Sejahtera; G = PT. Sentra Unggas Perkam; H = PT. Sinar Sarana Sentosa; I = PT. Star feed; IDR = Indonesian rupiah; BW = Body weight.

plasma which is incorporated in the PT F Partnership is more efficient in the use of production factors. The highest average production costs are breeders who are members of the PT. E 18,414 IDR/kg/period, due to variable costs impact of poor feeding management.

Revenue is the result of the sale of the resulting output, total revenue is the total product of the output with the selling price of production which is expressed in a certain amount of money. Revenue from the broiler farm business is obtained from the sale of broiler chickens, husks, manure, sacks of feed, and bonuses provided by the company. However, the income earned by farmers is dominated by livestock sales compared to others. The majority of revenue from broiler farming comes from the sale of livestock. This is by Zentiko *et al.* (2015) that the revenue from the main livestock business is revenue from the sale of chickens, the results of selling chickens are very dependent on the body weight of the chickens produced. With high chicken weight, accompanied by feed efficiency, the breeder will get good sales results. The average farm income can be seen in Table 1.

Revenue (profit) is the result of subtraction between the total incoming revenue and the total production costs incurred. The opinion of Jaelani *et al.* (2013) is that income is the difference between total revenue and total costs. The data in Table 1 shows that the highest average income of farmers in the partnership pattern is the breeder with the partnership of PT. F, which is 3,119 IDR/kg BW, happens because the production costs are very low with the selling price of chicken which is not much different from the partnerships.

3.2   *Broiler Productivity Performance*

3.2.1   *Break Even Point*

Table 2 shows that the average BEP value of the lowest price is the breeder with the partnership of PT. F, which is 15.509 IDR/kg, while the highest BEP value is owned by the breeder with the partnership of PT. E, which is 18,414 IDR/kg. The difference in the BEP value for each breeder is due to differences in the amount of production and the amount of total production issued each period. Even though there is a difference in the BEP value on the farm in each partnership, the selling price of the livestock contract that has been agreed upon by the breeder and the partner companies of all the breeders has exceeded the BEP value so that the farmer experiences a profit. This is by Rahayu *et al.* (2020) that for all broiler breeders to benefit from the partnership, they must sell chickens at prices above the BEP value.

Table 2.   BEP, mortality, FCR, and IP.

Company	BEP (IDR/kg/BW)	Mortality	FCR	IP
PT.A	16.918	4,17	1,56	384,55
PT.B	17.277	2,97	1,49	405,97
PT.C	17.163	3,06	1,53	422,59
PT.D	15.971	4,85	1,78	318,97
PT.E	18.414	3,83	1,66	341,49
PT.F	15.509	5,85	1,56	367,71
PT.G	17.285	3,42	1,63	374,62
PT.H	15.812	5,16	1,60	368,35
PT.I	17.931	3,05	1,59	371,14

Source: primary data processed 2022Note: A = PT. Anugrah Kartika Agro; B = PT. Intan Permata; C = PT Charoen Pokphand Indonesia; D = PT. Andalan Ternak Makmur; E = PT. Andalan Yasa Mitra; F = PT. Jaguar Sejahtera; G = PT. Sentra Unggas Perkam; H = PT. Sinar Sarana Sentosa; I = PT. Star feed; IDR = Indonesian rupiah; BW = Body weight; BEP = Break Event Point; FCR = Feed Conversion Ratio; IP = Performance Index.

3.2.2 Mortality

Table 2 shows that the highest average mortality value is farmed in partnership with PT. F (5.25%). There were more rejected chickens (*culling*) on farms in partnership with PT. H compared to PT. F, so the depletion rate is higher. The high mortality rate in addition to natural factors (climate/weather) and disease attacks, is also influenced by the behavior of farmers who become a habit by reducing the level of vaccines used and drugs whose goal is production cost efficiency (Febrianto *et al.* 2018).

3.2.3 Feed Conversion Ratio (FCR)

Table 2 shows that the lowest FCR value is breeder PT. B with an average value of 1.49 and the highest FCR value is breeder PT. D with an average value of 1.78. A high FCR value needs to be monitored for feed quality and DOC quality. The opinion of Marom *et al.* (2018) if the FCR is above the standard (1.63), which means more attention should be paid to the quality of the feed given. Marom *et al.* (2018) stated that FCR is used to measure livestock productivity, the higher the FCR, the more feed is needed to increase animal body weight per unit weight. A high feed conversion value indicates that the efficiency of feed utilization is not good, whereas a low feed conversion value indicates that more feed is used by livestock.

3.2.4 Performance Index (IP)

Table 2 shows that the average IP value is above 300, which means it is good. Mahardika *et al.* (2020) explained the IP assessment criteria for PT. B (405.97) and PT. C (422.59) is at a special level, which means broiler performance at PT. B and PT. C is very good, while the PT. D has the lowest average IP score of 318.97, which is at a sufficient level. A higher production index value indicates a more efficient and good broiler rearing. Fadilah (2007) in Susanti *et al.* 2016) stated that the greater the IP value obtained, the more efficient the use of feed.

4 CONCLUSIONS

Based on economic performance, it shows that the broiler farming business is still profitable. Based on production performance it is still by production standards, although management needs to be improved.

REFERENCES

Febrianto N., Putritamara J. A. and Hartono B. (2018). Analisis Kelayakan Usaha Peternakan Broiler di Kabupaten Malang. *Agriekonomika*, 7(2), 168–175.

Jaelani A., Suslinawati and Maslan. (2013). Analisis Kelayakan Usaha Peternakan Ayam Broiler di Kecamatan Tapin Utara Kabupaten Tapi. *Jurnal Ilmu Ternak*, 13(2), 42–49.

Mahardika C.B.D.P., Pello W.Y. and Pallo M. (2020). Performa Usaha Kemitraan Ayam Ras Pedaging. *PARTNER*, 25(1), 1270–1281.

Marom A.T., Kalsum U. and Ali U. (2018). Evaluasi Performans Broiler pada Sistem Kandang Close House dan Open House dengan Altitude Berbeda. *Dinamika Rekasatwa*, 2(2), 1–10.

Putri R.K., Sari R.I., Wahyuningsih R. and Meikhati E. (2020). Efek Pandemi Covid 19: Dampak Lonjakan Angka PHK Terhadap Penurunan Perekonomian Di Indonesia. *Jurnal Bisnis Manajemen dan Akuntansi (BISMAK)*, 1(2), 50–55.

Rahayu L., Widodo W. and Dyah P.S. (2020). Analisis Break Event Point Usaha Ternak Ayam Broiler Pola Kemitraan di Kecamatan Kedawung Kabupaten Sragen. *In Seminar Nasional Pertanian Peternakan Terpadu*, 4(3), 549–562.

Sihaloho E.D. (2020). Impacts of Regional Economic Factors on the Transmission of Coronavirus Disease 2019 (Covid-19) In Indonesia. *Journal of Economics and Business*, 4, 397–403.

Susanti E.D., Dahlan M. and Wahyuning D. (2016). Perbandingan Produktivitas Ayam Broiler Terhadap Sistem Kandang Terbuka (Open House) dan Kandang Tertutup (Closed House) di Ud Sumber Makmur Kecamatan Sumberrejo Kabupaten Bojonegoro. *Jurnal Ternak: Jurnal Ilmiah Fakultas Peternakan Universitas Islam Lamongan*, 7(1), 1–7.

Wakhidati Y.N., Sugiarto M., Aunurrohman, H., Einstein, A. and Muatip, K. (2020). Dampak Pandemi Covid-19 pada Restrukturisasi Tenaga Kerja pada Usaha Ayam Broiler Pola Kemitraan di Kabupaten Banyumas. *In Prosiding Seminar Teknologi Agribisnis Peternakan (STAP) Fakultas Peternakan Universitas Jenderal Soedirman*, 7, 278–279.

Zentiko B.D., Handayani M. and Santoso S.I. (2015). Analisis Break Even Point Usaha Peternakan Ayam Broiler Di Kecamatan Limbangan Kabupaten Kendal. *Animal Agriculture Journal*, 4(1), 15–21.

Developing Modern Livestock Production in Tropical Countries – Adli et al. (eds)
© *2023 The Authors, ISBN 978-1-032-44025-5*
Open Access: www.taylorfrancis.com, CC BY-NC-ND 4.0 license

Physical quality of nano-transfersome formulation of moringa leaf extract (*Moringa oleifera*) and honey

Yudhistira Aryo Pamuncak & Agus Susilo*
Faculty of Animal Science, Universitas Brawijaya, Malang City, East Java, Indonesia

Miftakhul Cahyati
Department of Oral Medicine, Faculty of Dentistry, Universitas Brawijaya, Malang City, East Java, Indonesia

Nurjannah
Department of Statistics, Faculty of Mathematics and Natural Sciences, Universitas Brawijaya, Malang City, East Java, Indonesia

Dodyk Pranowo
Department of Agroindustrial, Faculty of Agricultural Technology, Universitas Brawijaya, Malang City, East Java, Indonesia
Faculty of Animal Science, Universitas Brawijaya, Malang City, East Java, Indonesia

ABSTRACT: The purpose of this study was to determine the physical quality of the use of Moringa leaf extract and honey in the manufacture of transfersome as an oral gel. The method used is a laboratory experiment with a completely randomized design using six treatments and three replication. The transfersome was made using the vortexing sonicator method. The results of statistical analysis showed that the use of Moringa leaf extract and honey in transfersome formulations with different levels did not have a significant effect ($p>0.05$) on pH, total dissolved solids (TDS), and color intensity L*a*b*, but is having a significant impact ($p<0.05$) on the value of electrical conductivity. The study concludes that the use of Moringa leaf extract and honey with a ratio of 3:2 (F3) showed the best results in the transfersome formulation so F3 can be used as an excellent transfersome gel material.

Keywords: honey, moringa leaf extract, transfersome

1 INTRODUCTION

Many drug delivery systems have been developed, one of which is the transfersome delivery system. Transfersomes are phospholipid, surfactant, and water-based delivery systems that enhance transdermal penetration. Chaudhadya *et al.* (2013) stated that transfersomes could be used to deliver drugs transdermally (low or high molecular weight based on the excellent penetration strength and flexibility used. Transfersomes can penetrate the entire stratum corneum through intracellular or transcellular pathways. Transfersomes have several advantages, namely biocompatible, biodegradable, easy to manufacture, can protect drugs from environmental degradation, able to deliver medicines from narrow gaps between cells properly, and have been used for various materials such as peptides, proteins, analgesics, and natural product compounds (Ramadon & Abdul 2016). Nanotransfersomes have a smaller

---

*Corresponding Author: agussusilo@ub.ac.id

DOI: 10.1201/9781003370048-40
This chapter has been made available under a CC BY NC ND license

particle size than transfersomes. Nano is a particle measuring from 10 to 1000 nm (Lalotra *et al.* 2020). Nanotransfersomes enhance the delivery of a drug across the membrane. Nanotransfersomes have the potential to leave the vascular stem and enter the inflamed area due to their small size. Nanotransfersomes have been widely used to increase the penetration of drugs derived from natural ingredients.

2 MATERIALS AND METHODS

2.1 *Materials*

The transfersome is made from tween 80, phosphate buffer saline, lectins, honey, and moringa leaf extract. Honey is taken from the Apis mellifera bees which are cultivated in kapok trees area in Central Java, Indonesia. Moringa leaf extract is extracted from moringa leaf powder using the UAE method. The equipment used is a measuring cup, spatula, electric stirrer, film pot, and ultrasonicator (Biomaisen). The sample testing equipment consists of a colorimeter CS-10 (CHN Spec®), pH and EC meter (pH/EC-9853), and TDS meter (TDS-3).

2.2 *Methods*

The transfersome was made using the vortexing sonicator. The method used is a laboratory experiment using a completely randomized design (CRD). The factors used were variations in the different ingredients with 6 treatments and 3 replications, consisting of:

T1 = Moringa : Honey (5 : 0)
T2 = Moringa : Honey (4 : 1)
T3 = Moringa : Honey (3 : 2)
T4 = Moringa : Honey (2 : 3)
T5 = Moringa : Honey (1 : 4)
T6 = Moringa : Honey (0 : 5)

3 RESULT AND DISCUSSION

3.1 *Result*

The results of statistical analysis showed that different formulations had a significantly different effect ($p < 0.05$) on the value of electrical conductivity, while did not have a significant effect ($p > 0.05$) on color intensity, pH, and total dissolved solids. The results of the analysis of color intensity are in Table 1 and the results of the analysis of pH, electrical conductivity, and total dissolved solids are in Table 2.

Table 1. The effect of different formulations on color intensity L*a*b* ($p > 0,05$).

| Treatment | Color Intensity L*a*b* | | |
	L*	a*	b*
T1	66,96 ± 2,78a	−4,46 ± 1,55a	25,1 ± 2,559a
T2	70,23 ± 0,07c	−2,85 ± 0,51b	28,52 ± 0,631c
T3	64,75 ± 30,1a	−2,75 ± 0,51b	28,0 ± 3,42b
T4	67,27 ± 4,26b	−2,37 ± 1,89c	29,4 ± 7,142d
T5	67,93 ± 24,86c	−1,79 ± 0,821c	31,4 ± 3,183e
T6	67,23 ± 5,88c	−1,86 ± 0,136c	30,9 ± 0,366f

Table 2. The effect of different formulations on pH (p>0,05), EC (p<0,05), and TDS (p>0,05).

Treatment	Average ± SD (pH)	Average ± SD (EC)	Average ± SD (TDS)
T1	7,05 ± 0,003c	0,33 ± 0,0008c	121,33 ± 352,3b
T2	6,78 ± 0,256a	0,23 ± 0,001a	102,6 ± 9,3a
T3	7,06 ± 0,001c	0,34 ± 0,0004d	128,3 ± 101,3c
T4	7,02 ± 0,004c	0,34 ± 0,00009d	120,3 ± 17,3b
T5	6,81 ± 0,005b	0,34 ± 0,0007d	120,3 ± 102,3c
T6	6,67 ± 0,013a	0,31 ± 0,0002b	117 ± 139c

3.2 Result and discussion

The results of statistical analysis showed that the use of Moringa leaf extract and honey in transfersome formulations with different levels did not have a significant effect (p>0.05) on pH, total dissolved solids (TDS), and color intensity L*a*b*, but has a significant effect (p<0.05) on the value of electrical conductivity. In this color intensity analysis, color points are marked through three coordinates, namely L* which is the coordinate of light starting from no reflection, namely black (L value is 0) to perfect reflection, namely white (L value is 100). The second is the a* coordinate, namely the reddish coordinate starting from a negative value for green to a positive for red. The third is the b* coordinate, which is the yellowish coordinate starting from negative for blue and positive values for yellow (Kurniawan 2020).

4 CONCLUSIONS

This study concludes that the use of Moringa leaf extract: honey with a ratio of 3: 2 (F3) showed the best results in the physical quality of nano-transfersome formulation with the most optimal in terms of L*a*b* color intensity, pH, electrical conductivity, and total dissolved solids. Therefore, the formulation has the potential to be used as active ingredients for transdermal drug, which can then be developed for chemical and sensitivity testing.

ACKNOWLEDGEMENT

Thanks to the university of brawijaya through the Hibah Dana Penelitian strategies LPPM 2022 with contract number 1665.34/UN.01/UB/2022 which has provided facilities for this research.

REFERENCES

Chaudhary H., Kohli K., and Kumar V. (2013). Nano-transfersomes as a Novel Carrier for Transdermal Delivery. *International Journal of Pharmaceutics*, 454(1), 367–380.

Girindra F.G., Rosdiana E., and Suhendi A. (2019). Rancang Bangun Sistem Pengukuran Konduktivitas Listrik Larutan Hidroponik Berbasis Mikrokontroler. *eProceedings of Engineering*, 6(2).

Irwan F., and Afdal A. (2016). Analisis Hubungan Konduktivitas Listrik Dengan Total Dissolved Solid (TDS) dan Temperatur Pada Beberapa Jenis Air. *Jurnal Fisika Unand*, 5(1), 85–93.

Isnan W., and Muin N. (2017). Ragam Manfaat Tanaman Kelor (Moringa oleifera Lamk.) Bagi Masyarakat. *Buletin Eboni*, 14(1), 63–75.

Kurniawan H. (2020). Pengaruh Kadar Air Terhadap Nilai Warna Cie Pada Gula Semut Effect of Moisture Content On Cie Color Values in Granulated Palm Sugar. *Jurnal Teknik Pertanian Lampung*, 9(3), 213–221.

Lalotra A.S., Singh V., Khurana B., Agrawal S., Shrestha S., and Arora D. (2020). A Comprehensive Review on Nanotechnology-Based Innovations in Topical Drug Delivery for the Treatment of Skin Cancer. *Current Pharmaceutical Design*, 26(44), 5720–5731.

Legowo G. (2015). Manfaat Madu Sebagai Antioksidan Dalam Melawan Radikal Bebas Dari Asap Rokok Untuk Menjaga Kualitas Sperma. *Jurnal Majority*, 4(8), 41–46.

Mutia T., Novarini E., and Gustiani R.S. (2020). Preparasi dan Karakterisasi Membran Serat Nano Polivinil Alkohol/gelatin dengan Antibiotika Topikal Menggunakan Metode Electrospinning. *Arena Tekstil*, 35(2), 95–106.

Novenpa N.N., and Dzulkiflih D. (2020). Alat Pendeteksi Kualitas Air Portable dengan Parameter pH, TDS dan Suhu Berbasis Arduino Uno. *Inovasi Fisika Indonesia*, 9(2).

Omar M.M., Hasan O.A., and El Sisi A.M. (2019). Preparation and Optimization of Lidocaine Transferosomal Gel Containing Permeation Enhancers: A Promising Approach for Enhancement of Skin Permeation. *International Journal of Nanomedicine*, 14, 1551.

Oprescu E.E., Enascuta C.E., Radu E., Ciltea-Udrescu M., and Lavric V. (2022). Does the Ultrasonic Field Improve the Extraction Productivity Compared to Classical Methods–Maceration and Reflux Distillation? *Chemical Engineering and Processing-Process Intensification*, 179, 109082.

Putra I.W.D.P., Dharmayudha A.A.G.O., and Sudimartini L.M. (2016). Identifikasi Senyawa Kimia Ekstrak Etanol Daun Kelor (Moringa oleifera L) di Bali. *Indonesia Medicus Veterinus*, 5(5), 464–473.

Ramadon D., and Mun'im A. (2017). Pemanfaatan Nanoteknologi Dalam Sistem Penghantaran Obat Baru Untuk Produk Bahan Alam. *Jurnal ilmu kefarmasian Indonesia*, 14(2), 118–127.

Ramadon D., Wirarti G.A., and Anwar E. (2017). Novel Transdermal Ethosomal Gel Containing Green Tea (Camellia sinensis L. Kuntze) Leaves Extract: Formulation and in vitro Penetration Study. *Journal of Young Pharmacists*, 9(3), 336.

Vallianou N.G., Gounari P., Skourtis A., Panagos J., and Kazazis C. (2014). Honey and its Anti-inflammatory, Anti-bacterial and Anti-oxidant Properties. *Gen Med (Los Angel)*, 2(132), 1–5.

Developing Modern Livestock Production in Tropical Countries – Adli et al. (eds)

Quality test of restaurant cooking oil waste in terms of moisture content, specific gravity, and energy as a feed supplement

M. Rachman & Hartutik*
Faculty of Animal Science, Universitas Brawijaya, Malang, Indonesia

ABSTRACT: The purpose of this research was to determine the quality of waste oil from a restaurant on moisture content, specific gravity, and energy as a feed supplement. Fresh oil sampling is only done 1 time at the beginning and waste oil sampling is done 3 times on different days every 3 days. The data obtained were tabulated and analyzed of variance according to a nested Randomized Block Design (RBD) for waste oil in 4 restaurants (Wong Solo, Ocean Garden, Yogyakarta, and H Slamet) with 3 groups using Microsoft Excel. The variables observed were water content, specific gravity, and energy in the new cooking oil and its waste. The analysis of moisture content and specific gravity was carried out at the Laboratory of Nutrition and Animal Feed, Faculty of Animal Science, Brawijaya University, Malang, and the energy content analysis was carried out at the Integrated Research and Testing Laboratory, Gadjah Mada University, Yogyakarta. The results showed that the types of oil used were bimoli oil (T1 and T2), dorang oil (T3), and tropical oil (T4). The new bimoli oil consists of a water content of 0.37%, specific gravity of 0.95 kg/L, and energy of 9488.89 kcal/kg. In dorang oil, the water content is 0.04%, specific gravity is 0.89 kg/L and energy is 9219.78 kcal/kg, while in tropical water content is 0.04%, specific gravity is 0.96 kg/L, and energy is 9230.50 kcal/kg. Based on the analysis of variance from the 4 restaurants, the results showed that the water content, specific gravity, and energy of waste oil in the four restaurants were not significantly different ($P > 0.05$). It concluded frying food but has the potential to be used as animal feed supplements for both ruminants and non-ruminants

Keywords: energy, moisture content. specific gravity, waste oil

1 INTRODUCTION

Cooking oil is one much needed by Indonesian people, and this is proven with a quantity of more than 290 million tons of oil consumed annually by public. If cooking oil is used continuously and repeatedly at high temperatures (160–180°C) and accompanied by contact with air and water on the frying process will result in complex degradation reactions occurring in oil and produce various reaction products. Cooking oil also changes color from yellow to darker color. This degradation reaction lowers the quality of the oil and finally, oil can no longer be used and must be discarded. Cooking oil can be used up to 3–4 times for frying (Kapitan 2013). However, if the cooking oil is used repeatedly, the fatty acids contained in the cooking oil will be more saturated and the cooking oil will change color. The used cooking oil is said to have been damaged or can be called used cooking oil and is not good for consumption (Lipoeto 2011). Waste cooking oil can be used as a mixture of animal feed because cooking oil contains high energy compared to other feed ingredients, besides

---

*Corresponding Author: hartutik@ub.ac.id

DOI: 10.1201/9781003370048-41

that cooking oil also contains fatty acids including essential fatty acids, namely omega-3 fatty acids. 6 and contains energy 3 metabolic energy is 8300 kcal/kg (NRC 2001) and the metabolic energy of the used cooking oil is 7.430 kcal/kg (Kusmanto et al. 2005). This is done to determine the quality of the waste cooking oil which will later be used as feed for livestock. Based on this, the researchers are interested in taking the title "Quality Test of Restaurant Cooking Oil Waste in Terms of Moisture Content, Specific gravity, and Energy as a Feed Supplement."

2 MATERIALS AND METHODS

The materials used in this study are waste oil (oil that has been used to fry chicken) and new oil (unused oil) which was taken from 4 restaurants in the Malang City area. The analysis of the nutritional content was carried out according to the AOAC (2005) procedure, the following are the tools used in this study, namely: a) water content; dropper, cup, exicator, oven, and scale, b) specific gravity; micropipette and scale, and c) energy; scale, bomb calorimeter tube, ignition tank, wire igniter, and oxygen. The data obtained were analyzed using analysis of variance (ANOVA) Randomized Block Design (RBD) and if there was a difference in influence, then continued with Duncan's Multiple Range Test (DMRT) using the following models $Y_{ij} = B_0 + B_1X_{ij} + e_{ij}$ (Adli et al. 2022; Ardiansyah et al. 2022).

3 RESULTS AND DISCUSSION

The results of this study indicate that restaurants around the city of Malang mostly use packaged palm oil, namely bimoli, dorang, and tropical cooking oils. The waste oil produced by the restaurant is usually used to make chili sauce or thrown away. In addition, the restaurant resells waste oil to collectors and is used by culinary food sellers. The results of the survey conducted in each restaurant can be seen in Table 1.

Table 1. Survey results in each restaurant.

Treatment	Group	Mark	Used cooking oil Total (liter/ day)	How many times used to fry (portion)	Generated waste oil Ratio (portion/ liter)	Total (liter)	Treatment
T_1	U_1	Bimoli	16.00	1900	118.75	3.00	Given to
	U_2	Bimoli	15.00	1700	113.33	3.00	collector
	U_3	Bimoli	18.00	2200	122.22	3.50	
	Mean		16.33	1933.33	118.10	3.16	
T_2	U_1	Bimoli	22.00	2400	109.09	5.00	Disposed
	U_2	Bimoli	20.00	2100	105.00	4.00	
	U_3	Bimoli	19.00	2050	107.89	4.00	
	Mean		20.33	2183.33	107.32	4.33	
T_3	U_1	Dorang	20.00	2200	110.00	3.50	Disposed
	U_2	Dorang	19.00	2000	105.26	3.00	
	U_3	Dorang	23.00	2500	108.68	4.00	
	Mean		20.66	2233.33	107.98	3.50	
T_4	U_1	Tropical	15.00	1600	108.66	3.00	Made into
	U_2	Tropical	13.00	1400	107.69	1.50	chili
	U_3	Tropical	14.00	1450	103.57	2.00	
	Mean		14.00	1483.33	106.64	2.16	

Based on the survey results in Table 1. it can be seen that restaurants T1 (Wong Solo) and T2 (Ocean Garden) use the same type of oil, namely Bimoli, while restaurant T3 (Yogyakarta) uses the type of Dorang oil and T4 (H. Slamet) uses Tropical oils. In restaurants T2 and T3, the amount of oil used per day tends to be more with an average of 20.33–20.66 liters/day than in restaurants T4 and T1 with an average of 14.00–16.33 litres/day so restaurants T2 and T3 produce more cooking oil waste compared to restaurants T4 and T1.

Table 2.   The results of the analysis of the nutrient content of new cooking oil.

Treatment	Used cooking oil	Water content (%)	Specific gravity (g/ml)	Energy (kcal/kg)
T_1	Bimoli	0.37	0.954	9488.89
T_2	Bimoli	0.37	0.954	9488.89
T_3	Dorang	0.04	0.895	9219.78
T_4	Tropical	0.04	0.962	9230.50
Mean		0.20	0.932	9357.01

Based on the results of the analysis of new cooking oil in Table 3, it is known that the water content in the type of Bimoli oil is relatively higher, which is around 0.37% when compared to the type of Dorang and Tropical cooking oil which is around 0.04% which is in accordance with Standard National Indonesia (SNI), namely $< 300\%$. Dorang cooking oil has a lower specific gravity than the others, which is around 0.895 which is in accordance with SNI, which is 0.900 Kg/L when compared to Bimoli and Tropical cooking oil which has a specific gravity ranging from 0.954 Kg/L and 0.962 Kg/L. Meanwhile, the energy content has relatively the same level with an average of 9357.01 kcal/kg. The results of the analysis of water content, specific gravity, and energy in each restaurant are shown in Table 3.

Table 3.   The results of the analysis of water content, specific gravity, and energy in each restaurant.

Treatment	Water content (%)	Specific gravity (Kg/L)	Energy (kcal/kg)
T_1	0.07 ± 0.11	1.001 ± 0.05	9421.39 ± 93.534
T_2	0.74 ± 0.54	0.991 ± 0.04	9411.27 ± 240.08
T_3	0.28 ± 0.29	0.969 ± 0.07	9531.19 ± 198.82
T_4	0.37 ± 0.35	1.005 ± 0.01	9530.57 ± 200.69
Mean	0.36 ± 0.33	0.992 ± 0.04	9471.36 ± 183.28

Based on Table 3, the water content showed that the treatment had no significant effect $(P>0.05)$. The water content of cooking oil repeatedly has no effect on the wastewater content of cooking oil. The results of the water content test in the new cooking oil used by the restaurant are 0.04%–0.37%, while the water content test results in the waste cooking oil increase in the range of 0.07%–0.74%. The results of the analysis of the water content have exceeded the requirements set by SNI, namely $< 0.300\%$. One of the factors that affect the increase in the water content of cooking oil waste is the large amount of water contained in T_2, T_3, and T_4 cooking oil waste as a result of fried foods containing a lot of water, for example, in frying chicken so that the cooking oil is contaminated by water. This is in accordance with the statement of Fanani and Ningsih (2018), the water content in cooking oil waste can be influenced by several factors including the length of the frying process, differences in the rate of the cooking process, the water content in varied foodstuffs and the composition of the oil used.

4 CONCLUSION

The quality of cooking oil waste which includes water content with an average of 0.36 ± 0.33 and specific gravity with an average of 0.992 ± 0.04 does not meet the requirements for cooking oil according to SNI because the water content in the waste is $< 300\%$ and the specific gravity is > 0.900 Kg/L for frying food but has the potential to be used as animal feed supplements for both ruminants and non-ruminants.

REFERENCES

Adli D.N., Sjofjan O., Irawan A., Utama D.T., Sholikin M.M., Nurdianti R.R. Nurfitriani R.A., Hidayat C., Jayanegara A., and Sadarman S. (2022). Effects of Fibre-rich Ingredient Levels on Goose Growth Performance, Blood Profile, Foie Gras Quality and its Fatty Acid Profile: A Meta-Analysis. *Journal of Animal and Feed Sciences*, 31(4):301–309.

Ardiansyah W., Sjofjan O., Widodo E., Suyadi S., Adli D.N. (2022). Effects of Combinations of α-Lactobacillus sp. and Curcuma Longa Flour on Production, Egg Quality, and Intestinal Profile of Mojosari Ducks. *Advance in Animal Veterinary Science*, 10(8):1668–1677.

Fanani N., and Ningsih E. (2018). Analisis Kualitas Minyak Goreng Habis Pakai yang Digunakan oleh Pedagang Penyetan di Daerah Rungkut Surabaya Ditinjau dari Kadar Air dan Kadar Asam Lemak Bebas (ALB). *Jurnal IPTEK*, 22(2):59–66.

Kapitan B.O. (2013). Analisis Kandungan Asam Lemak Trans (Trans Fat) Dalam Minyak Bekas Penggorengan Jajanan Di Pinggir Jalan Kota Kupang. *Jurnal Kimiaterapan*, 1(1):17–31.

Kusmanto D. (2005). Penggunaan Minyak Goreng Bekas dan Minyak Segar Dalam Pakan Ayam Petelur Terhadap Kualitas Fisik dan Kolesterol Telur. *Jurnal Penelitian*, 268.

Lipoeto E. (2011). Synthesis of Biodiesel via Acid Catalysis. *Indonesia Engineering Chemical Research*, 44 (14):5353–5363.

Sundari D., Alamsyhuri., Lamid A.(2015).Pengaruh Proses Pemasakan Terhadap Komposisi Zat Gizi Bahan Pangan Sumber Protein. *Media Litbangkes*, 25(4):235–242.

Developing Modern Livestock Production in Tropical Countries – Adli et al. (eds)
© 2023 The Authors, ISBN 978-1-032-44025-5
Open Access: www.taylorfrancis.com, CC BY-NC-ND 4.0 license

Birth weight and weaning weight of crossed Belgian Blue calves

K. Kuswati, I. Novianti, W.A. Septian & R. Prafitri
Faculty of Animal Science, Universitas Brawijaya, Malang, Indonesia

T. Wicaksono
The East Java Livestock Services, Jawa Timur, Indonesia

ABSTRACT: The aim of this study was to observe the birth and weaning weight of the crossed Belgian Blue, especially in East Java. There were 13 female calves and 12 male calves observed in this study. These observed calves were located in Situbondo, Lamongan, and Tuban districts, East Java. All of the calves were the offspring of Gatot Kaca, a purebred Belgian Blue bull that has produced its frozen semen, with the beef cattle breed existing on the small-scale farmers (Limousin, Simmental, etc). The results showed that the average birth weight and adjusted weaning weight of 205-day female calves were 38.15 ± 3.87 kg and $176,53 \pm 58.21$ kg, respectively. Meanwhile, the average birth weight and adjusted weaning weight of 205-day male calves were 40.75 ± 5.69 kg and 219.5 ± 60.85 kg, respectively. The coefficient of variation (CV) indicated that there were moderate and high variations among the birth weight and adjusted weaning weight 205 days, this might be due to the variation among the cow's breed.

Keywords: birth weight, crossed Belgian blue, double muscle, weaning weight

1   INTRODUCTION

Population growth and changing consumer preferences are factors that boost the demand for livestock products in developing countries. High population growth and economic progress are the major driving forces for the growing demand for animal sources of food in Indonesia (Agus & Widi 2018). With the majority of consumers being Muslim, beef is one of the most common meat proteins in Indonesia, besides chicken. Most farmers in Indonesia carry out traditional management with limited feed and knowledge. So, there has always been a gap between the supply and demand of beef. To fulfill the demand for meat, the Indonesian Government has tried some ways to improve beef production in Indonesia. Introducing Belgian Blue cattle, double muscle cattle, to Indonesia become one of the Indonesian Government's efforts. Belgian blue cattle are expected to be able to improve local breeds that basically have small body sizes and low daily weight gains (Purwantara *et al.* 2018). Livestock Embryo Transfer (ET) has started to apply embryo transfer technology and artificial insemination using Belgian Blue frozen semen. In 2017, the first calf of pure Belgian Blue was born as the result of ET. The calf is named "Gatot Kaca". Currently, Gatot Kaca has produced millions of doses of frozen semen that have been distributed to some districts in East Java. Although the introduction of Gatot Kaca frozen semen in several areas has been carried out, information regarding their progeny is still limited. The objectives of this research are to observe the birth weight and weaning weight (adjusted at 205 days) of crossed Belgian Blue in Lamongan, Situbondo, and Tuban.

DOI: 10.1201/9781003370048-42

2   MATERIALS AND METHODS

2.1   *Material*

There were 13 female calves and 12 male calves observed in this study. Those observed calves were located in Situbondo, Lamongan, and Tuban districts, East Java. All of the calves were the offspring of GatotKaca, a purebred Belgian Blue bull that has produced its frozen semen, with the beef cattle breed existing on the small-scale farmers (Limousin, Simmental, etc.).

2.2   *Method*

The method used in this research is the descriptive. The variables observed were data on birth weight, weaning weight, dam age, and weaning age. Measurement of birth weight and weaning weight was carried out when the cattle were in a normal standing position using a digital scale. Weaning weights were adjusted at 205 days of age. Weaning weights that have been adjusted are then compared with Limousin cattle, Simmental cattle, Bali cattle, and Peranakan Ongole (PO) cattle (Table 1).

Table 1.   Birth weight and adjusted weaning weight 205 days of Belgian Blue cattle.

	Birth Weight ± SD (kg)	CV	Adjusted Weaning Weight 205 Days ± SD (kg)	CV
Female calves	38.15 ± 3.87	0.10	176.53 ± 58.21	0.33
Male calves	40.75 ± 5.69	0.14	219.50 ± 60.85	0.28

3   RESULT AND DISCUSSION

The birth weight of Belgian Blue in this research was relatively higher than the birth weight of Simmental and Limousin based on Putra *et al.* (2020) research, the birth weight of Simmental was 37.50 ± 1.64 kg and Limousin 38.00 ± 2.24 kg. According to Lawrence and Fowler (2002), high birth weight occurs because of the availability of sufficient energy so that the fetus is able to adapt well. High birth weight can cause losses because it causes dystocia. Bohnert *et al.* (2013) added that Dam who received additional nutrition at the end of pregnancy were able to produce calves with high birth weights because the high nutrition given to the Dam would affect fetal growth during pregnancy.

According to Chenoweth and Sanderson (2005), birth weight has a high heritability value (48%) and is positively correlated with the next stage growth, so the selection of calves with birth weights above the population average can increase the calf growth rate. Selection of birth weight is rarely done because high birth weight is not expected by farmers. The adjusted weaning weight of 205 days of male calves was higher than that of female calves. Lawrence and Fowler (2002) explained that male cattle are able to achieve faster growth than female cattle because male cattle produce the hormone testosterone which can stimulate growth. According to Putra (2020), the weaning weight of Simmental at the breeding station was 197.69 ± 41.62 kg for the male calves and 186.21 ± 40.06 kg for the female calves, lower than the adjusted weaning weight at 205 days of Belgian Blue in this research. Field (2007) explains that cattle breed affects calf weaning weight.

4   CONCLUSION

The birth weight and the adjusted weaning weight at 205 days were higher in male calves than in female calves in Belgian Blue.

ACKNOWLEDGMENT

The authors wish grateful thanks to the Associate Professor grant (*Hibah Lektor Kepala*), Faculty of Animal Science, Universitas Brawijaya number year granted 2022.

REFERENCES

Agus A., and Widi T.S.M. (2018). Current Situation and Future Prospects for Beef Cattle Production in Indonesia—A review. *Asian-Australasian Journal of Animal Sciences*, 31(7), 976.

Ali I.E., Ishaq I., Ibrahim F.H., Magzoob A., and Ahmed M. (2015). Impact of Genetic and Non-genetic Factors on Birth Weight of Crossbred Red Angus and Simmental with Local Cattle. *American Journal of Agricultural Science*, 2(3), 80–84.

Bohnert D.W., Stalker L.A., Mills R.R., Nyman A., Falck S.J., and Cooke R.F. (2013). Late Gestation Supplementation of Beef Cows Differing in Body Condition Score: Effects on Cow and Calf Performance. *Journal of Animal Science*, 91(11), 5485–5491.

Habtamu A., Solomon A., and Yoseph M. (2012). Influence of Non-genetic Factors on Growth Traits of Horro (Zebu) and Their Crosses with Holstein Friesian and Jersey cattle. *International Journal of Livestock Production*, 3(7), 72–77.

Lawrence T.L.J., Fowler V.R., and Novakofski J.E. (2002). *Growth of Farm Animals*. CABI Publishing. UK. ISBN 0-85199-484-9.

Purwantara B., Parlindungan O., Siswanti Y., Imron M., and Setiawan Y. (2018). FA-8 Embryo Transfer and Artificial Insemination Program of Belgian Blue Cattle in Indonesia: Pregnancy Rate, Birth Weight and Calving Ease. *Hemera Zoa*.

Developing Modern Livestock Production in Tropical Countries – Adli et al. (eds)
© 2023 The Authors, ISBN 978-1-032-44025-5
Open Access: www.taylorfrancis.com, CC BY-NC-ND 4.0 license

Morphometric characteristics and rearing system of Poteh Goat in the semi-arid region of Indonesia

T.E. Susilorini, K. Kuswati, W.A. Septian & R.D. Wahyuni
Faculty of Animal Science, Universitas Brawijaya, Malang, Indonesia

ABSTRACT: The aims of this study were to reveal the morphometrics of Poteh Goat and characterize the rearing system of this goat. Data were collected from 200 female goats of different ages (1–3 years). Five morphometric characteristics measured including chest girth, body length, wither height, tail length, and ear length. The value of these characteristics was 59.94 + 11.02 cm, 51.29 + 8.64 cm, 59.09 + 9.10 cm, 15.82 + 3.25, and 19.35 + 2.40 cm, respectively. Poteh Goat has bright white color, short ears, square iris of eyes, and the udder type similar to the Saanen Goat. In regard to the rearing system, most farmers used a semi-intensive approach to raise goats and browsing in the dry season. The main source of nutrients was fodder, from grass, leaves, and woody shrubs. They browse twice per day during the dry season and eat mostly dry leaves from agricultural land, backyard, and marginal land in the hill or forest.

Keywords: Dairy goat, rural area, semi-arid area, goat rearing system

1 INTRODUCTION

Small ruminant in general and goat production, significantly contribute to the national and household economy and is considered as the most important agricultural activity in East Java. Goats have a significant impact on the socioeconomic life of human beings, particularly in rural areas in developing countries. It provides income for the most households which depend on agriculture and for many landless farmers, cultural and religious benefits (Kaumbata *et al.* 2020). In addition, goat became the source of protein for meat and milk. The total goat population of Indonesia in 2020 stood at 18,689,711, which increased to 19,229,067 in 2021 (BPS 2022). The largest goat population was recorded in Central Java Province (3.785 million), followed by East Java Province (3.763 million) and Lampung Province (1.573 million).

Poteh Goat, one of the indigenous goats of Indonesia, is raised by smallholder farmers for meat production. The fact Poteh Goat covers the semi-arid area of Indonesia, in Madura Island. Fewer studies on morphometric characteristics have been published so far. Numerous farm animal populations and breeds have had their traits studied using morphometric measures, which has helped classify indigenous animal genetic resources and identify their origins. Morphometric features including chest girth, body length, chest width, rump width, and chest depth, which are more closely related to bone or muscle growth, can be used to evaluate production performances, particularly the function of meat production. Additionally, planning the management of animal genetic resources at the local, national, regional, and global levels depends on the data produced by characterization studies (FAO 2012). Using linear body measures, morphometric indices might be computed to determine the breed and purpose of the goat. Using relationships between linear body measurements, morphometric indices can be utilized to define an animal's proportions and overall size.

These indices, which combine many linear body dimensions, let breeders choose potential breeding stock in the current production system by evaluating the type, mass, and function of various animal breeds (Chacón et al. 2011). Therefore, the aims of this study were to reveal the morphometrics of Poteh Goat and characterize the rearing system of this goat.

2 MATERIALS AND METHODS

The study was conducted on 200 female goats of different ages (1–3 years) owned by 41 farmers located in the Bangkalan District of Indonesia from July to September 2022. The research method was a survey with purposive sampling. Interviews and observations were conducted to collect the intended data. The variables investigated were morphometric characteristics and the rearing system of goats. Descriptive and variance analyses were adopted to analyze collected data.

3 RESULTS AND DISCUSSION

The standard deviation (SD) in this current study ranged from 2.40 to 11.02 cm, which indicates high variability of measurement (Table 1). It suggests that the selection program will be effective if the population has high morphometric characteristic variation. Additionally, the significant age difference could contribute to the higher SD (Melesse et al. 2022). The average of chest girth, body length, and wither height of the Poteh Goat, similar to the Kacang Goat, was approximately 56.28 ± 2.46, 50.23 ± 2.54, and 48.45 ± 2.17, respectively (Depison et al. 2020). On the other hand, Susilorini et al. (2022) stated that Pote Goat appears to have similarity to Saanen, but is genetically close to Ettawa and Senduro Goats. Regarding another characteristic, Poteh Goat has bright white color, square iris of eye, and udder type same as Saanen Goat. Poteh is a local language for "white" which means Poteh Goat has white color. In general, the shape of iris is circle/oval, meanwhile Poteh Goat has a square iris. This is quite uncommon and easier to distinguish. In addition for the udder type, it indicates the Poteh Goat potential for dairy goats (Susilorini et al. 2022). Rearing system of Poteh Goat, most farmers used a semi-intensive approach to raise goats, and keep them in the barn during the rainy season and browsing in the dry season. This is an example of the unique characteristic of goats in the tropical region to adapt to the environment that enables them to survive and become productive.

Table 1. The average of Poteh Goat morphometrics.

Variables	Value (cm)
Chest girth	59.94 ± 11.02
Body length	51.29 ± 8.64
Wither height	59.09 ± 9.10
Tail length	15.82 ± 3.25
Ear length	19.35 ± 2.40

4 CONCLUSION

Chitosan can be used as a new nomenclature for inhibitor additives in silage. It provided a beneficial effect on silage quality. Chitosan reduces fermentative losses so that it becomes positive silage preservation. In addition, chitosan increased the of DMDi in situ. It can be concluded the morphometric of Pote Goat was similar to Kacang Goat based on chest girth, body length, and wither height, most farmers used a semi-intensive approach to raise goats in the rainy season and browsing in the dry season.

REFERENCES

BPS. (2022). *Populasi Kambing menurut Provinsi (Ekor)*, 2019–2021. Indonesia: BPS.

Chacón E., Macedo F., Velázquez F., Paiva S.R., Pineda E., and McManus C. (2011). Morphological Measurements and Body Indices for Cuban Creole Goats and Their Crossbreds. *Revista Brasileira de Zootecnia*, 40(8), 1671–1679.

Depison D., Putra W.P.B., Gushairiyanto G., Alwi Y., and Suryani H. (2020). Morphometric Characterization of Kacang Goats Raised in Lowland and Highland Areas of Jambi Province, Indonesia. *Journal of Advanced Veterinary and Animal Research*, 7(4), 734–743.

FAO. (2012). Phenotypic Characterization of Animal Genetic Resources. In *FAO Animal Production and Health Guidelines*. Italy: FAO.

Kaumbata W., Banda L., Mészáros G., Gondwe T., Woodward-Greene M.J., Rosen B.D., Van Tassell C.P., Sölkner J., and Wurzinger M. (2020). Tangible and Intangible Benefits of Local Goats Rearing in Smallholder Farms in Malawi. *Small Ruminant Research*, 187, 106095.

Melesse A., Yemane G., Tade B., Dea D., Kayamo K., Abera G., Mekasha Y., Betsha S., and Taye M. (2022). Morphological Characterization of Indigenous Goat Population in Ethiopia Using Canonical Discriminant Analysis. *Small Ruminant Research*, 206, 106591.

Susilorini T.E., Kuswati, Wahyuni R.D., Surjowardojo P., and Suyadi. (2022). Production of Feed Crops for Local Dairy Goats Using an Integrated Farming System. *Agrivita*, 44(2), 344–354.

Developing Modern Livestock Production in Tropical Countries – Adli et al. (eds)
© 2023 The Authors, ISBN 978-1-032-44025-5
Open Access: www.taylorfrancis.com, CC BY-NC-ND 4.0 license

Phenotypic analysis for birth weight, weaning weight and yearling weight in Bali cattle

H.P.I. Sudarmawan, V.M.A. Nurgiartiningsih* & G. Ciptadi
Faculty of Animal Science, Universitas Brawijaya, Malang, Indonesia

ABSTRACT: Performance test in Bali cattle have been conducted for several years in Indonesia. Evaluation of this program is important to maintain and improve the performance of Bali cattle. The purpose of this study was to evaluate the phenotypic traits of the body weight in Bali cattle from year of 2017 to 2021. We analyzed 663 data on birth weight (BW), 547 data on weaning weight (WW), and 463 data on yearling weight (YW) in Bali cattle at the Breeding Centre of Bali Cattle, Denpasar. The data were analyzed using analysis of variance in a completely randomized design with a unidirectional pattern applying the R Studio software. The mean of BW, WW, and YW were 18.82 ± 2.17; 91.70 ± 16.96; 144.55 ± 24.06 for male and 18.77 ± 2.43; 91.35 ± 16.75; and 129.68 ± 18.98 for female. The results showed that sex type had no effect on BW and WW ($P>0.05$) but had a significant effect on YW ($P<0.01$). The year of birth gave significant effect on BW, WW, and YW ($P < 0.01$). The result of BW in 2017, 2018, 2019, 2020, 2021 were 19.55 ± 1.86; 19.75 ± 2.25; 18.26 ± 2.13; 18.41 ± 2.05; 19.14 ± 2.01, respectively. The trend for BW, WW and YW fluctuates between year. This condition indicates that selection program was conducted based on the performance, not based on breeding value.

Keywords: birth weight, weaning weight, yearling weight

1 INTRODUCTION

Various efforts to meet the national meat needs continue to be carried out. Efforts to increase livestock productivity are carried out by improving genetic quality and increasing livestock populations. Improving genetic quality requires a livestock selection process. Simultaneous selection of livestock can accelerate the rate of genetic development (Viana *et al.* 2020). Livestock selection aims to produce superior livestock. Selection can be based on quantitative phenotypic traits of livestock. Quantitative traits are characteristics of living things that can be measured and counted. These traits are determined by many pairs of genes and are strongly influenced by the environment. Livestock selection can be done through performance tests. The performance test is one of the test methods on livestock to determine the extent of the performance level of cattle to obtain the best appearance which is then passed on to their offspring (Patmawati *et al.* 2013). One of the agencies that conduct performance tests is the Breeding Center of Bali cattle (BPTU HPT Denpasar). BPTU HPT Denpasar is the center of excellence in Bali cattle breeding in Indonesia. BPTU HPT Denpasar also has an important role in carrying out the breeding, and development of Bali cattle breeds. BPTU HPT Denpasar conducted a performance test of Bali cattle, but in practice, there are still shortcomings that need to be improved. Several things should be improved, namely, 1) A more in-depth study or evaluation of the genetic progress of Bali

---

*Corresponding Author: vm_ani@ub.ac.id

DOI: 10.1201/9781003370048-44

cattle as a result of performance tests that have been carried out for several years needs to do; 2) selection of breeding stock should be based on the ranking of breeding values, not only based on the parameters of growth traits compared to the Indonesian National Standard. Depth research on evaluating beef cattle performance test activity needs to do. The purpose of this study was to evaluate the phenotypic traits of the body weight in Bali cattle. This research was expected to provide input on the implementation of the Bali cattle breeding program at BPTU HPT Denpasar, to improve the genetic quality of Bali cattle.

2 MATERIAL AND METHODS

The research material used was data recording the growth trait of male and female Bali cattle at birth as many as 663 heads (292 males and 371 females), 547 heads at weaning (276 males and 271 females), and 463 heads at one-year-old (229 males and 234 females). This research was analyzed using a completely randomized analysis of unidirectional patterns of variance (ANOVA). The quantitative phenotypic data observed were body weight at birth (BW), weaning (205 days old/WW), and one-year-old (365 days old/YW). Data correction needs to do because it minimizes or reduces the influence of environmental factors (non-genetic) so that the results of the analysis truly describe the genetic potential of the livestock. The effect of the birth year on body weight of Bali cattle was analyzed using the analysis of variance (ANOVA) method. The statistical model used to analyze is as follows (Nurgiartiningsih 2011):

$$Yij = \mu + \tau_i + E_{ij}$$

where Y_{ij} = Quantitative trait measured (body weight) on individual j-th; μ = population mean; τ_i = fixed effect from year i-th; E_{ij} = random trial error.

3 RESULT AND DISCUSSION

The results at Table 1 show that the year of birth gave significant effect on BW, WW, and YW (P < 0.01). The result of BW in 2017, 2018, 2019, 2020, 2021 were 19.55 ± 1.86; 19.75 ± 2.25; 18.26 ± 2.13; 18.41 ± 2.05; 19.14 ± 2.01, respectively; WW were 110.18 ± 22.03; 87.75 ± 19.94; 87.50 ± 12.92; 94.32 ± 15.44; 93.27 ± 15.80; YW were 150.15 ± 27.78; 145.36 ± 28.21; 136.23 ± 20.07; 157.35 ± 21.03; 135.18 ± 19.26 for male, and BW 19.04 ± 2.60; 19.43 ± 2.62; 18.23 ± 2.40; 18.10 ± 1.81; 18.79 ± 1.97; WW were 100.24 ± 16.69; 88.42 ± 16.59; 87.03 ± 14.18; 91.54 ± 17.14; 92.10 ± 16.75; YW were 150.15 ± 26.88; 145.36 ± 22,32; 136.23 ± 15.00; 157.35 ± 18.53; 135.18 ± 19.85 for female.

The results of the analysis showed that sex type had no effect on BW and WW, but sex type had an effect on YW because male cattle had more dominant androgen and testosterone hormones than female cattle. Sampurna and Suatha (2010) said that the factors that affect the rate of animal growth include species, sex type, age, amount of food consumed, nutrients, genetics, and hormones. Androgen hormones in male cattle can stimulate growth so that male cattle are larger than female cattle. Growth is also influenced by sex type, as stated by Sumadi et al. (2014) that the body weight gain of male cattle is generally greater than female cattle, due to differences in the hormonal system. Testosterone hormone in male cattle can increase the *cytosol* binding capacity of the *gluteus muscle* which is associated with protein metabolism. The growth of female cattle is slower than that of male cattle because the estrogen hormone contained in female cattle limits the growth of pipe bones and the presence of androgen hormones that inhibit fat. The results of this study indicate that the mean of BW, WW and YW are higher than the results of study Kaswati, Sumadi, and Ngadiyono (2013) and Setiyabudi Muladno & Priyanto (2016) that is respectively as follows 17,8 ± 1,08;

Table 1. The mean of body weight of male and female Bali cattle by year of birth.

	Age		
Description	BW (kg) Mean ± SD	WW (kg) Mean ± SD	YW (kg) Mean ± SD
		Male	
n (head)	292	276	229
		Years	
2017	19.55 ± 1.86 b	110.18 ± 22.03 b	150.15 ± 27.78 bc
2018	19.75 ± 2.25 b	87.75 ± 19.94 a	145.36 ± 28.21 ab
2019	18.26 ± 2.13 a	87,.50 ± 12.92 a	136.23 ± 20.07 a
2020	18.41 ± 2.05 a	94.32 ± 15.44 a	157.35 ± 21.03 c
2021	19.14 ± 2.01 ab	93.27 ± 15.80 a	135.18 ± 19.26 a
		Female	
n (head)	371	271	234
		Years	
2017	19.04 ± 2.60 ab	100.24 ± 16.69 b	150.15 ± 26.88 cd
2018	19.43 ± 2.62 b	88.42 ± 16.59 a	145.36 ± 22.32 bc
2019	18.23 ± 2.40 a	87.03 ± 14.18 a	136.23 ± 15.00 ab
2020	18.10 ± 1.81 a	91.54 ± 17.14 a	157.35 ± 18.53 d
2021	18.79 ± 1.97 ab	92.10 ± 16.75 a	135.18 ± 19.85 a

88,59 ± 16,15; 131,12 ± 25,50 and 17,91 ± 1,26; 85,06 ± 16,55; 17,56 ± 19,40. This difference in mean value can be caused by differences in calculation time, besides that, it can be caused by environmental factors such as feed nutrition, livestock management, and climate change. The trend for BW, WW and YW fluctuates between years both male and female. The year of birth affects appearance due to fluctuations in feed availability from year to year or due to instability in management practices related to feeding methods, animal health management, and changes in climatic factors and parental influences (Setiyabudi et al. 2016).

4 CONCLUSION

Sex type had no effect on BW and WW, but had an effect on YW because in male cattle the androgen and testosterone hormones were more dominant than in female cattle. These hormones can stimulate growth so that male cattle are larger than female cattle. The year of birth affects BW, WW, YW due to instability in management practices related to feeding methods, changes in climatic factors and livestock selection which are not based on estimated breeding value (EBV), but are still based on phenotypic performance.

REFERENCES

Baiduri A.A. and Ngadiyono N. (2012). Pendugaan Nilai Heritabilitas Ukuran Tubuh Pada Umur Sapih dan Umur Setahun Sapi Bali di Balai Pembibitan Ternak Unggul Sapi Bali, Jembrana, Bali. *Buletin Peternakan*, 36(1), 1–4.
Kaswati, Sumadi and Ngadiyono N. (2013). Estimasi Nilai Heritabilitas Berat Lahir, Sapih, Dan Umur Satu Tahun Pada Sapi Bali Di Balai Pembibitan Ternak Unggul Sapi Bali. *Buletin Peternakan*, 37 (2), 74–78.

Nurgiartiningsih V.A. (2011). Peta Potensi Genetik Sapi Madura Murni di Empat Kabupaten di Madura. *Journal of Tropical Animal Production*, 12(2), 25–34.

Patmawati N.W., Trinayani N.N., Siswanto M., Wandia I.N. and Puja I.K. (2013). Seleksi Awal Pejantan Sapi Bali Berbasis Uji Performans Eary Selection of Bali Cattle Stud Based on Performance Test. *Jurnal Ilmu dan Kesehatan Hewan*, 1(1), 29–33.

Prihandini P.W., Hakim L., and Nurgiartiningsih V.A. (2011). Seleksi Pejantan Berdasarkan Nilai Pemuliaan Pada Sapi Peranakan Ongole (PO) di Loka Penelitian Sapi Potong Grati–Pasuruan. *Journal of Tropical Animal Production*, 12(2), 99–109.

Sampurna I.P. and Suatha I.K. (2010). Pertumbuhan Alometri Dimensi Panjang dan Lingkar Tubuh Sapi Bali Jantan. *Jurnal Veteriner*, 11(1), 46–51.

Setiyabudi R.J.W., Muladno M. and Priyanto R. (2016). Pendugaan Parameter Genetik Sifat Pertumbuhan Sapi Bali di BPTU HPT Denpasar. *Jurnal Ilmu Produksi Dan Teknologi Hasil Peternakan*, 4(3), 327–333.

Sudarwati H., Natsir M.H. and Nurgiartiningsih V.A. (2019). *Statistika dan Rancangan Percobaan: Penerapan dalam Bidang Peternakan*. Indonesia: Universitas Brawijaya Press.

Prajayastanda J. and Ngadiyono N. (2014). Estimasi Heritabilitas Sifat Pertumbuhan Domba Ekor Gemuk di Unit Pelaksana Teknis Pembibitan Ternak-hijauan Makanan Ternak Garahan. *Buletin Peternakan*, 38(3), 125–131.

Viana A.F.P., Rorato P.R.N., Mello F.C.B., Machado D.S., Figueiredo, A.M., Bravo A.P. and Feltes G.L. (2020). Principal Component Analysis of Breeding Values for Growth, Reproductive and Visual Score Traits of Nellore Cattle. *Livestock Science*, 241, 104262.

Developing Modern Livestock Production in Tropical Countries – Adli et al. (eds)
© 2023 The Authors, ISBN 978-1-032-44025-5
Open Access: www.taylorfrancis.com, CC BY-NC-ND 4.0 license

The effect of addition myristic acid and the levels of calliandra leaf meal in concentrates on nutrient content, feed digestibility, and nitrogen retention

S. Chuzaemi*, Mashudi, P.H. Ndaru & M. Mufidah
Faculty of Animal Science, Universitas Brawijaya, Malang, Indonesia

ABSTRACT: This research aimed to determine the effect of myristic acid and calliandra leaf meal on concentrate on nutrient digestibility and nitrogen retention. This study used a randomized block design with three treatments and five replications. The treatment consists of T0 (40% corn stover + 60% concentrate), T1 (40% corn stover + 50% concentrate + calliandra leaf flour 10%/Kg DM and myristic acid 30 g/Kg DM), and T2 (40% corn stover + 45% concentrate + calliandra leaf flour 15%/Kg DM and myristic acid 30 g/Kg DM). The measurable parameters were nutrient content, dry matter digestibility, crude protein digestibility, and nitrogen retention. The increasing level of calliandra leaf meal and myristic acid in the concentrate increases the crude protein content and decreases the crude fiber content. The average dry matter digestibility ranged from 77,32–78,06%, average crude protein digestibility ranged from 78,74–80,63%, and the last parameter is nitrogen retention ranged from 21,16–21,25 g/head/day. The result of this study showed that the increasing levels of calliandra leaf meal 15%/Kg DM + Myristic acid 30 g/Kg DM on the concentrate T2 give the best result on nutrient content but not a significant effect of nutrient digestibility and nitrogen retention.

Keywords: myristic acid, calliandra leaf flour, digestibility, nitrogen retention, thin-tailed sheep

1 INTRODUCTION

Sheep are one of the sources of animal protein other than cattle, which is essential in supporting national food security (Basyar 2021). Sheep belong to small ruminants where sheep have a perfect digestive system. Sheep have a fermentative digestive system, so rumen microbes influence the feed's digestibility level. Feed digestibility is an indicator used in assessing feed quality. Good feed quality allows the absorption of feed nutrients that are easily digested and will later be utilized in increasing livestock productivity and growth (Siswoyo 2020). The increasing demand for meat proves that public awareness of the importance of animal protein sources is also increasing. The production rate and population of sheep can be utilized to meet the national demand for meat. The thin-tailed sheep breed is one type widely bred and raised by the community. Sheep have a high level of productivity, easy maintenance, and can quickly adapt to the new feed. The obstacle that is often experienced by the community is the low nutrient content of feed given to livestock, resulting in less than optimal livestock productivity. Forage feed has the potential to maintain the sustainability of a sustainable livestock business, one of which is the use of agricultural

---

*Corresponding Author: schuzaemi@ub.ac.id

DOI: 10.1201/9781003370048-45

waste. Agricultural waste in the form of corn stover continues to increase yearly. Giving corn stover to ruminants is used as a source of feed for fiber. Feeding livestock is not enough if it only comes from forage so that other sources of feed can meet livestock's nutritional needs (Adli et al. 2018). Legume plants are plants that have a high level of plant productivity and have a fairly high crude protein content. Thus, the use of legume plants as animal feed has the potential to meet the needs of nutrients for livestock (Nurjannah et al. 2021). The crude protein content of calliandra leaf reaches 25.27% (Pranata et al. 2020). Adding calliandra in this research is expected to increase the feed's nutrient content, especially crude protein.

2 MATERIALS AND METHODS

The material used in this study was thin-tailed sheep as many as 15 males, calliandra leaf flour from ponco kusumo, Malang Regency, and myristic acid from Tuban. This study used an in vivo using randomized block design with three treatments and five replications. The treatments used in this study are: T0: 40% corn stover + 60% concentrate; T1: 40% corn stover + 50% concentrate + calliandra leaf flour 10% + myristic acid 30 g/kgDM; T2: 40% corn stover + 45% concentrate + calliandra leaf flour 15% + myristic acid 30 g/kgDM. A collection of feces and urine was carried out for the last 2 weeks of the maintenance period, then all samples obtained were composted, and nitrogen content tests were carried out to determine the nitrogen content in the feces and urine, then calculated the amount of nitrogen retention. The data in this study were tabulated and analyzed with an analysis of the variance of experiments using Randomized Block Design (RBD). If a significant or not significant different result is obtained, followed by the Duncan multiple range test.

3 RESULTS AND DISCUSSION

3.1 *Nutrient content*

In Table 1, the results of the analysis of nutritional content in the form of Dry Matter (DM), Organic Matter (OM), Ash, Crude Protein (CP), Extract Ether (EE), and Crude Fiber (CF) were obtained. The content of the T0, T1, and T2 treatment feed analysis experienced an increase in protein for each treatment due to an increase in the level of use of calliandra leaf flour in concentrates. The protein content of calliandra by 21.66% can increase the protein content of concentrate feed in the T1 treatment by 15.92% and T2 by 16.29% compared to the T0 treatment, which is 15.38%. The protein content in the feed added with calliandra

Table 1. Nutrient content of treatments.

Nutrient Content (% DM)	Treatment		
	T0	T1	T2
Dry Matter (DM)*	63.55	63.97	64.33
Organic Matter (OM)*	88.59	89.65	89.77
Ash*	11.41	10.35	10.23
Crude Protein (CP)*	15.38	15.92	16.29
Extract Ether (EE)*	4.01	5.32	5.23
Crude Fiber (CF)*	24.68	19.30	19.61

Feed Analysis results from Laboratory of Animal Feed and Nutrient, Faculty of Animal Science, University of Brawijaya (2021).

contains different proteins according to the level of use of calliandra leaf flour in concentrates. This follows the study by Akbar et al. (2018), which states that the complete feed substituted with calliandra leaf flour has the highest protein of 15.96%—proving that this study's results are better than those of previous studies.

3.2 Feed digestibility

Tahun et al. (2017) explained that the digestibility value of dry matter can be used as a reference in the assessment of feed quality and animal feed forage. In line with according to Sjofjan et al. (2020) explains that digestibility is the feed nutrient that is excreted in the feces or digestibility is the content of nutrients that are not found in the feces. The content of nutrients that are not found in the feces is considered to be completely absorbed and digested by the body of livestock. The digestibility of the feed can be seen based on the nutrient content. The nutrient content taken by the data in this study is the digestibility of dry matter and the digestibility of crude protein. The digestibility of the feed is the result of a reduction between the amount of consumption and the amount of feces excreted. The average digestibility value of the feed is shown in Table 2.

Table 2.   Average value of dry matter digestibility (DMD) and crude protein digestibility (CPD).

Treatments	DMD (%)	CPD (%)
T0	77.92 ± 2.45	80.63 ± 2.45
T1	77.32 ± 2.35	78.74 ± 1.31
T2	78.06 ± 3.25	78.74 ± 3.43

The results of statistical analysis showed no significant effect ($P>0.05$) on the average dry matter digestibility (DMD) and crude protein digestibility (CPD). Numerically, the dry matter digestibility (DMD) in treatment T0 (without the addition of myristic acid and use level of calliandra in concentrate) showed a decrease in the average dry matter digestibility value (DMD) when compared to treatment T1 (addition of myristic acid and use level of calliandra leaf flour at the 10% level in concentrate) which is 77.92% to 77.32%. Furthermore, the T2 treatment (addition of myristic acid and use level of calliandra leaf flour at the 15% level in concentrate) showed an increase in dry matter digestibility (DMD) from 77.32% to 78.06%. Furthermore, the results of statistical analysis of the average crude protein digestibility value (CPD) also showed results that were not significantly different ($P>0.05$). The average crude protein digestibility value of treatment (CPD) T0 (diet without the addition of myristic acid and use level of calliandra leaf flour in concentrate) showed a decrease in the value of crude protein digestibility (CPD) when compared to treatment T1 (Diet with the addition of myristic acid and use level of calliandra leaf flour at the 10% level in concentrate) which is 80.63% to 78.74%.

3.3 Nitrogen retention

One of the nitrogen retention values is influenced by the crude protein content of the treated feed. The higher the crude protein content of the treated feed, the greater the chance of precipitation of crude protein that did not do protein synthesis, resulting in an increased nitrogen retention rate. The results of this study showed that the nitrogen retention content in the T0 treatment was 21.25 g/head/day and showed an increase in the T1 treatment which was 21.31 g/head/day but decreased in the T2 treatment where the nitrogen retention content value was 21.16 g/head/day.

Table 3. Average value of nitrogen retention.

Treatments	Nitrogen Retention (g/head/day)
T0	21.25 ± 1.80
T1	21.31 ± 0.61
T2	21.16 ± 3.42

It is known that the value of crude protein digestibility is ordered from the smallest to the largest value, namely T1 of 15.32%, T0 of 15.46%, and T2 of 16.06% in line with the magnitude of the nitrogen retention value, i.e., if the digestibility of crude protein increases accompanied by a decrease in the value of nitrogen retention. In this case, the use of tannin source feed ingredients in livestock rations at the levels of 10% and 15% had a positive effect on nitrogen retention. The role of feed containing tannins is to protect feed protein so that it is protected from digestion in the rumen so that it escapes from the abomasum which will then carry out optimal absorption of feed nutrients in the small intestine (Faotlo et al. 2018).

4 CONCLUSION

The result of this study showed that the increasing levels of calliandra leaf meal 15%/Kg DM + Myristic acid 30 g/Kg DM on the concentrate T2 gives the best result on nutrient content but not a significant effect of nutrient digestibility and nitrogen retention.

REFERENCES

Adli D.N., Sjofjan O., and Mashudi M. (2018). A Study: Nutrient Content Evaluation of Dried Poultry Waste Urea Molasses Block (dpw-umb) on Proximate Analysis. *Jurnal Ilmu-Ilmu Peternakan*, 28(1), 84–89.

Akbar M., Chuzaemi S., and Mashudi. (2018). The Evaluation of Raw Material of Complete Feed Basedon Corn Stover with Calliandra Leaf (*Calliandra Calothyrsus*) and *Myristic Acid* Addition. *The International Journal of Engineering and Science (IJES)*, 7(8), 56–59.

AOAC. (1995). *Official Methods of Analysis.* Association of Official Analytical Chemists. Washington, DC, USA.

Basyar B. (2021). Beef Cattle Farm Development policies to Overcome Beef Distribution Problem in Indonesia: A Literature Review. *American Journal of Animal and Veterinary Sciences*, 16(1), 71–76.

Faotlo D.Y., Nikolaus T.T. and dan Jalaludin. (2018). Substitusi Konsentrat dengan Daun Kabesak Terhadap Kecernaan, Retensi Nitrogen dan Total Digestible Nutrient Ternak Kambing. *Jurnal Nukleus Peternakan*, 5(2), 118–125.

Nurjannah S., Rahman and Krisnan R. (2021). Digestibility of Calliandra, Indigofera sp. And the Mixture in the Ration as a Substitute for the Concentrate Given to the Tup Garut. *Advances in Biological Sciences Research*, 20(1), 244–249.

Pranata R. and dan Chuzaemi S. (2020). Nilai Kecernaan in Vitro Pakan Lengkap Berbasis Kulit Kopi (Coffea sp.) Menggunakan Penambahan Daun Tanaman Leguminosa. *Jurnal Nutrisi Ternak Tropis*, 3(2), 48–54.

Siswoyo P. 2020. Kecernaan Kambing Kacang Jantan Periode Pertumbuhan Dengan Pemberian Kombinasi Kaliandra (Calliandra calothyrsus) dan Rumput Lapangan. *Journal of Animal Science and Agronomy Panca Budi*, 5(2), 16–29.

Sjofjan O., Adli D. N. and dan Muflikhien F.A. 2020. Konsep Bahan Pakan Pengganti Bekatul dalam Pakan Itik Hibrida dengan Tepung Bonggol Pisang (Musa paradiciasa L.) terhadap Peningkatan Persentase Karkas, Organ Dalam dan Lemak Abdominal. *Jurnal Nutrisi Ternak Tropis dan Ilmu Pakan*, 2(2), 78–85. https://doi.org/10.24198/jnttip.v2i2.28561

Developing Modern Livestock Production in Tropical Countries – Adli et al. (eds)

Predicted phenotype parameters for body weight and body measurements at weaning and yearling in bali cattle as indigenous genetic resources

R. Azis, V.M.A. Nurgiartiningsih, G. Ciptadi, S. Wahjuningsih, Kuswati & H. Sudarwati
Faculty of Animal Science, Universitas Brawijaya Jl. Veteran, East Java, Indonesia

ABSTRACT: This study aimed to analyze the correlation between body weight and body measurements at 205 and 365 days of age in Bali cattle. The total samples used in this study were 437 Bali cattle consisting of 248 males and 189 females. The traits measured were hip height (HH), body length (BL), and chest girth (CG) at 205 days. The data were collected from 2018 to 2020 in the Breeding Centre of Bali cattle. The regression and correlation between body weight and body measurement were analyzed using SPSS version 26.0. The result showed that positive correlations were observed between BW and all body measurements. The highest positive correlation was found between BW and three variates (HH, BL, and CG), whereas the lowest correlation occurred between BW and HH. The reverse pattern was observed in the standard error of the mean (SEM). The traits with the highest correlation had the lowest SEM. In this study, the linear regression models for 205 were Y = −159.173 + 0.355 HH + 0.715 BL + 1.430 CG. This study concluded the BW at 205 days of age could be estimated from three variates (HH, BL, and CG) as the best linear regression models. For instance, the BW estimation accurately and easily based on CG could be done by everyone to accelerate and support the selection program of Bali cattle.

Keywords: Bali cattle, body weight, body measurement, correlation, genetic resource

1 INTRODUCTION

Bali cattle are native Indonesian cattle which has the good genetic potential to be developed as a source of animal protein in the future. Bali Cattle are able to live in tropical regions (Indonesia), able to produce well, and there are no disturbances in reproductive characteristics. Bali cattle also have an efficient production performance with a pregnancy and birth rate (80%) (Wawo 2018), daily body weight gain between 0.6 kg/day (female) and 0.7 kg/day (male), meat-bone ratio ranges from 51.5 to 59.8% and has a low-fat content of meat (Biscarini *et al.* 2015; Tahuk *et al.* 2018). Bali cattle contribute (26.92%) to the fulfillment of national meat needs. The need for meat in Indonesia continues to increase according to the population, income, and consumer tastes (Sutarno & Setyawan 2015).

Live body weight estimation is also used to determine the amount of feed for Bali cattle. Estimation of cattle live body weight is technically an obstacle in the field and often cannot be weighed due to the scale limitations. Traditional farms in determining the selling price of cattle in traditional markets do not weigh body weight. One of the methods to estimate the cattle's live body weight is through body measurements such as hip height, body length, and chest girth (Shirzeyli *et al.* 2013). Based on the research report, the live body weight estimation based on body measurements proved positive and could be applied without a scale

DOI: 10.1201/9781003370048-46

(Martins *et al.* 2020). However, the most accurate correlation of body measurements to estimate live body weight at different ages is still limited. The purpose of this study is to analyze the correlation between live body weight and body measurements at different ages in the Bali cattle breeding center.

2 MATERIALS AND METHODS

The research was conducted at the Bali cattle Breeding Center, where the institution focus on breeding and developing Bali cattle in Indonesia. Bali cattle (male and female) were not separated into one paddock. Each paddock was filled with about 30–40 Bali cattle of relatively the same age. The number of Bali cattle in the paddock was determined based on the potential of the pasture that could be accessed by each Bali cattle. Bali cattle could graze at any time, while additional feed (concentrate and forage) was presented in the morning (07.00–08.00 am) and afternoon (15.00–16.00 pm) and the amount was determined based on the average body weight. The total sample used in this study was 437 (males: 248 and females: 189). Phenotypic data in the form of live body weight, body length, hip height, and chest girth. Data collection in the form of live body weight (BW) was obtained by weaning-yearling each Bali cattle and carried out routinely every month. The scales used were digital scales and calibrated every 6 months. Measurement of hip height (HH) was measured from the ground to the hip bone (cm), and body length (BL) was measured from the shoulder blades to the pin-bone (cm), while chest girth (CG) was measured as the girth behind the exactly forelegs using tape (cm). The linear measurements were subjected to linear regression analysis which was performed in SPSS ver. 26.0. The linear regression equation was used based on the model suggested by Vanvanhossou *et al.*, (2018), where LW = the live body weight, X = the body measurement, b_0 = intercept, b_1 = regression coefficients of LW on X, and ε = error.

Live body weight is the most important characteristic and gets attention in the beef cattle industry, due to its traits being selection criteria and profit from the economic aspect. Phenotypic traits can change due to aspects of management, environment, feed conditions, and genetics. Live body weight can also change due to gender factors, where males are generally heavier than females due to the influence of hormonal status on livestock (Suwiti *et al.* 2017). Based on the results of this study (Table 1), the highest CV was body weight (205 days of age), which was probably influenced by genetic factors and environmental factors (age, sex, feed, and health). It was proven that the environment, especially feeding, could increase live body weight and body measurement even though there were differences caused by genetic factors. Genetic and environmental factors determine growth and were able to optimally express genetic potential. The correlation between BW and body measurements at 205 days of age in Bali cattle was summarized in Table 2. The correlations were positive and higher than 0.70. The R^2 ranged from 0.543 to 0.805.

Table 1.   A number of observations (n), means, SD, CV, minimum and maximum for body weight (BW), hip height (HH), body length (BL), and chest girth (CG) at 205 days of age in Bali cattle.

Trait	N	Mean	SD	CV	Minimum	Maximum
BW (kg)	437	92.18	19.01	0.21	57	167
HH (cm)	437	92.83	5.40	0.06	70	111
BL (cm)	437	86.82	5.72	0.07	70	103
CG (cm)	437	109.32	8.65	0.08	81	134

Table 2. Correlation between body weight and body measurements at 205 days of age in Bali cattle.

Trait	Linear Regression Model	SEM (%)	R^2
BW-HH	Y = −148.631 + 2.594 HH	12.84	0.543
BW-BL	Y = −124.706 + 2.498 BL	12.52	0.565
BW-CG	Y = −117.589 + 1.919 CG	9.25	0.763
BW-HH, BL, CG	Y = −159.173 + 0.355 HH + 0.715 BL + 1.430 CG	7.70	0.805

BW: body weight, HH: hip height, BL: body length, CG: chest girth

3 DISCUSSION

Correlation is one of the most commonly used ways to describe the relationship between two or more variables. In particular, this research was applying the concept of correlation to explain the relationship between BW and body measurements (HH, BL, and CG) of Bali cattle. The results of statistical calculations of correlation and simple regression between BW and body measurement in Bali cattle obtained a correlation coefficient (r) and a coefficient of determination (R^2) on weaning and yearling. The strongest r in the estimation of BW using three variables of body measurements (HH, BL, and CG) on weaning (0.897) and yearling (0.923). The correlation (r) between BW-CG both on weaning (0.873) shows a higher relationship with live body weight when compared to other body measurements, where BW-HH = 0.737, BW-BL = 0.752 and 0.873. The results of the linear regression equations are shown in Table 2. Generally, the three variables of body measurement could be used to predict live body weight accurately. The best model used to estimate BW at weaning was Y = −159.173 + 0.355 HH + 0.715 BL + 1.430 CG. All body measurements in this study could be used to predict live body weight. The CG measurement was proven to be sufficient to estimate BW using algometric regression models. In addition, the CG measurement could be easily and accurately performed by everyone for BW estimation. Therefore, these models could be used by farmers and researchers to efficiently predict and monitor BW in Bali cattle.

4 CONCLUSION

The correlation between body weight and body measurements was positive and high at weaning and yearling in Bali cattle. BW could be estimated by all traits of body measurements using multivariate analysis. Alternatively, CG could be used to estimate BW simply. In the field, CG was the easiest to measure among the traits.

ACKNOWLEDGMENTS

The author would like to thank Universitas Brawijaya for funding this research through PNBP Universitas Brawijaya and according to the DIPA Universitas Brawijaya with Number: DIPA-023.17.2.677512/2021. The authors also thank BPTU-HPT Denpasar for facilitating this research.

REFERENCES

Biscarini F., Nicolazzi E.L., Stella A., Boettcher P.J., and Gandini G. (2015). Challenges and Opportunities in Genetic Improvement of Local Livestock Breeds. *Frontiers in Genetics*, 6, 33.

Martins B.M., Mendes A.L.C., Silva L.F., Moreira T.R., Costa J.H.C., Rotta P.P., and Marcondes M.I. (2020). Estimating Body Weight, Body Condition Score, and Type Traits in Dairy Cows Using Three Dimensional Cameras and Manual Body Measurements. *Livestock Science*, 236, 104054.

Shirzeyli F.H., Lavvaf A., and Asadi A. (2013). Estimation of Body Weight From Body Measurements in Four Breeds of Iranian Sheep. *Songklanakarin Journal of Science and Technology*, 35(5).

Sutarno S., and Setyawan A.D. (2015). Genetic Diversity of Local and Exotic Cattle and Their Crossbreeding Impact on the Quality of Indonesian Cattle. *Biodiversitas Journal of Biological Diversity*, 16(2).

Suwiti N.K., Besung I.N., and Mahardika G.N. (2017). Factors Influencing Growth Hormone Levels of Bali Cattle in Bali, Nusa Penida, and Sumbawa Islands, Indonesia. *Veterinary World*, 10(10), 1250.

Tahuk P.K., Budhi S.P.S., Panjono P., and Baliarti E. (2018). Carcass and Meat Characteristics of Male Bali Cattle in Indonesian Smallholder Farms Fed Ration with Different Protein Levels. *Tropical Animal Science Journal*, 41(3), 215–223.

Vanvanhossou S.F.U., Diogo R.V.C., and Dossa L.H. (2018). Estimation of Live Bodyweight From Linear Body Measurements and Body Condition Score in the West African Savannah Shorthorn Cattle in North-West Benin. *Cogent Food and Agriculture*, 4(1), 1549767.

Wawo A.A. (2018). Effect of Bulls on Birth Rate and Birth Weight by Using Semi-intensive Bali Cattle Maintenance. *Chalaza Journal of Animal Husbandry*, 3(1), 24–28.

Developing Modern Livestock Production in Tropical Countries – Adli et al. (eds)
© 2023 The Authors, ISBN 978-1-032-44025-5
Open Access: www.taylorfrancis.com, CC BY-NC-ND 4.0 license

The difference in heat tolerance coefficient and sweating tate between *Bos sondaicus* and *Bos taurus* bulls

I.W. Nursita & N. Cholis
Faculty of Animal Science, Universitas Brawijaya, Malang, Indonesia

ABSTRACT: *Bali* cattle (*Bos sondaicus*) are the direct result of the domestication of wild *banteng* (*Bos banteng*). The purpose of this study was to determine the difference in heat tolerance coefficient and sweating rate between *Bos sondaicus* (*Bali* cattle) and *Bos taurus* (Limousin and Simmental) bulls. The research method was a case study and used 6 *Bali*, 6 Limousin, and 6 Simmental bulls. The data obtained were tested statistically by unpaired t-test. The average t rectal, respiration frequency, and HTC of animals in this study ($p > 0.05$) were 38–39.2°C, 32.2–33.2 times/minute, and 2.4–2.46, respectively. Both animals experienced slight heat stress (HTC>2). The average sweating rates of *Bali*, Limousin, and Simmental bulls were 516.8 ± 19.06, 408.1 ± 24.93, 436.1 ± 12.58 g/m^{2}h ($p < 0.05$), respectively. The conclusion of this study is that *Bos taurus* had difficulties in releasing body heat to the environment through the skin which is indicated by the lower sweating rate than *Bos sondaicus*.

Keywords: Bali cattle, heat tolerance, sweating rate, temperature

1 INTRODUCTION

Bali cattle (*Bos sondaicus*) are pure-blooded cattle because they are the result of domestication directly from wild bulls (B*anteng*) (*Bibos banteng*). This B*anteng* can still be found in the forests of the West Bali National Park, Ujung Wetan (East Java), and Ujung Kulon (West Java). Bali cattle, male and female, have a white color on the canon bones, white semi-circles on the rump and black lines or hair along the back (Susilawati 2017). Bali bulls experience a change in skin color from brick red to black after reaching sexual maturity, but the female does not change. Limousin and Simmental cattle have been widely developed in Indonesia. Farmers like to cross them with local cattle because will produce larger and higher body weight gain calves, These *Bos taurus* originated from temperate climates so they are less resistant to tropical hot environments.

Bos taurus kept in areas with hot air temperatures and high air humidity will quickly experience heat stress and increase body temperature (Gantner *et al.* 2011). Heat release by evaporation occurs when the release of insensible heat (conduction, convection, and radiation) for a long time cannot compensate for the body's heat stress (Kadzere 2002). Livestock is said to have good heat resistance if the value of HTC = 2 (Montsma 1984). `The purpose of this study was to determine the difference in Heat Tolerance Coefficient (HTC) and Sweating Rate (SR) between Bos sondaicus (Bali) and Simmental bulls, or between Bali and Limousin bulls.

DOI: 10.1201/9781003370048-47

2 MATERIAL AND METHODS

The study was conducted at private cattle fattening farm in Tasikmalaya, West Java, using 6 bulls each of Bali, Limousin, and Simmental breeds aged of 2 years, have a bodyweight of ± 300 kg, and have permanent teeth already. The initial stage of the research was preparing measuring equipment in the form of a thermohygrometer, digital body thermometer, hand tally counter, stopwatch, and Cobalt Chloride Disc (CCD). After that, the filter paper was dried again in the oven at 80°C for 2 hours. Next, the paper is made into a circle with a perforator and placed on a glass object with three circles and then covered with clear tape with a distance of 5 mm between the discs (Nursita *et al.* 2020). The procedures performed in collecting Heat Tolerance Coefficient (HTC) data are as follows: HTC observations were carried out when the maximum ambient temperature ranged from 11.00–11.30. The temperature and humidity of the cage were measured at maximum ambient temperature by placing a thermohygrometer in the cage. Cattle body temperature is measured with a thermometer inserted into the rectum for 60 seconds.

$$HTC = \frac{Tb}{Ti} + \frac{Fr}{Fi}$$

where Tb is the measured body temperature (°C); Ti is the standard body temperature (38.3°C); Fr is the measured frequency of respiration (times /minute); and Fi is the standard frequency of respiration (23 times/minute (Benezra 1954). The research method used in this research is a case study with observational implementation. The process of taking sample subjects based on certain characteristics that are already known. Sampling was done deliberately based on certain purposes, with the same quantity of the two samples. The data obtained were analyzed by unpaired t-test (Sudarwati Natsir & Nurgiartiningsih 2019).

$$t = \frac{|X_A - X_B|}{\frac{\sqrt{(n_A)(s^2A) + (n_B)(s^2B))}}{n_A + n_B} \times (1/n_A + 1/n_B)}$$

(Sudarwati *et al.* 2019

X_A: Average *Bos sondaicus* (Bali) / Limousin cattle
X_B Average *Bos taurus* (Limousin / Simmental) / Bali cattle
n_A: Amount of *Bos sondaicus* (Bali) / Limousin cattle data
n_B: Amount of Bos taurus (Limousin / Simmental) and Bali cattle data
s^2A: Variance of *Bos sondaicus* (Bali) / Limousin cattle
s^2B: Variance of Bos taurus (Limousin / Simmental) / Bali cattle

3 RESULT AND DISCUSSION

All domestic livestock are warm-blooded animals (homeotherms), which means that livestock will try to maintain their body temperature in the most suitable range for optimal biological activity. The location where the research was conducted had high rainfall intensity with average daily temperature and relative humidity during the day ranging from 26–35°C and 48–99%, respectively. Kurihara and Shioya (2003) stated that at a temperature of 28°C and an environmental humidity of 40–89%, body temperature, and respiratory rate are still normal, but more than that will affect feed consumption and body heat release.

Cattle are livestock with a body temperature regulation mechanism (thermoregulation) that relies on heat production in the body, which means that cows will obtain body temperature from the results of the body's metabolism. Rectal temperature can be used as an indicator of livestock body temperature because it is relatively more consistent than other body parts. Statistical test results showed no difference (P>0.05) between Bali cattle and

Table 1. The average and unpaired t-test results of rectal temperature/TR (°), respiratory rate/RR *(times/min)*, Heat Tolerance coefficient/HTC values, and Sweating Rate [g/(m^2.h)] for *Bos sondaicus* (Bali) and *Bos taurus* (Limousin and Simmental) cattle during the study.

Variable	Bali vs Limousin	Bali vs Simmental	Limousin vs Simmental
TR (°C)	38 ± 1.04 vs. 39.2 ± 0.86	38 ± 1.04 vs. 39.0 ± 1.14	39.2 ± .86 vs. 39.0 ± 1.14
RR (times/min)	32.3 ± 1.37 vs. 32.7 ± 1.40	32.3 ± 1.37 vs. 33.2 ± 2.32	32.7 ± 1.40 vs. 33.2 ± 2.32
HTC	2.4 ± 0.67 vs. 2.5 ± 0.05	2.4 ± 0.67 vs. 2.4 ± 0.09	2.5 ± 0.05 vs. 2.4 ± 0.09
SR [g/(m^2.h)]	516.8 ± 19.06^a vs. 408.1 ± 24.93	516.8 ± 19.06^a vs. 436.1 ± 12.58	408.1 ± 24.93 vs. 436.1 ± 12.58

Limousin, Bali cattle and Simmental or Limousin cattle and Simmental. The average rectal temperature in this study ranged from 38–39.2°C (Table 1). Brown-Brandl *et al.* (2006) stated that the body temperature of cattle ranges from 38.1–40.5°C. In searching for heat-tolerant livestock, it is necessary to measure physiological characteristics such as body temperature and respiratory rate (Carabano *et al.* 2019).

4 CONCLUSION

Based on the study results, it can be concluded that the Heat Tolerance Coefficient of *Bos sondaicus (Bali)* and *Bos taurus* (Limousin and Simmental) is the same, but *Bos taurus* had difficulties in releasing body heat to the environment through the skin which is indicated by lower sweating rate than *Bos sondaicus* bulls.

REFERENCES

Benezra M.V. (1954). A New Index for Measuring the Adaptability of Cattle to Tropical Conditions. *Journal of Animal Science*, 13(4), 1015–1015.

Brown-Brandl T.M., Eigenberg R.A., Nienaber J.A., and Hahn G.L. (2005). Dynamic Response Indicators of Heat Stress in Shaded and Non-shaded Feedlot Cattle, Part 1: Analyses of Indicators. *Biosystems Engineering*, 90(4), 451–462.

Carabaño M.J., Ramón M., Menéndez-Buxadera A., Molina A., and Díaz C. (2019). Selecting for Heat Tolerance. *Animal Frontiers*, 9(1), 62–68.

Collier R.J., and Gebremedhin K.G. (2015). Thermal Biology of Domestic Animals. *Annual Rev Animal Bioscience*, 3(1), 513–532.

Gantner V., Mijić P., Kuterovac K., Solić D., and Gantner R. (2011). Temperature-humidity Index Values and Their Significance on the Daily Production of Dairy Cattle. *Mljekarstvo: Časopis za Unaprjedenje Proizvodnje i Prerade Mlijeka*, 61(1), 56–63.

Jian W., Duangjinda M., Vajrabukka C., and Katawatin S. (2014). Differences of Skin Morphology in Bos indicus, Bos taurus, and Their Crossbreds. *International Journal of Biometeorology*, 58(6), 1087–1094.

Kadzere C.T., Murphy M.R., Silanikove N., and Maltz E. (2002). Heat Stress in Lactating Dairy Cows: A Review. *Livestock Production Science*, 77(1), 59–91.

Kurihara M., and Shioya S. (2003). *Dairy Cattle Management in a Hot Environment*. Food and Fertilizer Technology Center.

Nursita I.W., Pratiwi H., Cholis N., and Taufiqi Y. (2020, April). The Comparison of Sweating Rate and Sweat Gland Anatomy between Simmental and Its Crossing with Ongole Crossbred (Simpo) Bulls. In *IOP Conference Series: Earth and Environmental Science* (Vol. 478, No. 1, p. 012047). IOP Publishing.

Sudarwati H., Natsir M.H., and Nurgiartiningsih V.A. (2019). *Statistika dan Rancangan Percobaan: Penerapan dalam Bidang Peternakan*. Universitas Brawijaya Press.

Susilawati T. (2017). *Sapi Lokal Indonesia: Jawa Timur dan Bali*. Indonesia: UB Press.

Developing Modern Livestock Production in Tropical Countries – Adli et al. (eds)

The effect of using cassava leaf hay and pineapple wastes in complete feed on feed consumption and digestibility of crossbred Brahman heifers

Kusmartono, Mashudi, P.H. Ndaru & S. Retnaningrum
Faculty of Animal Science, Brawijaya University, Veteran Street, Malang, Indonesia
Great Giant Livestock, Co.Ltd. Lampung, Indonesia

ABSTRACT: An in vivo study was done to determine the effects of using various levels of cassava leaf hay and pineapple wastes in complete feed on feed intake and digestibility. The materials used were cassava leaf hay, pineapple waste, cassava waste, copra meal, cassava meal, mineral mix, and molasses. Forty-five crossbred Brahman heifers were used and given five treatments with three replications. The feed treatments consisted of T0 (cassava meal 25% + pineapple waste 20% + copra meal 10% + cassava waste 10% + cassava leaf hay 30% + molasses 5%), T1 (cassava meal 25% + pineapple waste 20% + copra meal 15% + cassava waste 10% + cassava leaf hay 25% + molasses 5%), T2 (cassava meal 25% + pineapple waste 20% + copra meal 20% + cassava waste 10% + cassava leaf hay 20% + molasses 5%), T3 (cassava meal 25% + pineapple waste 20% + copra meal 25% + cassava waste 10% + cassava leaf hay 15% + molasses 5%), and T4 (cassava meal 25% + pineapple waste 20% + copra meal 30% + cassava waste 10% + cassava leaf hay 10% + molasses 5%). Data on nutrient feed intake and digestibility were analyzed using a randomized block design (RBD). The results showed that T4 tended to give the best results on DM and OM Intake.

Keywords: brahman cross heifers, cassava leaf hay, pineapple waste, feed intake

1 INTRODUCTION

The total population of beef cattle in Indonesia reached 18,053,710 heads in 2021 (Directorate General of Livestock and Animal Health 2021). This figure was higher than the beef cattle population in 2020, which was only 17,440,393 heads. This insignificant increase in cattle population was mainly due to the method of raising beef cattle which is still traditional and the lack of knowledge, especially on good feeding systems. Brahman Cross cattle have been reported to have a high tolerance for various types of forage and have good adaptability to various environmental conditions, especially tropical environments such as Indonesia. Currently, Brahman Cross cattle have good prospects in supporting the Meat Self-Sufficiency Program as the national demand for meat has kept increasing. One of the important factors determining the success of beef cattle production is the feeding system using as maximum local feed resources as possible in the ration. Local feed resources in general consist of agricultural and industrial waste/by-products. For example, cassava leaves (*Manihot utilissima*, Pohl) are available abundantly and have high crude protein content (±20%). However, cassava leaves contain an anti-nutritive substance called cyanide acid (HCN) which may give a negative effect on ruminants when the HCN consumed is upper the limit. This requires processing or technology that can reduce the content of anti-nutrient substances such as drying (hay) or silage making. The CP and OM contents of cassava hay were 22.2 and 86.7%, respectively (Ndaru *et al.* 2014); Similar results were reported by

DOI: 10.1201/9781003370048-48

Kusmartono (2007) that the OM content of cassava leaves was 86.1% and 90.5%, respectively, Based on the description above, a study is needed to determine the effect of a cassava leaf and pincapple supplementation in complete feed on the nutrient consumption and digestibility of Brahman Cross Heifers cattle. The purpose of this study was to determine the effect of the amount of cassava leaf hay and pineapple waste in complete feed on consumption and digestibility in Brahman Cross heifers.

2 MATERIAL AND METHODS

An in vivo experimental method consisting of 5 feed treatments with 9 replications was done. The treatments given in this study were as follows:

T0: cassava meal 25% + pineapple waste 20% + copra meal 10% + cassava waste 10% + cassava leaf hay 30% + molasses 5%)
T1: cassava meal 25% + pineapple waste 20% + copra meal 15% + cassava waste 10% + cassava leaf hay 25% + molasses 5%)
T2: cassava meal 25% + pineapple waste 20% + copra meal 20% + cassava waste 10% + cassava leaf hay 20% + molasses 5%),
T3: (cassava meal 25% + pineapple waste 20% + copra meal 25% + cassava waste 10% + cassava leaf hay 15% + molasses 5%),
T4 (cassava meal 25% + pineapple waste 20% + copra meal 30% + cassava waste 10% + cassava leaf hay 10% + molasses 5%).

The feeds were given twice a day, namely in the morning at 08:00 and in the afternoon at 15:00 According to the feed treatments given and water was available at all times. The experiment was arranged in a randomized block design (RBD) and the variables measured were feed intakes (dry matter and organic matter) (Table 1), digestibility of dry matter, and organic matter. The data obtained were subjected to statistical analysis using the SAS program.

Table 1.   Nutrient content of feed materials.

Feedstuffs	Nutrient Contents	
	DM (%)	OM* (%)
Cassava Meal	87.90	98.07
Pineapple Waste	27.22	94.67
Copra Meal	90.21	95.50
Cassava waste	86.92	91.64
Cassava Leaf Hay	89.67	93.40
Molasses	70.25	92.18

*DM basis

3 RESULT AND DISCUSSION

Statistical analysis showed that feed treatments significantly affected DM, OM, and CP intakes (P<0.05) of crossbred Brahman heifers (Table 2). The highest DMI value was achieved by cattle that received T0 (85.48 g/kg $BW^{0.75}$/d) and the lowest DMI has observed in cattle that received P1 (77.55 g/kg$BB^{0.75}$/d). There seems to be an indication that a higher

Table 2. Consumption of DM and OM.

Consumption of Nutrient (g/kgBW$^{0.75}$/d)	Treatments				
	T0	T1	T2	T3	T4
Dry Matter	85.48 ± 4.46^d	77.55 ± 3.29^a	78.69 ± 1.50^b	81.54 ± 3.01^{cd}	80.75 ± 2.95^{bc}
Organic Matter	78.51 ± 4.47^c	71.14 ± 3.29^a	73.00 ± 1.50^b	74.90 ± 3.01^c	74.91 ± 2.96^{bc}
Dry Matter Digestibility (%)	55.17 ± 3.62^a	54.18 ± 1.64^a	51.38 ± 1.85^a	51.22 ± 0.96^a	56.29 ± 1.22^a
Organic Matter Digestibility (%)	60.41 ± 3.33^a	58.87 ± 2.32^a	58.34 ± 1.69^a	57.34 ± 1.11^a	60.14 ± 1.0^a

Superscript with different notation within rows is significantly different (P<0.05)

level of cassava leaf hay in complete (P0) resulted in higher DMI which means that complete feed P0 was more palatable than the other feed treatments. Feed intake is influenced by the proportion of forage in the ration, the rate of passage and environmental (Jati et al. 2019). The presence of anti-nutritive factors such as tannin as reported in cassava products (Wanapat et al. 1997) will affect the palatability, intake and digestibility as cattle prefer more digestible feeds compared to the fewer ones which account for tannin content in the ration (Wanapat et al. 2000). A similar phenomenon was also observed in OMI value where the cattle that received T0 had the highest OMI (78.51 g/kg BW$^{0.75}$/d), followed by T4 (74.91 g/kg BW$^{0.75}$/d), T3 (74.90 g/ kg BW$^{0.75}$/d), T2 (73 g/ kg BW$^{0.75}$/d), and T1 (71.14 g/ kg BW$^{0.75}$/d). A higher provision of cassava leaf hay in complete feed increased the amount of feed consumed and this may be related to the presence of condensed tannin that allowed the protein of cassava leaf hay to be ungraded in the rumen and contributed bypass protein in the abomasum (Despal et al. 2019).

4 CONCLUSIONS

From the research that has been done, it can be concluded that the use of cassava leaf hay at 30% in the complete feed did not reduce palatability indicated by the highest nutrient intake. A reduction in cassava hay level below 30% in the complete feed resulted in lower feed intake, as well as digestibility values.

ACKNOWLEDGMENTS

The authors wish to thank Great Giant Livestock, Co. Ltd for providing cattle and other facilities to conduct the experiment.

REFERENCES

Despal I.G.P.T., Toharmat and Amirroennas D.E. (2019). *Feeding Dairy Cattle*. Bogor: PT Publisher IPB Press.
Jati S.L., Sobang Y.U.L., and Yunus M. (2019). The Effect of Feeding Concentrates Containing Moringa Leaf Powder on Consumption of BK, BO, PK· and Energy for Bali Cattle in Breeder Patterns. *Journal of Dry Land Animal Husbandry*, 1(3): 403–409.
Kusmartono K. (2002). Effect of supplementing Jackfruit (Artocarpus heterophyllus L) Wastes With Urea or leaves of Gliricidia Sepium on Feed Intake and Digestion in Sheep and Steers. Malang, Indonesia. *Livestock Research for Rural Development*, 14(2).

Ndaru P.H., Kusmartono K., and Chuzaemi S. (2014). Pengaruh Suplementasi Berbagai Level Daun Ketela Pohon (Manihot utilissima. Pohl) Terhadap Produktifitas Domba Ekor Gemuk Yang Diberi Pakan Basal Jerami Jagung (*Zea mays*). *Jurnal Ilmu-Ilmu Peternakan (Indonesian Journal of Animal Science)*, 24(1), 9–25.

Wanapat M., Pimpa O., Petlum A. and Boontao U. (1997). Cassava Hay: A New Strategic Feed for Ruminants During the Dry Season. *Livestock Research for Rural Development*, 9(2).

Wanapat M., Puramongkon T. and Siphuak W. (2000). Feeding of Cassava Hay for Lactating Dairy Cows. *Asian-Australian Journal Animal Science*, 13, 478–482.

Developing Modern Livestock Production in Tropical Countries – Adli et al. (eds)
© 2023 The Authors, ISBN 978-1-032-44025-5
Open Access: www.taylorfrancis.com, CC BY-NC-ND 4.0 license

The effect of water availability on the growth pattern of Redbead tree (*Adenanthera pavonina* L.) seedlings based on the accumulation of dry matter, organic matter, and ash

S.N. Kamaliyah*, H.E. Sulistyo & I. Subagiyo
Faculty of Animal Science, Universitas Brawijaya, Malang, Indonesia

ABSTRACT: The research aimed to find out the effects of different levels of water availability on the contents and accumulation of DM, OM, and Ash in the Redbead tree (*Adenanthera pavonine* L.) seedling biomass and its growth pattern. A nested fully randomized design was employed. The treatment comprised 4 levels of water availability (100, 80, 60, and 40% of the field capacity of the planting media) with 4 replications. Fresh weight of the seedlings biomass was measured at 4, 8, 12, 16, 20, and 24 weeks after planting (wap) and the harvested materials were subjected to DM, OM, and Ash content analysis. The results were used to calculate DM, OM, and Ash accumulation. It was found that at 24 wap, reduced water availability has a more substantial effect on the accumulated amount of DM, OM, and Ash than on their concentration in the seedlings' biomass. The exponential growth pattern of the DM and OM accumulation indicates that the best growth rate of Readbed seedlings up to 24 wap is obtained under water availability at 80% of the planting media Field Capacity.

Keywords: Adenanthera pavonina, growth pattern, accumulation of DM, OM, ash, seedling, water availability

1 INTRODUCTION

The Redbead (*Adenanthera pavonina* L.), in Indonesia, called Saga, is a tree legume with great potential to produce forage, especially in the dry season. Kamaliyah *et al.* (2019) reported that a 2-year-old tree plantation, planted at a 1×1 m distance and harvested every 3 months, produced edible materials of 21.1 t $ha^{-1}y^{-1}$ of Dry Matter (DM), 19.6 t $ha^{-1}y^{-1}$ of Organic Matter (OM), and 3.43 t $ha^{-1}y^{-1}$ of Crude Protein (CP). It was also observed that the tree produced a higher quantity and quality of forages in the dry season than in the rainy season.

Availability of water is substantively needed from the initial phase of plant development, i.e., germination and seedling formation up to the establishment phase in the field (Jaleel *et al.* 2009). A shortage of water can lead to the dehydration and death of seedlings (da Siva *et al.* 2013). Vigorous plant seedlings are important as they will affect the growth of the plant; hence, the optimal level of water availability is necessary to be provided (Benlloch-González *et al.* 2015.; Farooq *et al.* 2009; Lipiec *et al.* 2013; Seleiman *et al.* 2021). Water availability is the proportion of water to the Field Capacity (FC) of the planting media of certain plants which are commonly regarded as the level of water stress (Herdiawan 2013). Evidence regarding the required water availability for the growth of Readbead trees as

---

*Corresponding Author: snkamaliyah@ub.ac.id

DOI: 10.1201/9781003370048-49
This chapter has been made available under a CC BY NC ND license

forage resources for ruminant animals is still hardly found. Therefore, this research was formulated to study the effects of water availability in the soil on the contents and accumulation of DM, OM, and Ash in the Redbead tree (*Adenanthera pavonina* L.) seedling biomass and its growth pattern.

2 MATERIALS AND METHOD

The experiment was conducted from May 11th to October 26th, 2018, at the Greenhouse of Field Laboratory of the Faculty of Animal Science, Universitas Brawijaya located in the Dau district of Malang Regency at $112^0 54'34"$ East Longitude and $7^0 92'97"98$ South Latitude with an altitude of 630 m asl. The Redbead tree seeds were scarified and soaked for 24 hours in hot water (100°C) until the water became cold then the seeds were planted in media consisting of soil, compost, and sand in a ratio of 1:1:1 that filled in 15 × 20 cm polybag.

The experiment followed a Nested Fully Randomized Design. The treatments were 4 levels of water availability, i.e., W100 (100% of media FC), W80 (80% of media FC), W60 (60% of media FC), and W40 (% of media FC); each was replicated 4 times. The treatments were started on day 7 after the seeds were planted. Each replication consisted of 12 plants; each grown in a polybag. The field Capacity (FC) of the planting media was determined by the Gravimetry method (Herdiawan 2013). The fresh weight of the aerial part of seedlings biomass was measured at 4, 8, 12, 16, 20, and 24 weeks of age using the destructive method and the harvested materials were subjected to DM, OM, and Ash content analysis. Accumulated DM, OM, and Ash were calculated as DM, OM, and Ash content time fresh biomass. The growth pattern of the seedlings was analyzed using regression and correlation between the accumulated DM, OM, and Ash against its observation time.

3 RESULT AND DISCUSSION

3.1 *Water availability effects on DM, OM, and ash contents and their accumulation in the seedling biomass*

It was found that seedlings' survival was a hundred percent at all treatments. This may be because the lowest level of water availability in this experiment is still above the seedlings permanent wilting point. Figure 1 shows that the content and accumulated DM, OM, and Ash in seedlings biomass exhibited a significant response to water availability 24 weeks after

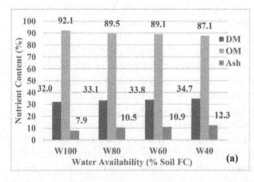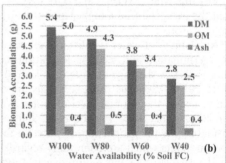

Figure 1.   Nutrient content (a) and biomass accumulation (b) of DM, OM, and Ash of Readbead seedlings under different water availability at 24 wap. (Notes: FC = Field Capacity; DM = Dry Matter; OM = Organic Matter).

planting (wap). Figure 1a shows that the decreasing level of water availability significantly (P<0.05) increased DM and Ash contents but reduce OM content (P<0.05) of the seedlings. From W100 to W40, the DM, and Ash content respectively increased by 8.4% and 55.6% while OM content decreased by 4.8%. Such a phenomenon was also reported by Benlloch-González et al. (2015) and Hou et al. (2021) who found that low water availability at vegetative stage will impair turgor and stomatal conductance as well as increase the solute level inside cytosol. The ash content increased as the water availability decreased. The seedlings' ash content at W40 was 55.5% higher than that at W100. This is quite in line with the finding of Hou et al. (2021) that the concentration of inorganic ions of potassium, Sodium, and Chlor in leaves and roots increased substantially in a plant grown under drought conditions. Waraich et al. (2011) also indicated that some macronutrients (nitrogen, phosphorus, potassium, calcium, and magnesium), micronutrients (Zinc, Boron, and Copper), and silicon absorbed by plants reduce the adverse effects of drought in crop plants. As the ash content increased, consequently the OM content of the seedling in this experiment decreased as shown in Figure 1a.

Figure 1b shows that in terms of accumulation of respectively DM, OM, and Ash in the seedling biomass was decreased when water availability was decreasing. From W100 to W40, the DM, OM, and Ash accumulation decreased by 53%, 50%, and 18.4%, respectively. The relatively sharp decrease of DM and OM accumulation shown in Figure 1b indicates that the decreasing level of water availability significantly inhibits photosynthesis in plants by closing stomata and damaging the chlorophyll contents and photosynthetic apparatus. Thus, the seedling biomass decreased substantially (da Silva et al. 2013; Seleiman et al. 2021; Waraich et al. 2011). A woody perennial like Adenanthera pavonina had capacity to store nutrients such as N and others as well as carbohydrates in woody tissues (twigs, buds, stems, bark, and roots). In recent research, exposure to 25% of field water holding capacity in soil for 3 months significantly decreased the biomass of all organs, photosynthetic rate, and enzyme activities related to N assimilation (Yang et al. 2020). Both Figure 1a and 1b suggested that at 24 wap, reduced water availability from W100 to W40 has a more substantial effect in decreasing the DM, OM, and ash accumulation than altering the contents of DM, OM, and ash in the seedling biomass. Among DM, OM and ash contents, reduced water availability had a greater effect on increasing the ash content.

3.2 Growth and biomass accumulation pattern of Adenanthera pavonina L. seedlings

Seedling is the initial plant growth stage where seed sprouts and plants develop roots, stems, and their first true leaves. All the growth of these plant components can be represented by the accumulation of DM, OM, and Ash. In Figure 2, the growth of the aerial part of

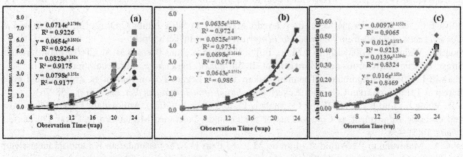

Notes: ━■━ W100; ⋯✦⋯W80; ─ ·▲· · W60; ─ ·●· ─ W40

Figure 2.   Growth pattern based on DM (a), OM (b), and Ash (c) biomass accumulation in different water availability.

Readbed tree seedlings from 4 to 24 wap under different treatments according to their DM, OM, and Ash accumulation as observed in this experiment are presented.

Figure 2a to 2c show that the coefficient of determinants between wap and respectively of DM, OM, and Ash accumulated in the aerial part of Readbed at all treatments was above 90% except that between wap and Ash accumulation under W40 which was 84%. Such a high correlation between the two variables supports the exponential regression curve between the two variables at all treatments applied.

The regression equations presented in Figure 2a to 2c indicated that the highest growth rate of DM and OM accumulation were found at W80 treatment (0.1831 g/week and 0.1897 g/week, respectively) while for Ash was at W100 (0.1553 g/week). Apart from explaining the slow growth of Read bed trees for up to 2 years as previously observed by Kamaliyah et al. (2019), it also indicated that Red bead tree seedlings prefer to grow at water availability of 20% below field capacity. As red bead trees provide forage for ruminants, their DM and OM accumulation are more important variables than Ash accumulation. It is because the DM and OM contain all the necessary materials that provide nutrients and energy for the ruminants. Hence, this experiment suggests that in order to get the best seedling accumulation rate of DM and OM up to 24 warp is to provide the seedlings with water up to 80% of the FC of the planting media.

4 CONCLUSION

It was concluded that the decreasing level of water availability will increase DM and Ash content, but decrease OM content of the Readbed tree seedlings. The highest accumulation of DM and OM of the seedling was obtained at water availability of 100% of planting media FC but the highest ash accumulation was at water availability of 80% of planting media FC. The growth of OM and Ash accumulation followed an exponential pattern and the highest DM and OM accumulation rate of seedlings were found underwater availability of 80% of the planting media FC.

REFERENCES

Asghar M.G. and Bashir A. (2020). *Protagonist of Mineral Nutrients in Drought Stress Tolerance of Field Crops*. Intech Open.

Benlloch-González M., Quintero J.M., García-Mateo M.J., Fournier J.M., and Benlloch M. (2015). Effect of Water Stress and Subsequent Re-watering on K+ and Water Flows in Sunflower Roots. A Possible Mechanism to Tolerate Water Stress. *Environmental and Experimental Botany*, 118, 78–84.

Da Silva E.C., de Albuquerque M.B., de Azevedo Neto A.D., and da Silva Junior C.D. (2013). Drought and its Consequences to Plants—From Individual to Ecosystem. *Responses of Organisms to Water Stress*, 18–47.

Da Silva E.C., de Albuquerque M.B., de Azevedo A.D. and da Silva Junior C.D. (2013). *Drought and its Consequences to Plants-from Individual to Ecosystem (Ch.2)*. In Tech Open.

Farooq M., Wahid A., Kobayashi N.S.M.A., Fujita D.B.S.M.A., and Basra S.M.A. (2009). Plant Drought Stress: Effects, Mechanisms and Management. In *Sustainable agriculture*. Dordrecht: Springer.

Herdiawan I. (2013). Pertumbuhan Tanaman Pakan Ternak Legum Pohon Indigofera Zollingeriana Pada Berbagai Taraf Perlakuan Cekaman Kekeringan. *Jurnal Ilmu Ternal dan Veteriner*, 8(4), 258–264.

Hou P., Wang F., Luo B., Li A., Wang C., Shabala L., and Chen L. (2021). Antioxidant Enzymatic Activity and Osmotic Adjustment as Components of the Drought Tolerance Mechanism in Carex Duriuscula. *Plants*, 10(3), 436.

Jaleel C.A., Manivannan P., Wahid A., Farooq M., Al-Juburi H.J., Somasundaram R., and Panneerselvam R. (2009). Drought Stress in Plants: A Review on Morphological Characteristics and Pigments Composition. *International Journal of Agriculture and Biology*, 11(1), 100–105.

Kamaliyah S.N., Ifar S., Kusmartono and Chuzaemi. (2019). Effect of Cutting Interval and Cutting Methods on *Adenanthera pavonina* L. Annual Forage Yield. *Journal Global Biosciences*, 8(12), 6642–6654.

Lipiec J., Doussan C., Nosalewicz A., and Kondracka K. (2013). Effect of Drought and Heat Stresses on Plant Growth and Yield: A Review. *International Agrophysics*, 27(4), 463–477.

Seleiman M.F., Al-Suhaibani N., Ali N., Akmal M., Alotaibi M., Refay Y., and Battaglia M.L. (2021). Drought Stress Impacts on Plants and Different Approaches to Alleviate its Adverse Effects. *Plants*, 10(2), 259.

Waraich E.A., Ahmad R., and Ashraf M.Y. (2011). Role of Mineral Nutrition in Alleviation of Drought Stress in Plants. *Australian Journal of Crop Science*, 5(6), 764–777.

Yang S., Shi J., Chen L., Zhang J., Zhang D., Xu Z., and Zhong Y. (2020). Physiological and Biomass Partitioning Shifts to Water Stress Under Distinct Soil Types in Populus Deltoides Saplings. *Journal of Plant Ecology*, 13(5), 545–553.

Developing Modern Livestock Production in Tropical Countries – Adli et al. (eds)
© 2023 The Authors, ISBN 978-1-032-44025-5
Open Access: www.taylorfrancis.com, CC BY-NC-ND 4.0 license

Animal feed accessibility level goats in the Bireuen district

Y. Yusriani, Fitriawaty, S.Y. Hayanti & N. Qomariyah
Research Center for Animal Husbandry, Research Organization for Agriculture and Food, National Research and Innovation Agency (BRIN), Cibinong Sciences Center, Cibinong, Bogor, Indonesia

N. Usrina
Laboratory of Parasitology, Faculty of Veterinary Medicine, Syiah Kuala University, Banda Aceh, Indonesia

D.N. Adli
Faculty of Animal Science, Universitas Brawijaya, Malang, Indonesia

ABSTRACT: The sustainability of livestock business development cannot be separated from the support of various resources, one of which is feed accessibility. This study aimed to determine the accessibility or difficulty of goat breeders obtaining animal feed. The method of sampling farmers intentionally (purposive sampling) is a sampling method with a specific purpose, with the consideration that the farmer sample has the information needed for the research. Respondents were 40 breeders with the ownership of 2–3 goats and had at least 2 years of experience raising livestock. Accessibility to the observed feed sources is related to the origin of the feed, the distance to the location of the feed source and travel time, the purchase of feed, the availability of labor, and the time required to search for feed. The results of the study were reported descriptively. The results showed that the average of the five observed variables, namely the origin of feed, distance and travel time, availability of labor, and time to search and purchase feed, obtained a score of 0.82, 0.75, 0.80, 0.85, and 0.81, respectively, so that the total score is 4.02. The conclusion is that the accessibility of goat feed sources in July Keudee Dua Village, Juli District, is good.

Keywords: accessibility, feed, breeders, July sub-district

1 INTRODUCTION

Goat farming in Indonesia is still small in scale and needs to be commercially managed in line with population growth and increasing people's purchasing power (Batubara *et al.* 2012). Small ruminants (goats and sheep) have a significant role in the life of rural communities and religious celebrations in Indonesia (Budisatria *et al.* 2007). Goats have beneficial advantages for small farmers, including high adaptability to a bad environment, high reproduction (quickly reaching sexual maturity), increased production output with lower inputs, and contribution to the household economy of rural communities (Namonje-Kapembwa *et al.* 2022). Regency Bireuen has the potential to support effort development farms with available forage feed cattle that have not optimized for effort cattle goat that is available land and from results side agriculture (Yusriani *et al.* 2020). Areas of productive agricultural land provide abundant harvests followed by agricultural by-products (Yusriani *et al.* 2020). The Indonesian Central Statistics Agency recorded three groups of livestock cultivated in this region: large livestock (cows, buffaloes, and horses), small livestock (goats, sheep, and pigs), and poultry. Goats themselves experience an increase in population every

DOI: 10.1201/9781003370048-50
This chapter has been made available under a CC BY NC ND license

year. In 2020, the goat population was 70.976 individuals, and experienced an increase in population in 2021, namely 73,525 individuals (Vanvanhossou *et al.* 2021). Accessibility of feed is one of the determinants of the availability of feed for livestock which includes several aspects, including forage sources, land ownership, distance and travel time of labor, feed processing, and feed production costs (Susilorini *et al.* 2022). Based on this, this study aims to determine the accessibility or difficulty of goat breeders in the Bireun Regency in obtaining animal feed.

2 MATERIAL AND METHODS

Respondent's farmers consist of 40 people who own 2–3 goats and have more than 2 years of experience raising livestock. The method of intentionally sampling breeders (purposive sampling) is a method of taking with a specific purpose, considering that the sample of farmers has the information needed for research. Determination of the number of respondents carried out with consideration of location access (technically, it can be used as a sampling location), time, effort, and cost, as well as following a participatory research model so that with certain conditions determined from the number of respondents it has been able to provide a picture that is close to the truth. Each instrument must have a scale to measure the value of the variables studied in producing accurate qualitative data. The measurement scale uses the Guttman Scale to get a firm answer that is easy to difficult, which is made in the form of a score. The highest score is 1 (easy) and the lowest score is 0 (difficult). The total score in the study was 5 which was obtained from the sum of the five criteria (variables) where the interval of each of the criteria was the same (Table 1).

Table 1. Accessibility level with an assessment score.

Accessibility Level	Total Score	Tiers
Very easy	5	Very high
Easy	4	Tall
Enough	3	Enough
Difficult	2	Low
Very difficult	1	Very low

3 RESULT AND DISCUSSION

3.1 *Goat feed accessibility in Kab. Bireuen*

In the management of goat rearing, breeders provide feed from several sources, including cultivated forage, natural grass, and legumes are widely available in paddy fields and community gardens (Table 2). By utilizing natural food sources accessibility in the price category is classified as easy to obtain or at low prices—tree legumes such as lamtoro, turi, and gamal, as well as agricultural and agro-industrial products. Lamtoro tarramba (*Leucaena leucocephala*) cv. is a superior quality forage that contributes to the development of animal feed in several regions in Indonesia (Nusa Tenggara, Sumatra, Kalimantan, Java) and neighboring countries (Timor Leste) (Susilorini *et al.* 2022). In overcoming the limitations of forage in the dry season by utilizing agricultural and agro-industrial products (rice straw, corn cobs, cocoa husk, soybean straw), formulated in the form of complete feed (Vanvanhossou *et al.* 2021). The distance and travel time to obtain feed are quite easy for goat breeders, and this is supported by the area's topography, road infrastructure that is easy to travel, and means of transportation. The distance traveled also affects the foraging time.

Table 2. Animal feed accessibility score goat.

No	Feed type	Origin	Distance	Availability	Search time	Purchase of feed	Amount	Average
1	Natural grass	40	35	40	40	40	195	5.57
2	Odot	35	30	30	35	40	170	4.86
3	Gamal	36	30	30	30	35	161	4.60
4	Indigofera	35	3 0	35	35	35	170	4.86
5	Rice straw	3 7	35	35	35	20	162	4.63
6	Soy Straw	3 5	35	37	30	35	172	4.91
7	corn straw	30	30	33	32	35	160	4.57
8	Banana leaves and stems	36	38	30	33	35	172	4.91
9	Concentrate	20	15	15	35	20	105	3.00
10	Tofu Dregs	22	20	34	34	30	140	4.00
	Total score	326	298	319	339	325	1607	45.91
	Minimum score	400	400	400	400	400	2000	
	Average score	0.82	0.75	0.80	0.85	0.81	4.02	

4 CONCLUSION

Based on the study results, it can be concluded that the accessibility of goat feed in Bireun Regency is easy in terms of several categories, namely origin of feed, distance and travel time, time of search, and purchase of feed. Judging from the accessibility of feed, the development of goat farming in this area is still very possible.

REFERENCES

Batubara A., Mahmilia F., Inounu I., Tiesnamurti B., and Hasinah H. (2012). Rumpun Kambing Kacang di Indonesia. *Badan Penelitian dan Pengembangan Pertanian Kementerian Pertanian Republik Indonesia: Rumpun Kambing Kacang di Indonesia*. Jakarta: IAARD.

Budisatria I.G.S., Udo H.M.J., Eilers C.H.A.M., and Van der Zijpp A.J. (2007). Dynamics of Small Ruminant Production: A Case Study of Central Java, Indonesia. *Outlook on Agriculture*, 36(2), 145–152.

Namonje-Kapembwa T., Chiwawa H., and Sitko N. (2022). Analysis of Goat Production and Marketing Among Smallholder Farmers Zambia. *Small Ruminant Research*, 208, 106620.

Susilorini T.E., Kuswati K., Wahyuni R.D., Surjowardojo P., and Suyadi S. (2022). Production of Crops as Feeds of Three Local Dairy Goats Under the Integrated Farming System. *AGRIVITA, Journal of Agricultural Science*, 44(2).

Vanvanhossou S.F.U., Dossa L.H., and König S. (2021). Sustainable Management of Animal Genetic Resources to Improve Low-Input Livestock Production: Insights into Local Beninese Cattle Populations. *Sustainability*, 13(17), 9874.

Yusriani Y., Andriani R., and Sabri M. (2020). Introduksi Pakan Basal dan Indigofera untuk Meningkatkan Performa Kambing di Kabupaten Bireun. *Jurnal Peternakan Indonesia (Indonesian Journal of Animal Science)*, 22(3), 267–276.

Developing Modern Livestock Production in Tropical Countries – Adli et al. (eds)
© 2023 The Authors, ISBN 978-1-032-44025-5
Open Access: www.taylorfrancis.com, CC BY-NC-ND 4.0 license

The quality and amino acid profile of liquid whole eggs using acetic acid

Y.M.L. Simbolon, H. Evanuarini & I. Thohari
Faculty of Animal Science, Brawijaya University, Malang, East Java, Indonesia

ABSTRACT: The aim of this study is to determine the percentage of the best addition of acetic acid in pasteurized liquid whole eggs. The materials used were pasteurized liquid whole eggs from 64 fresh eggs, which were homogenized and pasteurized (in a water bath at 60°C for 3.5 minutes), and acetic acid (commercial vinegar). The method used is a laboratory experiment, with a completely randomized design. The treatments were using 0% (control), 0.5%, 1%, and 1.5% acetic acid. Data were analyzed by analysis of variance (ANOVA) and continued with Duncan's Multiple Range Test (DMRT). The addition of acetic acid had a very significant effect ($P<0.01$) on the yield, acidity, reducing sugar, and organoleptic values. In conclusion, the addition of 1.5% acetic acid resulted in the best quality and amino acid profile of pasteurized liquid whole eggs.

Keywords: acetic acid, amino acid, denaturation, discoloration, egg

1 INTRODUCTION

Eggs are one type of food that has a complete and balanced nutritional content, with a biological value of protein 94%. The nutritional content of eggs includes proteins, fats (lipids), carbohydrates, minerals, and vitamins that play an important role in the growth and development of the human body from the age of children, adolescents, to adults (Liu *et al.* 2020). Eggs are a source of high-quality protein and have other advantages, including complete essential amino acid content and high digestibility (Bakhtra *et al.* 2016). Protein in fresh or raw eggs has a digestibility of 51%, while in cooked eggs the digestibility of protein is 91% (Adeyeye *et al.* 2012). The disadvantages of fresh eggs include a short shelf life and the shell tends to crack or break easily and is easily contaminated by microorganisms that enter through the pores of the eggshell. The quality and freshness of fresh eggs will decrease after more than 7 days of storage, with signs of the yolk breaking and mixing with the egg white (Widyantara *et al.* 2017). This can cause losses during storage and distribution. Preservation and processing need to be done to maintain the quality and extend the shelf life of eggs, one of which is through thermal treatment.

This study aims to determine the percentage of the best use of acetic acid in pasteurized liquid whole eggs (LWE) based on the amino acid profile.

2 MATERIAL AND METHODS

The research material used was 64 fresh laying hens (weighing 60 ± 2 g). The research method used is a laboratory experiment, using a completely randomized design (CRD). The treatment given was the addition of acetic acid with various percentages, namely 4 treatments and 4 replications as follows: T0 (control): Pasteurized liquid whole eggs + 0% acetic acid; T1:

DOI: 10.1201/9781003370048-51

Pasteurized liquid whole eggs + 0.5% acetic acid; T2:Pasteurized liquid whole eggs + 1% acetic acid; and T3:Pasteurized liquid whole eggs + 1.5% acetic acid. Microsoft Excel is used to tabulate the data obtained from the test results of each research variable. The method used to analyze the data is the analysis of variance (ANOVA). Duncan's Multiple Range Test (DMRT) is a further test if there is a significant difference between each treatment group.

3   RESULT AND DISCUSSION

Table 1.   The amino acid profile of the pasteurized liquid whole eggs.

			Treatment groups	
No.	Amino acid	Unit	T_0	T_3
1.	Arginine	mg/kg	7459.09	7514.20
2.	Valine	mg/kg	6803.01	6849.00
3.	Leucine	mg/kg	10297.19	10355.73
4.	Threonine	mg/kg	7126.99	7185.32
5.	Fenilalanin	mg/kg	7392.54	7422.81
6.	Isoleucine	mg/kg	5450.42	5492.40
7.	Lysine	mg/kg	8026.41	8104.55
8.	Histidine	mg/kg	2929.19	2966.82
9.	Glutamic acid	mg/kg	14224.83	14317.09
10.	Aspartic acid	mg/kg	10879.10	10967.04
11.	Glycine	mg/kg	4948.04	4982.36
12.	Serine	mg/kg	10802.04	10875.00
13.	Proline	mg/kg	4381.81	4399.75
14.	Alanine	mg/kg	6406.35	6459.73
15.	Tyrosine	mg/kg	5001.86	5033.93

Egg whites are added to increase the protein content of eggs, and the taste is obtained from the glutamic acid (Evanuarini 2010). Kong et al. (2017) stated that the HPLC system was used to compare 17 free amino acids between 10 brands of vinegar. Seventeen types of amino acids are divided into 4 groups of taste content. The amino acids Asp and Glu belong to the umami taste; Ser, Pro, Gly, Thr, and Ala are classified as sweet; Val, Met, Ile, Phe, Lys, Leu, Arg, His, and Tyr are bitter tastes; Cys-Cys, which only accounted for less than 2.97% of the total amino acids in our tests, was identified as an unsour amino. Some of these kinds of vinegar contain the highest sweet and bitter amino acids, followed by umami amino acids. According to Santoso et al. (2015), the addition of weak acids such as citric acid is thought to cause the amino acid content of protein to increase. Increasing the concentration of citric acid is thought to result in an increase in the number of citric acid molecules in the solution. This will continue until there is an increase in molecular weight, expansion, and breaking of the covalent bonds connecting the amino acids.

4   CONCLUSION

The conclusion of this study is based on the results and discussion of the addition of acetic acid with different levels can be used as a food additive to maintain the physicochemical quality of whole eggs that have been pasteurized. The addition of 1.5% acetic acid to pasteurized liquid whole eggs resulted in the best treatment with a yield of 100.89%, acidity of 0.17%, reducing sugar of 0.16%, amino acid profiles, and organoleptic quality.

REFERENCES

Adeyeye E.I., Adebayo W.B., and Ayejuyo O.O. (2012). The Amino Acid Profiles of the Yolk and Albumen of Domestic Duck (Anasplatyrhynchos) Egg Consumed in Nigeria. *Elixir Food Science*, 52(1), 11350–11355.

Bakhtra D.D.A., Rusdi and Mardiah A. (2016). Penetapan Kadar Protein Dalam Telur Unggas Melalui Analisis Nitrogen Menggunakan Metode Kjeldahl. *Jurnal Farmasi Higea*, 8(2), 143–150.

Evanuarini H. (2010). Kualitas Chicken Nuggets Dengan Penambahan Putih Telur. *Jurnal Ilmu dan Teknologi Hasil Ternak*, 5(2): 17–22.

Kong Y., Zhang L.-L., Sun Y., Zhang Y.Y., Sun B.G., and Chen H.T. (2017). Determination of the Free Amino Acid, Organic Acid, and Nucleotide in Commercial Vinegars. *Journal Food Science*, 82(5), 1116–1123.

Liu T., Lv B., Zhao W., Wang Y., Piao C., Dai W., Hu Y., Liu J., Yu H., and Sun F. (2020). Effects of Ultrahigh Temperature Pasteriuzation on the Liquid Components and Functional Properties of Stored Liquid Whole Eggs. *BioMed Research International*, 1(1), 1–10.

Santoso C., Surti T., and Sumardianto. (2015). Perbedaan Penggunaan Konsentrasi Larutan Asam Sitrat Dalam Pembuatan Gelatin Tulang Rawan Ikan Pari Mondol (Himantura gerrardi). *Jurnal Pengolahan dan Bioteknologi Hasil Perikanan*, 4(2), 106–114.

Widyantara P.R.A., Dewi G.A.M.K., and Ariana I.N.T. (2017). Pengaruh Lama Penyimpanan Terhadap Kualitas Telur Konsumsi Ayam Kampung dan Ayam Lohman Brown. *Majalah Ilmiah Peternakan*, 20(1), 5–11.

Developing Modern Livestock Production in Tropical Countries – Adli et al. (eds)

The combination of nano zeolite and natural feed additives as mycotoxin binders in corn feed materials

I. Ibrahim, M.H. Natsir, O. Sjofjan & Y.F. Nuningtyas
Faculty of Animal Science, Universitas Brawijaya, Malang, East Java, Indonesia

ABSTRACT: Aflatoxins commonly found in animal feed are aflatoxins B1 and B2 produced by the fungus *Aspergillus flavus*. The purpose of this study was to determine the levels of aflatoxins in corn feed given natural additives. This study used a combination of treatments P0 (corn), P1 (corn + zeolite 1.2%), P2 (corn + galactomannan 1.2%), and P3 (corn + herbio 1.2%). The variable observed was aflatoxin levels in corn combined with additives using UV (ultraviolet) light exposure. The result of this study showed that the aflatoxin levels in the P0 treatment were 38 ppb, P1 20 ppb, P2 44 ppb, and P3 treatment 14 ppb. The conclusion of this study showed that the aflatoxin content of corn feed did not exceed the maximum limit of the standard quality (SNI) requirement of 50 ppb.

Keywords: Aflatoxin, corn, feed additive, mycotoxin

1 INTRODUCTION

Mycotoxins are secondary metabolites from fungal metabolism because they can produce toxins for humans and livestock. Aflatoxin is one type of dangerous poison. Aflatoxin is a carcinogenic metabolite from fungal metabolism because it causes toxic effects in humans and livestock. Aflatoxin is one type of dangerous poison. Aflatoxin is one of the toxins that can cause cancer. Aflatoxins B1 and B2 are made by *Aspergillus flavus*, while *Aspergillus parasiticus* makes aflatoxins G1 and G2. *A. parasiticus* usually contaminates corn cereals and other foods with aflatoxins B1 and B2 (Rajarajan *et al.* 2013). Furthermore, feed additives known as mycotoxin adsorbents or binders are one of the most commonly used approaches to prevent and treat mycotoxins in poultry (Ibrahim & Usman 2019; Siloto *et al.* 2013). The negative impact is that chemical drugs given to poultry will produce levels of drug residues and chemicals that are very disturbing (Adli *et al.* 2022). Moreover, aflatoxin prevention can be done by using feed additives mixed in feed ingredients so that, in vivo, the feed additives will be active against mycotoxins. So far, the glucomannan purchased as a binder is glucomannan from the cell wall of the fungus *Sacchromyces cereviseae* and has been shown to be able to bind aflatoxins (Mogadam & Azizpour 2011). The source of glucomannan is porang tubers (iles-iles), whose glucomannan content varies depending on the species, with a range of glucomannan content between 5% and 65%. It was also reported that aluminosilicates (zeolite and bentonite), indigestible complex carbides (cellulose), and bacteria such as glucomannan have the ability to chemically absorb aflatoxins from dissolution (Liu *et al.* 2018; Whitlow 2014). In humans, consumption of aflatoxin can cause acute and carcinogenic aflatoxicosis (IARC 2002) and is usually associated with stunted growth. To date, alternative binding with binding agents, also called "mycotoxin binders," is the most well-known method of reducing the effects of mycotoxins in humans and animals. Besides, herbal spices and their extracts have been used as natural additives as sources of antioxidants that can protect and reduce mycotoxins in food/feed ingredients contaminated with these

DOI: 10.1201/9781003370048-52

aflatoxins. But the goal of this study was to find out how much aflatoxins were in corn feed that had natural additives.

2 MATERIAL AND METHODS

The materials used in this study were corn, zeolite, galactomannan derived from the porang plant, and bioherbal from natural spices. The tools used in this study were 365 nm UV (ultraviolet) light, trays, tweezers, and scales. The study used a sample of 200 grams with a combination of treatments T0 (maize), T1 (corn + zeolite, 1.2%), T2 (corn + galactomannan, 1.2%), and T3 (corn + herbio, 1.2%).

3 RESULTS AND DISCUSSION

Table 1 shows that the amount of aflatoxin levels in the sample of 200 grams of corn was T0 = 38 ppb, T1 = 20 ppb, T2 = 44 ppb, and T3 = 14 ppb. This is in line with the maximum contamination limit for feed, which is 50 ppb (SNI 2015). Martindah *et al.* (2015) stated that the incidence of aflatoxin contamination (AFB1) in broiler and laying hens was high, namely 91% and 82.73%, but the level of contamination was relatively low, still under the regulation of SNI aflatoxin in 50 bpd feed (SNI). 2009) and also still below the maximum limit of AFB1, 20 ng/g (ppb).

In Figure 2, it can be seen that the aflatoxin detection test device was able to show that the corn kernels suspected of containing aflatoxin were more likely to emit a characteristic greenish fluorescent color when exposed to ultraviolet (UV) light. Corn is viewed under ultraviolet light (365 nm) and can emit a greenish-yellow fluorescence, which correlates with aflatoxin contamination in corn kernels (Chavez *et al.* 2020; Hamzah 2019). Widiyanti (2020) stated that aflatoxin B can fluoresce under ultraviolet light to become blue (blue), while aflatoxin G is green (green). Furthermore, Zhu *et al.* (2016) stated that, under UV

Table 1. The results of the analysis of aflatoxin levels.

Aflatoxin Treatment (ppb)	Aflatoxin Level (200 gr)	SNI Quality Requirements (ppb)
T0	38	50
T1	20	50
T2	44	50
T3	14	50

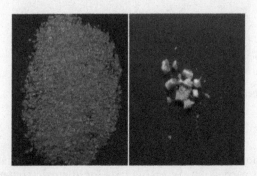

Figure 1. Corn (control).

excitation, kernels with higher contamination levels have fluorescence peaks at longer wavelengths with lower intensities. This is not only suspected to be due to handling factors (room temperature), but also because storage conditions can stimulate the growth of the *A. flavus* mold (Figure 1,3,4).

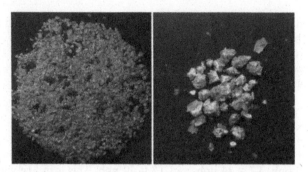

Figure 2.   Corn + Zeolite.

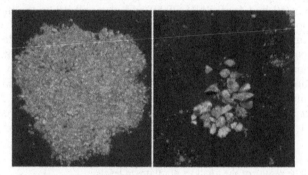

Figure 3.   Corn + galactomannan.

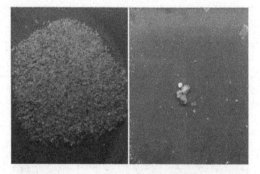

Figure 4.   Corn + Bio herbal.

3   CONCLUSION

Aflatoxin contamination in feed ingredients and feed in Indonesia can occur at any time, whenever inspection is carried out. Screening tests for aflatoxin content in feed ingredients and using ultraviolet light need to be studied in depth for their correlation with standard quantitative methods, such as Thin Layer Chromatography (TLC), High-Performance Liquid Chromatography (HPLC), or Enzyme-Linked Immunosorbent Assay (ELISA).

REFERENCES

Adli D.N., Sjofjan O., Irawan A., Utama D.T., Sholikin M.M., Nurdianti R.R. Nurfitriani R.A., Hidayat C., Jayanegara A., and Sadarman S. (2022). Effects of Fibre-rich ingredient Levels on Goose Growth Performance, Blood Profile, Foie Gras Quality and its Fatty Acid Profile: A Meta-analysis. *Journal of Animal and Feed Sciences*, 31(4):301–309.

Chavez R.A., Cheng X., and Stasiewicz M.J. (2020). A Review of the Methodology of Analyzing Aflatoxin and Fumonisin in Single Corn Kernels and the Potential Impacts of These Methods on Food Security. *Foods*, 9(3), 297. https://doi.org/10.3390/foods9030297

Hamzah I. (2019). Penggunaan Level Energi Dan Protein Yang Berbeda Terhadap Efisiensi Pakan, Pendapatan, Dan Income Over Feed and Chick Cost Pada Ayam Kampung Super Fase Pertumbuhan. *Mitra Sains*, 7(1), 1–10.

IARC. (2002). *International Agency for Research on Cancer (Some traditional herbal medicines, some myco-toxins, naphthalene and styrene)*. IARC Press World Health Organization.

Ibrahim I., and Usman U. (2019). Efisiensi Ransum Dengan Penggunaan Dedak Padi Fermentasi Pada Ayam Kampung Fase Pertumbuhan. *Tolis Ilmiah: Jurnal Penelitian*, 1(2).

Liu N., Wang J., Deng Q., Gu K., and Wang J. (2018). Detoxification of Aflatoxin B 1 by Lactic Acid Bacteria and Hydrated Sodium Calcium Aluminosilicate in Broiler Chickens. *Livestock Science*, 208, 28–32.

Martindah E., Maryam R., Wahyuwardani S., and Widiyanti P.M. (2015). Studi Pendahuluan Epidemiologi Kontaminasi Aflatoksin B1 Pada Pakan Ayam. *Prosiding Seminar Nasional Teknologi Peternakan Dan Veteriner*, 30, 525–531.

Mogadam N., and Azizpour A. (2011). Ameliorative Effect of Glucomannan-containing Yeast Product (Mycosorb) and Sodium Bentonite on Performance and Antibody Titers Against Newcastle Disease in Broilers During Chronic Aflatoxicosis. *African Journal of Biotechnology*, 10(75), 17372–17378.

Rajarajan P.N., Rajasekaran K.M., and Asha Devi N.K. (2013). Aflatoxin Contamination in Agricultural Commodities. *Indian Journal of Pharmaceutical and Biological Research*, 1(04), 148–151.

Siloto E.V., Oliveira E.F.A., Sartori J.R., Fascina V.B., Martins B.A.B., Ledoux D.R., Rottinghaus G.E., and Sartori D.R.S. (2013). Lipid Metabolism of Commercial Layers Fed Diets Containing Aflatoxin, Fumonisin, and a Binder. *Poultry Science*, 92(8), 2077–2083.

SNI B.S.N. (2015). Pakan Ayam Ras Pedaging (broiler) ⊠ Bagian 2: Masa Awal (starter). In *Badan Standarisasi Nasional Indonesia SNI* (p. 9).

Whitlow L.W. (2014). *Evaluation of mycotoxin binders* (Issue January 2006). North Carolina State University.

Widiyanti M. (2020). Deteksi Aflatoksin B1 Dalam Bahan Pakan dan Pakan Secara Enzyme Linked Immunosorbent Assay. *Prosiding PPIS*, 225–230.

Zhu F., Yao H., Hruska Z., Kincaid R., Brown R. L., Bhatnagar D., and Cleveland T. E. (2016). Integration of Fluorescence and Reflectance Visible Near-infrared (VNIR) Hyperspectral Images for Detection of Aflatoxins in Corn Kernels. *American Society of Agricultural and Biological Engineers*, 59(3), 785–794. https://doi.org/10.13031/trans.59.11365

Author index